THE
RN
FIRST ASSISTANT

An Expanded Perioperative Nursing Role

THIRD EDITION

THE
RN
FIRST ASSISTANT

An Expanded Perioperative Nursing Role

THIRD EDITION

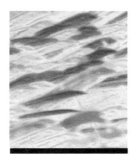

Jane C. Rothrock, DNSc, RN, CNOR
Professor, Perioperative Nursing
Delaware County Community College
Media, Pennsylvania

With 12 additional contributors

Lippincott
Philadelphia • New York

Q09 1879

Acquisitions Editor: Susan M. Glover, RN, MSN
Coordinating Editorial Assistant: Bridget Blatteau
Production Editor: Virginia Barishek
Production Manager: Helen Ewan
Production Service: P.M. Gordon Associates, Inc.

Compositor: Pine Tree Composition
Printer/Binder: R.R. Donnelley & Sons/Crawfordsville
Cover Designer: Melissa Walter
Cover Printer: Lehigh Press

Third Edition

Library of Congress Cataloging-in-Publication Data

The RN first assistant : an expanded perioperative nursing role /
 [edited by] Jane C. Rothrock : with 12 additional contributors.—
 3rd ed.
  p. cm.
 Includes bibliographical references and index.
 ISBN 0–7817–1501–6
 1. Operating room nursing. 2. Surgical nursing. I. Rothrock,
Jane C., 1948– .
  [DNLM: 1. Perioperative Nursing—methods. WY 162 R627 1999]
 RD32.3.R6 1999
 610.73′677—dc21
 DNLM/DLC
 for Library of Congress   98–20816
                                              CIP

Care has been taken to confirm the accuracy of the information presented and to describe generally accepted practices. However, the authors, editors, and publishers are not responsible for errors or omissions or for any consequences from application of the information in this book and make no warranty, express or implied, with respect to the contents of the publication.

The authors, editors and publisher have exerted every effort to ensure that drug selection and dosage set forth in this text are in accordance with current recommendations and practice at the time of publication. However, in view of ongoing research, changes in government regulations, and the constant flow of information relating to drug therapy and drug reactions, the reader is urged to check the package insert for each drug for any change in indications and dosage and for added warnings and precautions. This is particularly important when the recommended agent is a new or infrequently employed drug.

Some drugs and medical devices presented in this publication have Food and Drug Administration (FDA) clearance for limited use in restricted research settings. It is the responsibility of the health care provider to ascertain the FDA status of each drug or device planned for use in their clinical practice.

DEDICATION

The third edition of this book is dedicated to

Sergius Pechin, MD, FACS

As his colleague and friend, I am humbled by what I have learned

from him. His courageous conscience, depth of insight, and true

caring have changed the lives of hundreds of RNFA students and

faculty colleagues. He wears a purple heart; he lives in our hearts.

CONTRIBUTORS

ARTHUR S. BROWN, MD
Professor and Head
Division of Plastic and Reconstructive Surgery
Robert Wood Johnson Medical School at Camden
Camden, New Jersey

RUDOLPH C. CAMISHION, MD, FACS
Professor of Surgery
Robert Wood Johnson Medical School at Camden
Camden, New Jersey

NANCY B. DAVIS, RN, BSN, NP, CNOR, CRNFA
RN First Assistant
Nurse Practitioner
Cardiovascular and Chest Surgical Associates, P.A.
Boise, Idaho

CHRISTINE C. ESPERSEN, RN, CNOR, CRNFA
RN First Assistant
Division of Cardiac Surgery
Buffalo General Hospital
Buffalo, New York

CHRISTOPHER C. HLOZEK, BSN, RNFA
Cardiovascular Specialist
Ethicon Endo-Surgery, Inc.
A Johnson & Johnson Company
Cincinnati, Ohio

CECIL A. KING, RN, BSN, CNOR, MS(C)
Assistant Nurse Manager—OR
Surgical Services
University of Washington Medical Center
Seattle, Washington

SERGIUS PECHIN, MD, FACS
Faculty, RN First Assistant Program
Delaware County Community College
Media, Pennsylvania

JAMES E. RASINSKY, DO, MSW
Anesthesiologist
Department of Anesthesia
North Kansas City Hospital
North Kansas City, Missouri

PATRICIA C. SEIFERT, RN, MSN, CNOR, CRNFA
Manager, Open Heart Surgery
Operating Room
Halifax Medical Center
Daytona Beach, Florida

DALE A. SMITH, RN, CNOR, RNFA
RN First Assistant
Maine Medical Center/Brighton Surgical Center
Portland, Maine

BRENDA COLE ULMER, RN, MN, CNOR
Senior Clinical Educator
Valley Lab, Inc.
Stone Mountain, Georgia

BARBARA M. WILSON, RN, CNOR, CRNFA
RN First Assistant
Clinical Consultant
Atlanta, Georgia

LIST OF REVIEWERS

CANDYCE L. BRIGHT, MSN/NP, RN, CNOR, RNFA
Adjunct Professor, School of Nursing
Atlantic Community College
Mays Landing, New Jersey

MARLENE CRADEN, RN, CNOR, CRNFA
RN First Assistant
Millard Fillmore Health System
Buffalo, New York

VICKI J. FOX, MSN, RN, ACNP, CRNFA
Acute Care Nurse Practitioner
Trinity Mother Frances Health System Trauma
  Services
Tyler, Texas

THOMAS Z. LAJOS, MD
Associate Professor
Division of Cardiac Surgery
State University of New York at Buffalo
Buffalo, New York

JOANNE V. MCLAUGHLIN, RN, CNOR, CRNFA
RN First Assistant
Margaretville Memorial Hospital
Margaretville, New York

ROBIN MOZENTER, PA
Physician Assistant, Department of Surgery
Crozer Chester Medical Center
Upland, Pennsylvania

JOHN J. PADAVANO, DO
Orthopedic Center of New England
Portland, Maine

ELIZABETH PEARSALL, RN, CNOR, RNFA
Staff Nurse
Taylor Hospital Division of Crozer Chester Medical
  Center
Ridley Park, Pennsylvania

KAREN L. RITCHEY, MSN, RN, CNOR
Assistant Director, Education
NCQA, Washington, DC
and
Faculty Member, RNFA Program
Delaware County Community College
Media, Pennsylvania

CANDACE L. ROMIG, MA
Legislative Program Coordinator
Association of Operating Room Nurses
Denver, Colorado

PREFACE

In 1925, M. Adelaide Nutting noted:

> We need to realize and affirm anew that nursing is one of the most difficult arts. Compassion may provide the momentum, but knowledge is our only working power. Perhaps, too, we need to remember that growth in our work must be preceded by ideas, and that any conditions that suppress thought, must retard growth. Surely we will not be satisfied in perpetuating methods and traditions. Surely we shall wish to be more and more occupied with creating them.

The third edition of *The RN First Assistant: An Expanded Perioperative Nursing Role* intends to help RNFAs with the working power of knowledge as they move toward a new tomorrow. In each of the chapters, the authors have shared knowledge that leads to skill acquisition by the RNFA. They have focused on a topic essential to the knowledgeable RNFA, elucidated critical concepts related to the topic, and included information that builds competence. The resulting synergy of the book is thus obvious and real.

RNFAs characteristically carry out the work of nursing and collaborate with others on the heath care team in a way that adds considerable value to patient care and the organization as a whole. It is the confluence of what is in their heads, hearts, and hands—knowledge, compassion, and technical acumen—that makes them exemplary. They understand that adding value is not just in going above and beyond their work requirements, but consists in being who they are—their experiences, ideals, and dreams. RNFAs have never tolerated professional obsolescence; instead, they accept and even embrace accountability for maintaining leading-edge knowledge and skills. Inherently, they have a natural feeling, deep down inside, that they will serve their patients' highest-priority needs. This third edition of *The RN First Assistant: An Expanded Perioperative Nursing Role* has the clear intention of helping them do just that.

JANE C. ROTHROCK, DNSc, RN, CNOR

ACKNOWLEDGMENTS

The third edition of this book, like the ones before it, represents a testimonial to the art and science of assisting at surgery. Anyone who reads it must understand that it was not written by me, but by nurses and surgeons who are clinically talented and willing to share that talent with me and the book's readers. Each of them, along with the panel of reviewers listed at the front of the book, understands that something as simple as a stitch requires intellect, skill mastery, and even caring—caring that the stitch is the right one for the right tissue with the right material that has the right outcome, both technically and aesthetically. So, too, do the individuals at Lippincott–Raven Publishers, with special thanks to Bridget Blatteau, who worked on this edition and committed to making it "right," both editorially and artistically. These multiple contributions have guided this edition, as we have all worked together to achieve a shared goal—a book that adds value, prizes the valuable knowledge and skills of RNFAs, and makes a positive difference in accelerating effectiveness in patient care.

Contents

5.   The Diagnostic Process   105

Jane C. Rothrock

6.   Perioperative Patient Preparation   127

Jane C. Rothrock

7.   Anesthesia and Patient Positioning   153

James E. Rasinsky

8.   Principles of Tissue Handling   181

Rudolph C. Camishion
Arthur S. Brown

9.   Providing Exposure: Retractors and Retraction   201

Nancy B. Davis

10.   Suturing Materials and Techniques   223

Nancy B. Davis

11.   Wound Healing   259
Jane C. Rothrock

12.   Using Grasping Instruments   287
Sergius Pechin

13.   Providing Hemostasis   297
Nancy B. Davis
Brenda C. Ulmer

14.   The RN First Assistant and Collaborative Practice   343
Patricia C. Seifert

15.   Clinical Applications   365
Dale A. Smith
Christine C. Espersen
Barbara M. Wilson
Christopher C. Hlozek

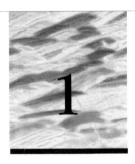

HISTORY OF THE RN
FIRST ASSISTANT ROLE

JANE C. ROTHROCK

■

Each regiment in this civilian army had brought its own physician. Medical and surgical treatment by these men—known as regimental surgeons—seemed even less likely of success than that of their military brothers. They were hometown doctors of varied ability, and needed only the approval of the regimental commander and a rubber stamp from the colonial legislature before receiving their commissions.[1]

The origins of the nurse's role as assistant during surgery are evidenced throughout history. For centuries, nurses have assisted physicians during surgical procedures in the home and the hospital. The evolution of medicine and surgery is paralleled by the development of professional nursing and the presence of the nurse in the operating room.[2] In particular, wounds inflicted during war and the new technology needed to repair these wounds created the opportunity and the need for the nurse to act as a surgical assistant.

In the 18th century there was little formal education available for nurses or surgeons. In 1775, during the Revolutionary War, fewer than 300 of the 3,500 regimental surgeons had received a medical degree. Most physicians in colonial times were apprentice trained. The primary qualification for these apprentice "doctor's boys" was the ability to stand the sight of blood.[3] Apprenticeships lasted from 3 to 6 years, after which the fledgling new physician was ready to do bloodletting, tooth-pulling, wound dressing, and minor surgery. Advanced skills were learned on the battlefield, where wounds, burns, and fractures were treated and amputations and the trepanning of skull fractures were undertaken. The surgeon was attended by a "surgeon's mate." Nurses, who were females, were kept from the battlefield and waited to attend the soldiers as they were removed to a hospital.

In this era, preparation for the role of "nurse" was even less standardized than the apprenticeship system for surgeons. Throughout the colonial era, caring for friends and relatives was an important societal role for women. Nursing was often taught from mother to daughter or learned by a domestic servant as part of her job. Ministering to the sick was expected of all women in the family. Nursing was a woman's duty, and as the economy began to expand, older widows and spinsters from the working class "professed" themselves as nurses. Also known as "natural-born" nurses, these women often came to their profession when other forms of employment were closed to them; nursing then became their obvious choice for work.[4] Working either in the home or hospital, many of these nurses were devoted women who demonstrated caring and concern in their duties. However, the quality of their efforts and their skills were more disparate than similar; some blundered badly beyond their capabilities or knowledge.[5]

Advances in science, the work of Florence Nightingale, and the introduction of formal training for nurses furthered the development of the role of nurse as first assistant.[6] Nightingale defined nursing as "putting the patient in the best condition for nature to act upon him."[7] She emphasized cleanliness, quiet, and environmental control as part of her understanding of the importance of patients' environments on their illness, all of which are important to both the caring and the curing roles of nursing and vital to effective surgical intervention.[8] Believing strongly that both maturity and a deep understanding of the character traits necessary to care for the sick were attributes of good nurses, Nightingale established the basis for scientific training while also acknowledging that science alone would not nurture the art of good nursing.[9]

■ IMPACT OF WARTIME

Crimean War

During the Crimean War, from 1854 to 1856, Florence Nightingale and her staff of 125 nurses provided nursing services at the Barrack Hospital in Turkey. The hospital, with 4,000 patients in a facility designed to care for 1,700, was infested with maggots, lice, rats, and other vermin.[10] There were no clean dressings, clothing, or bedding. Food and water were extremely limited; there was no soap or water for cleaning either the patients or the hospital. Physicians were in drastically short supply, nurses were essentially nonexistent, and patients cared for one another.

Emphasizing cleanliness and environmental control, Nightingale instituted sanitation measures and obtained needed food, water, and supplies. She stressed the importance of the nurse's role in managing and supervising patient units and the operating room. Under her guidance, cleanliness in infection control and environmental sanitation became basic principles for managing a hospital as well as critical elements in nursing interventions in the operating room. She cautioned the surgical nurse to "be ever on the watch, ever on guard, against want of cleanliness, foul air, want of light, and of warmth."[11]

The role of nurse as first assistant was initially conceived during Nightingale's tenure. At the physician's side, the nurse prepared wounds for surgery and assisted during the surgical procedure. Meticulous care of the surgical site and prevention of infection were of paramount importance. Perioperative role nursing functions, from preoperative sanitation and care of the sick on the patient ward to accompanying the patient to the operating room and acting as a nurse participant to resuming care activities of the postoperative patient and wound, became the basis for role evolution. Thomas Eakins's painting, *The Agnew Clinic,* portrays Mary Clymer, recipient of the Nightingale Medal from the Hospital of the University of Pennsylvania's School of Nursing in 1889. Clymer is in a shaft of light in a portrait of a surgical amphitheater. Lynaugh notes that by portraying her this way, Eakins sought to convey a new ideal of professional training and competence.[12] RN first assistants have continued to symbolize the optimism and promise memorialized in that painting.

American Civil War

During the Civil War, 1861 to 1865, conditions in hospitals and operating rooms were similar to those found in the Crimea. Dorothea Dix, Florence Nightingale's American counterpart, and a nursing force of 10,000 provided care to thousands of wounded soldiers. Cleanliness and infection control were the primary nursing directives. Dix adopted and practiced many of the principles established by Nightingale, and this war again saw the nurse assuming the responsibilities of the first assistant in surgery. Amputation was the predominant surgical procedure.[13] Abdominal surgery was extremely high risk; hemorrhage and infection were grave complications. Postoperative infection and bleeding were of such magnitude that nurses continuously concerned themselves with tying off bleeders and cauterizing blood vessels with heat. The primary disinfectant used by the nurse was alcohol, although in 1865 Lister began to use carbolic acid to soak dressings, slowly reducing the 45.7% surgical mortality rate associated with limb amputation.[14]

Nurses of the Civil War era left important legacies as they worked to improve patient welfare and influence wartime health policies. Nursing care in the United States was revolutionized during this war, and nurses were influential in creating the impetus for change. With its incredible demands for the care of hospitalized soldiers, the Civil War triggered the beginning of respectable, well-educated women extending their knowledge of nursing care outside their own circle of family and friends. Social barriers were breached as more women knowledgeable in the principles of nursing care began to practice nursing in hospitals. This was not accomplished without overcoming the prejudices of chief surgeons in the hospitals, however. Woolsey related these prejudices in her diary:

> Hardly a surgeon of whom I can think received or treated them [women nurses] with even common courtesy. Government had decided that women should be employed, and the army surgeons—unable, therefore, to close the hospitals against them—determined to make their lives unbearable that they should be forced in self-defense to leave. . . . Some of the bravest women I have ever known were among the first company of army nurses. They saw at once the position of affairs, the attitude assumed by the surgeons, and the wall against which they were expected to break and scatter; and they set themselves to undermine the whole thing.[15]

In the Confederate army, Lucy Wilhelmina Otey organized a corps of women to serve as nurses. The surgeon who served as director of the city's hospitals in Lynchburg rebuffed her with the admonition that "hospitals were no place for women or flies."[16] Undaunted, Otey met with President Jefferson Davis, who commissioned her; with the official acknowledgment of the War Department, she established the Ladies Relief Hospital. By the end of the war, her hospital had the lowest death rate of any of the military hospitals in Lynchburg.

The nurses of the Civil War won the grudging respect of surgeons and were often idolized by their patients. Although army surgeons initially wished to bar them from hospitals, these nurses went on to become regional and national heroes. Using perseverance, plain talk, and political power, they radically transformed the care of hospitalized soldiers.[17] In battlefield stations, they were innovative and resourceful. Clara Barton, in the battle of Fredericksburg, had to find a way to keep wounded soldiers warm during the night before surgeons could attend them. She had fires lit, dismantled a chimney, heated bricks, and placed them around the wounded to keep them warm until the surgeons could operate in the daylight.[18] Despite the rigor of their duties, these nurses further developed the concept of caring. In his diary, Walt Whitman described a nurse he especially admired: "I noticed how she sat a long time by the fellow who just had, that morning, in addition to his other sickness, bad hemorrhage—she gently assisted him, relieved him of the blood, holding a cloth to his mouth, as he coughed it up—he was so weak he could only just turn his head over on the pillow."[19]

Spanish-American War

The Spanish-American War, in 1898, had one major land battle that resulted in 968 casualties and 5,438 deaths from disease due to poor sanitation and yellow fever.[20] An all-graduate nursing staff replaced medical corpsmen in caring for the war victims. Although surgery was limited, advances were made in preventing transfer of disease and infection. These epidemiological discoveries helped both to advance surgical recovery and to expand the role of the nurse first assistant. After the war, government investigations led to the founding of the Army and Navy Nurse Corps. These corps helped stabilize the role of the nurse as first assistant and led to advanced specialization in operating room nursing.

World War I

During World War I, 8,587 American nurses cared for 184,000 wounded and sick soldiers on the European front. This war also saw a large volume of amputations for which the nurse acted as first assistant. The nature of the wounds mandated the need to remove much dead and devitalized tissue. Frequently, stretchers were placed directly on the operating table. With clothing quickly cut away, one nurse would begin to administer chloroform and ether while another nurse, functioning as first assistant, cleaned the wound with gasoline, then iodine, and began the procedure of wound debridement.[21]

The use of gas warfare created new problems. The gas destroyed lung tissue and caused massive burns; in particular, the eyes, face, and hands were severely affected by first-degree burns.[22] Again in a first assistant role, the nurse assumed primary responsibility for burn dressing, wound debridement, and pinch grafting. Wounds of the head were very common and some so disfiguring that the field of plastic reconstructive surgery developed; research on skin grafting, orthopedic surgery, and casting also made great strides.[23] The nursing emphasis on infection prevention continued to direct care activities.[24]

The nursing literature of the era generated ideas regarding the changing focus of nursing roles. Themes that emerged related to, in part, the nature of nursing education. The need for educational preparation that developed the individual, allowed for the acquisition of general knowledge, educated the nurse for citizenship and social reform, and developed patterns of critical thinking would eventually have a strong influence on the nursing profession and on the education of its practitioners.[25]

World War II

During World War II, more and more nurses functioned as first assistants in both civilian and military facilities. On the civilian front, 23% of the available patient beds and operating rooms were not used because nursing personnel were scarce. Student nurses represented 80% of the work force in the 1,300 hospitals with schools of nursing or affiliated with schools of nursing. By 1944, casualties numbered as high as 1,750 per day.[26] "Give us nurses; 10,000 needed overnight" became the national call.[27] By June 1945, 29% of all graduate nurses were on duty with the armed forces.[28] The nursing profession had been alerted to the kinds of health problems to anticipate at war from their experiences in World War I, and those who engaged in military service were able to respond to a new and challenging requirement for their knowledge and skills.[29] In her book, Juanita Redmond described her experience on Corregidor:

> Inside, we heard the screaming of the shells. All the doctors and nurses hurried to duty, as the gates were opened and corpsmen ran out with stretchers to bring in the wounded. The shells had done their work well. We worked all that night. . . . Endless, harrowing hours of giving injections, anesthetizing, ripping off clothes, stitching gaping wounds of amputation, sterilizing instruments, bandaging, settling the treated patients in their beds, covering the wounded that we could not save. . . .[30]

The combination of personnel shortages and high casualty rates gave impetus to the continued need for the RN to act as first assistant. In this role, nurses opened and closed wounds; the surgeon performed the internal interventions. Tying and clamping of bleeding vessels was a routine nursing function. Nursing experience with abdominal and chest surgery was increasing, and nurses sometimes performed procedures such as tracheostomy and chest tube insertion. New sorting and treatment possibilities—such as triage, antibiotic therapy, transfusions, and rehabilitation—led both nursing and medicine into the fledgling technological era of health care. Air evacuation and flight nursing was an important innovation. Since flight surgeons rarely were on the airplanes, flight nurses were responsible for the care of patients until a hospital could be reached.[31] At no other time in American history were nurses in greater demand. Nursing roles expanded in response to this demand, and the RN first assistant filled a patient care need with efficiency and acumen.

World War II also brought important changes in American society that affected nurses. The changing roles of women, increasing levels of education among the general population, advances in medical science, and altered economic conditions contributed to changing patterns of nursing practice. Nursing in the home increasingly shifted to clinics and hospitals as a result of the public health movement. Nursing curricula began to accommodate advances in science, especially medical science, to prepare nurses not only with knowledge but also with an understanding of both the what and why of changes in nursing practice. This upgrading of nursing's educational standards was opposed by many physicians and hospital administrators, who were concerned about possible reductions in nursing school enrollments, the possibility of nurses becoming more independent in their actions and less obedient to the demands of physicians, the threat of competition from highly educated nurses taking over aspects of the physician's role, and the possibility of such educated nurses passing judgment on physicians' work. Despite such opposition, however, the need for a strong science background and critical thinking and judgment abilities would continue to make itself felt in the educational preparation of the RN first assistant. Unquestioning obedience was no longer compatible with standards of nursing behavior or with the practice of nurses who met the rigorous demands of perioperative patient care during the war.

Korean War

The Korean War, 1950 to 1953, witnessed the expansion of the nurse's role as first assistant in mobile army surgical hospitals. These MASH units were each staffed with 16 skilled nurses who perfected the role of first assistant. Skill and knowledge were essential; nurses worked long hours assisting in complex procedures under adverse conditions. Triage became a nursing responsibility during this war. Nurses assessed patient injury, prioritized casualties for surgery, provided initial emergency intervention, and administered emergency medical services. Eventually, the role of the medical corpsman evolved as a part of wartime medicine, but this did not deter some nurses from holding on to the role and responsibility that had evolved for the RN first assistant. This role continued to be important to the military forces in both Vietnam and the Middle East during Desert Storm.

Vietnam War

Active U.S. involvement in Vietnam began in 1961. Approximately 7,500 military women served in this war, with about 80% being members of the military Nurse Corps.[32] The severity of wounds and injuries during this war was staggering. Because mines, booby traps, and high-velocity bullets were used, multiple mutilating wounds were often sustained. Incendiaries complicated the casualties, resulting in massive, smoldering burns. The combination of helicopter shuttle to hospitals and trauma care, however, saved many injured who would have died in previous wars. Despite the fact that the rate of multiple amputations was triple what it was in World War II, survival rates for lower extremity amputation were 300% better than they had been in that war. At the beginning of the 1968 Tet offensive, the operating room was reserved for patients with head and chest wounds; amputations were done in a roped-off area of a sidewalk.[33] Experienced operating room nurses were in great demand and their responsibilities encompassing. In her book, Van Devanter relates,

Some doctors were frustrated with my performance and angry that I didn't already know everything they had been taught in their residencies. Others were more patient. One of the most understanding teachers was a thoracic surgeon named Carl Adams. If you want good help, he said, you've got to be willing to teach them. He taught me to tie off blood vessels and even talked me through my first splenectomy, when I had to remove what remained of one of the soldier's spleen, while he worked lower in the belly on more pressing problems.[34]

Marshall is even more explicit:

> I did all kinds of surgery. Sometimes I actually had to function as a surgeon. Like, guys would come in with wounds all over their bodies. Maybe they'd hit a mine and there would be all these little pellet injuries. My job then was to make an incision and cut away the dead muscle and dead tissue. . . . And we would do this for hours . . . on just one guy . . . with hundreds of wounds all over his body. So what we did was divide the body up and the surgeon would work on one half of the body and I'd work on the other half. . . . When it was chest or bowel surgery . . . [I'd] tie off blood vessels and suture. . . . I had to learn to do everything with one hand that I used to do with two.[35]

Surgeons who worked with nurses such as Marshall, and the Vietnamese operating room nurses who similarly demonstrated such surgical skill, returned home with new perspectives on the possible roles for perioperative nurses. In 1968, Rogers, an orthopedic surgeon who served in Vietnam, pondered,

> With the present and ever increasing shortage of doctors, the use of physicians as surgical assistants in hospitals where there is no house staff is a wasteful activity and relatively nonproductive . . . an assistant with the background and training of a registered nurse who has gained experience in orthopedic nursing is usually of greater help during surgery than the physician [as an] assistant. . . . I am personally convinced that this is the coming place for the operating room nurse in surgery . . . the nurse's background enables her not only to assist the physician in the technical procedures, but also to supervise those activities in the operating room where we physicians rely on our surgical nurse . . . the reasons for which are not understood by casual workers or less qualified technicians. [36]

▇ THE STUDENT NURSE AS FIRST ASSISTANT

From 1873 until the early 1930s, hospital nursing staffs often consisted of a superintendent of nurses (who was a graduate nurse) and nursing students. As late as 1926, 549 nursing schools had no full-time graduate teachers; the remaining 894 schools had from one to six graduate teaching faculty.[37] In 1927, as many as 73% of the hospitals with nursing schools had no graduate nurses employed for general duty. Hospitals without schools were staffed by attendants.[38] Graduate nurse staffs increased slightly during the 1930s but decreased again in the 1940s. Even from 1944 to 1945, student nurses provided nearly 80% of the nursing services in hospitals affiliated with schools.[39] Consequently, hospital operating room nurses were often students.

Various early nursing texts referred to the nursing role in the operating room, describing the perioperative nurse as a provider of indirect and direct nursing care and as a first assistant. Weeks, who wrote an early textbook on nursing, in 1890 stated that two nurses should be in attendance at the operating table and emphasized the participant nature of their roles: "You are present not as a spectator, but as an assistant."[40] In 1901 Luce described the role of the operating room nurse: "The operating room nurse assists the surgeon with sponges, ligatures, and sutures; she keeps the instruments clean and ready for use, and is sometimes required to hold retractors or specula."[41]

Usually four nurses participated in a surgical procedure; these nurses were sometimes referred to as a permanent operating room nurse, a senior operating room nurse, and two junior operating room nurses.[42] The nurse in charge of the room, called the circulating nurse in later years, prepared and draped the patient in the etherizing room while the surgeon completed another patient procedure. Two nurses were in attendance with the surgeon at the operating table. One of these two nurses was to retract viscera, assist during the surgery, and attend to the routine of closure.[43–46] The other nurse was often referred to as the "sponge" nurse. Senn described the practice of sponging: "If asked to do the sponging, she [the nurse] does not wipe but merely compresses the bleeding parts, allowing the sponge to absorb what it will."[47] The fourth nurse administered anesthesia.[48–50]

Over the years, the vital nature of anesthesia administration and of the role of first assistant became recognized, and students were not permitted to fill these roles. By the 1930s, anesthesia was administered only by graduate nurses. By the 1960s, only graduate nurses were permitted to act as first assistants.

■ THE PRIVATE DUTY NURSE AS FIRST ASSISTANT

From 1873 to the late 1920s, private duty nursing was the primary area of employment for the graduate nurse. A limited amount of this private duty was performed by students, who were sent into private homes by proprietary hospital schools to render nursing service. During this time, and even until the late 1920s, many surgical procedures were performed in the home. Wound morbidity and mortality were lower for persons undergoing surgery in the home than for those undergoing surgery in a hospital.

The early nursing literature described processes used to prepare the home for surgery. Descriptions included precise suggestions for creating suitable conditions for operating. Instructions were offered for converting the kitchen and stove into a good operating room and sterilizer.[51] DeLee, in another early nursing textbook, provided a detailed description of how to prepare the home for obstetric procedures, including vaginal forceps delivery, craniotomy, decapitation, and abdominal cesarean section.[52] DeLee advised that "a kitchen or library table makes an excellent operating table; a sewing table does well for the instruments and basins; a euchre table gives additional space. Two kitchen chairs with a table board on them makes an excellent side table."[53]

In her textbook, Weeks described in detail the practice of cauterizing vessels with nitrate of silver and tying off bleeders. This was an essential part of the nurse first assistant role. According to Weeks, "the artery is picked up by a pair of forceps, and a ligature tucked firmly about it. A ligature should be about eighteen inches long. . . . Test its strength well, so as to leave no chance of its breaking when strained; and if you have to tie, be sure and make it a firm knot."[54] She went on to detail how to make the surgeon's reef knot, the surgeon's knot, and the cat's paw, complete with diagrams and the dictate that nurses practice these knots. Murphy describes a nurse entrepreneur in 1905 who "offered her services as a surgical specialist to surgeons who performed procedures in patients' homes. She charged $5 per procedure if the procedure did not require certain supplies or if the surgeon provided the supplies; she charged $25 if she furnished supplies."[55]

■ EDUCATION OF THE NURSE
FOR THE OPERATING ROOM

Formal schools of nursing in the United States originated in 1873 and were modeled on the Nightingale schools in England. In the early years of nursing education, the theory component included the use of surgical instruments, hemostasis, and preparation of the patient for surgery. The contributions of the nurse in the operating room were widely acknowledged as vital to the success of the operation and to the surgical patient's welfare. The number of hours in theory instruction gradually increased, and the National League for Nursing Education began publishing curriculum guides for schools. The 1937 edition of this publication recommended that operating room theory and practice be covered in the second year of 3-year diploma programs and that students be prepared to assist in operations and emergencies.[56]

In 1933 the Committee on the Grading of Nursing Schools reported that nursing schools placed a high priority on operating room nursing and that most schools included the recommended 6- to 8-week clinical rotation for this specialty. Objectives for the curricular undertaking in operating room nursing included an understanding of the relationship between the procedure and the patient's safety, an improvement in skill in nursing patients in the operating room, and an understanding of operating room techniques and their scientific basis.[57] In 1942 the National League for Nursing Education, in an attempt to alleviate the nursing shortage and prepare practitioners in a shorter time, proposed three different plans to reduce the 36-month diploma program. Consistently, the high priority given to operating room nursing resulted in the recommendation that this experience be increased from 6 weeks to 8 weeks.[58] Beginning in 1945, nursing education made earnest efforts to transform the role of the student as nonpaid hospital employee to that of academic participant. Essential to this transformation was the use of full-time, qualified nurse faculty to guide academic development. These changes had a negative impact on operating room nursing. The expense of the small ratio of faculty to students in the operating room was not cost-effective, and students' clinical experience in the operating room began to decrease in schools.

Compounding this problem was the emergence of specialization among surgeons and operating room nursing staffs. As early as 1961, a surgical nursing textbook stated that "in these days of specialization, it is essential that knowledge be built on a foundation of sound basic science, for then it does not matter whether work is done in a plastic, thoracic, or general surgery unit."[59] The rapid development of new surgical treatments and new knowledge required operating room nurses to become versatile members of the surgical team. The role of circulating nurse became increasingly complex; this nurse simultaneously became instructor, supervisor, and patient care manager in the assigned operating room. The scrub nurse of the 1970s needed "above all else, experience. This must be intelligent experience, based on a thorough understanding of each proposed surgical procedure and a careful observation and anticipation of each step in the operation."[60] To help students fully appreciate the importance of these nursing roles, authors specified various assignments and purposes for the student nurse's first, second, third, and fourth operating room experiences.[61] Based on the view that only highly trained and experienced personnel could fulfill the complicated and highly responsible functions of operating room nurse, it was believed that student nurses should be advanced slowly and progressively during their surgical experiences. Nursing curricula, on the other hand, could ill afford the time required for this slow progression. "Scrubbing up to assist the surgeon" was a duty that a ward nurse should be familiar with, but that was performed by nurses who specialized in the operating room.[62] Soon, the goals of student rotations also became more oriented toward familiarization with the role than toward skill or competency in it.

Despite the efforts of the Association of Operating Room Nurses (AORN), with its well-designed and patient-focused learning modules for nursing educators who oversaw curricular content for nursing in the operating room, by the 1980s experience for students in the perioperative nursing role had all but disappeared from basic nursing curricula. The long-term impact of this change led to a shortage of perioperative nurses in 1997. Even with the advance of managed care and its anticipated downsizings, mergers, and acquisitions, demand for perioperative interventions and nurses to care for those patients will remain stable.[63] The RN first assistant will be needed in hospitals, where patients are more aged, sicker, with high-tech demands; as surgical care shifts outside of the hospital, RNFAs will be needed to integrate ambulatory patient care. An emerging cohort of RNFAs prepared as advanced practice nurses will compensate for the decrease in numbers of surgical residents as graduate medical education funds are diverted to prepare primary care physicians.

▓ FACTORS INFLUENCING THE FIRST ASSISTANT ROLE, 1945 TO 1998

The period following World War II was marked by major increases in hospital construction, increases in elective surgery procedures, and a continued severe nursing shortage. The preferred solution to the health care personnel emergency was to free the nurse to nurse, a solution proposing that specific tasks and nonnursing duties could be performed by less skilled personnel. Brown was the primary originator and long-term advocate of this concept. Writing in 1948, she stated that "the graduate staff nurse should be freed, or should free herself, to the maximum degree from those relatively unimportant duties still performed by her in order that she may concentrate her whole attention, within the voluntary hospital, upon the acutely ill and those in greatest need of total care."[64]

Brown also emphasized that no institution should pay for nursing services that could be performed as effectively by a person with shorter preparation than the RN. The Brown Report, as her study became known, called for increasing use of practical nurses, licensing of practical nurses, use of paid aides to take the place of volunteers who had been used during the war years, and use of a new group of nonnursing personnel classified as technicians.[65] The Brown Report was readily accepted by hospital administrators, third-party payers, and unemployed military corpsmen. The practical nurse entered the operating room and was rapidly followed by the operating room technician. Both of these workers quickly began to replace the RN at the operating table, as scrub nurse and as first assistant.

By 1965 the use of operating room technicians had become an accepted practice. The mid–1960s also brought the return of large numbers of independent duty corpsmen. These persons had received the equivalent of practical nurse training in their military programs. They were also proficient in the execution of emergency medical measures. Increasing numbers of these corpsmen entered the civilian job market each year. Coupled with a physician shortage, these events abetted the emergence of yet another health care worker who entered the operating room. These workers have become the physician's assistant in today's market. By 1970, the physician's assistant was functioning as first assistant during surgery. With the advent of the technician and the physician's assistant, the roles of the professional nurse in the operating room, as scrub person and first assistant, were seriously threatened.

The 1970s and 1980s were marked by articulate debate and concerted attempts to clarify the role of the professional nurse in the operating room. The philosophical premise on which the operating room nurse has explored role ambiguity and role clarification is the concern with providing safe, economical patient care. It is this concern with the patient that has driven and continues to drive the activity surrounding research on the perioperative role, scope of practice for RN first assistants, and third-party reimbursement.

By 1980 the American College of Surgeons (ACS) had defined the duties of the first assistant. In this definition the role of the RN as provider of first assistant services was affirmed. However, the ACS emphasized that when the RN functions in this capacity, those assigned duties must fall within the scope of the nurse's State Nurse Practice Act.

In 1980 AORN developed guidelines for the RN functioning as first assistant. These guidelines also emphasized that when the RN serves as first assistant, the first assistant functions must fall within the scope of the pertinent Nurse Practice Act.[66]

By 1983 the RN was permitted to function in the role of first assistant in 17 states. However, only the state of Washington clearly stated that the RN could function as a first assistant and still function within the scope of the Nurse Practice Act. The majority of states considered first assistant practice to be a delegated medical function or a function regulated by hospital policy. Twelve states firmly stated that the RN could not function as a first assistant because this function was not clearly identified within the scope of their nurse practice acts. Many other states continued to study the question.[67]

In 1983 AORN appointed a task force to study and clarify the role responsibilities and qualifications of the RN first assistant. The task force issued its report and presented its findings as guidelines for position assumption; in 1984, the AORN House of Delegates approved the first Official Statement on the RN First Assistant. Thus a landmark movement to return nurses to their rightful role as first assistant took shape in this country. Committed to and energized by the issue, perioperative nurses became politically active patient advocates.

An event in Pennsylvania captured what was occurring across the nation. On June 19, 1980, the Pennsylvania State Board of Nurse Examiners ruled that RNs could not function as first assistants and further stated that any nurse who did function as a first assistant would be liable for malpractice. As the RN first assistant movement swept the country, Pennsylvania nurses began taking steps to reverse the board's position. AORN members contacted board members and set up a process of dialogue and debate. These nurses extensively interviewed and surveyed practicing operating room nurses and clearly identified for the state board what nonnurses were doing as first assistants and the inherent danger of such practice for the consumer. A detailed plan of action was developed. Information relative to the AORN goal was disseminated to other nursing organizations in an attempt to gain and solidify professional nursing support. In November 1984, representatives of the Pennsylvania Council of Operating Room Nurses met with the State Board of Nurse Examiners to discuss proposed changes in the interpretation of the Nurse Practice Act.

During the November meeting of the Pennsylvania State Board of Nurse Examiners, the previous ruling concerning first assistant practice was withdrawn. The state board ruled that first assisting did fall within the scope of nursing practice under the Professional Nurse Act. This decision was made possible because the board stated that according to the Pennsylvania Professional Nursing Law's definition of nursing, nursing practice is allowed if it provides for "provision of care supportive to or restorative of life and well being and executing medical regimens as prescribed by a licensed physician or dentist."[68] In addition, provision for allowing the RN to function as a first assistant was covered under rules and regulations relating to the responsibilities of the RN in Section 21.11, General Functions, specifically:

> Carries out nursing care actions which promote, maintain, and restore the well being of individuals.
> The Board recognizes standards of practices and professional codes of behavior as developed by appropriate nursing organizations as the criteria for assuring safe and effective practice.[69]

Since 1985 there have been rapid, persistent, and promising efforts and events that have clearly confirmed the importance of the role of the RN first assistant. As first assistant educational courses began to flourish, the ranks of perioperative nurses prepared to assist at surgery swelled. Legislative efforts were initiated, seeking third-party reimbursement from both private and federal payers; initiatives at the state level began in Florida and are continuing to be introduced into state legislatures. *A Core Curriculum for the RN First Assistant* was published by AORN, and activities were undertaken to develop a certification examination for RN first assistants in 1992. Repeated surveys of boards of nursing indicated that by 1992, no states ruled that assisting at surgery by the RN was outside the scope of nursing practice. Instead, all states had either rendered an opinion that the RN could first assist or had declined to render an opinion. The RN First Assistant Specialty Assembly was formed in 1992, with a mission of providing a coalition dedicated to the advancement of the RNFA.

In testimony of AORN on reimbursement for nonphysician providers before the Physician Payment Review Commission, it was noted that

> The RN first assistant is a very versatile professional whose contribution to the patient is not limited to intraoperative "assisting" the surgeon. Preoperatively, the RN first assistant is involved in taking the patient history and doing the physical examination. They also teach the patient, order routine laboratory tests, check the x-rays, evaluate the patient's emotional status, and check on last-minute details of the surgery schedule. Immediately before the surgery, the RN who will later assist the surgeon assists the anesthesiologist with insertion of intraoperative monitoring lines and preliminary procedures. Intraoperatively, the RN first assistant assists the surgeon with the surgical procedure itself. Specific tasks are directly related to the specialty, training, and education of the RN first assistant. Virtually every surgical specialty uses RN first assistants. More than 40% work in general surgery, with 24% evenly split between orthopedic and cardiovascular specialties. Plastic surgery, gynecology, and ophthalmology are also popular specialties who utilize the services of an RN first assistant. RN first assistants are experts in their area of practice. For example, those who are employed by cardiovascular surgeons may in fact harvest veins for cardiac bypass surgery. The specific procedures for which an RN first assistant is credentialed would be determined by the in-

dividual hospital credentialing procedure. All RN first assistants do not do the same procedures, but they do share common skills such as retraction, tying sutures, clamping bleeding vessels, and closing incisions. Postoperatively, the RN first assistant makes rounds to evaluate the patient's condition and remove sutures, chest tubes, central monitoring lines, and in some cases intra-aortic balloons. Many RN first assistants also see patients in the physician's office postdischarge, at which time they do a great deal of patient teaching.[70]

The window of opportunity for RN first assistants is wide open. The nursing literature has provided cumulative evidence that nurses deliver cost-effective care that can be substituted for a physician's care in many instances. Studies have been done linking surgical volume with lower inpatient mortality and indicating that hospitals with a larger proportion of RNs provide better care as measured by lower mortality rates. The problem with many of these studies, however, is that they do not isolate or measure the specific nursing contributions to improvements in patient care. The clarion call for the next millennium must be the development of a body of research that validates the contributions of the RN first assistant. Such research should focus on operating room productivity, quality and outcomes of care, intraoperative contributions, practice settings, roles and responsibilities, effects of collaboration, nurse-generated innovations, cost-effectiveness, utilization, and reimbursement patterns. As RN first assistants develop this body of knowledge, what is now only intuitively and experientially known will become visible and evident to all who seek to confirm the value of the RN first assistant to the efficient and effective care of perioperative patients. RNFAs must continue to interface with the political system if they are to influence public policy and assist in moving forward with the nursing profession's goals. In order to do this, RNFAs, already clinical experts, will need to also become expert in health care economics, clinical decision making, organization of health care systems, financing of health care, clinical outcomes research, quality and accountability, informatics, care of populations and communities, social justice and issues of access, and ethics of health care decisions.[71]

CONCLUSION

The role of first assistant has always been an integral part of perioperative nursing. Although specific aspects of role dimension have been modified throughout history, the vital nature of the knowledge base and the skill level possessed by the perioperative nurse have always pointed to this person as the member of the nursing team best prepared to provide care to the surgical patient. For a time this role, as well as the quality of health care provided to the consumer, was at risk. By 1985 the role of the RN as first assistant had made a full historical circle and repeated itself. The future will determine the full importance of the RN first assistant role as well as its impact on quality perioperative patient care. Nursing's social contract has always been to provide care to those in need, and this underpins the RNFA's commitment to the person undergoing an operation or other invasive procedure.

Review Questions

Please select the best response to the following questions. Answers are provided at the conclusion of the review questions section.

1. During colonial development in the United States:
   a. Nursing service had a distinctive role.
   b. Nursing of the sick was done by women in the home.
   c. Colonial medicine was in the hands of educated physicians.
   d. Boards of health instituted important sanitation measures.

2. In the early part of the 18th century, hospitals became so crowded that cleaning was impossible in a hospital ward. This furthered the belief that:
   a. It was a disgrace for respectable people to send a relative to the hospital.
   b. Educated women and women of the upper class should participate in hospital nursing.
   c. It was a woman's social responsibility to change these deplorable conditions.
   d. Nurses should be paid higher wages, considering their working conditions.

3. The service of nursing began its slow climb up the ladder of respectability when Florence Nightingale sailed for Scutari in the Crimea in 1854. The results of her efforts are well known and proved the value of
   a. Accepting female nurses in a military hospital.
   b. Nursing collaboration with medical staff.
   c. Having social contacts to purchase resources for care of the ill.
   d. Using prepared individuals (her 38 nurses) in the care of the ill.

4. In her *Notes on Nursing,* Nightingale depicted nursing as
   a. Performance of household and laundering chores.
   b. The proper use of fresh air, light, warmth, and cleanliness.
   c. Unfailing loyalty and obedience to the physician.
   d. The duty of devoted women, despite their subordinate position.

5. At the beginning of the Civil War, there were no organized nursing groups, no ambulances, and no field hospital service. The woman appointed Superintendent of the Female Army of Nurses was
   a. Mary Ann Bickerdyke.
   b. Louise Schuyler.
   c. Dorothea Dix.
   d. Louisa May Alcott.

6. The goals of nursing leaders of the late 19th century focused on
    a. Subverting medical opposition to female doctors.
    b. Developing schools of nursing in universities.
    c. Trying to contain hospital costs for nursing service.
    d. Improving nursing service and widening opportunities for women.

7. During World War I:
    a. Clara Barton became Superintendent of the Army Nurse Corps.
    b. Some nurses served with surgical teams close to the front lines.
    c. Nursing care continued to consist of routine care and comfort.
    d. Nurses were forbidden assignment in camp, evacuation, or mobile hospitals.

8. The nursing profession emerged from World War I with:
    a. A deep sense of pride in its accomplishments.
    b. Little eagerness for a more independent status for nurses.
    c. A sad lack of increased prestige in the eyes of the public.
    d. A renewed zeal for private duty nursing.

9. In the first third of the 20th century, nursing began to think of protecting those needing nursing service. Nurses realized that one way to do this was by
    a. Organizing labor unions to improve working conditions.
    b. Using students, rather than graduates, to keep costs down.
    c. Changing the 24-hour work day to a 12-hour work day.
    d. Advocating nurse registration.

10. There were 1,619 nurses serving in World War II who received medals for their service. For perioperative nursing and RN first assistants, one of the most important outcomes of this war was their
    a. Replacement in operating rooms on the home front by practical nurses.
    b. Demonstrated ability in front-line aid stations and field hospitals.
    c. Development of psychosocial skills to keep up the morale of the wounded.
    d. Assignment to bedside nursing in war zones, which added a pre-operative dimension to their practice.

11. At the close of the 1970s, nurses were finding themselves in conflict with demands from physicians to take on tasks once done only by physicians. For the RN first assistant, an example of such task conflict was
    a. Performing blood pressure measurement.
    b. Expanding into labor and delivery to assist at complicated births.
    c. Tying surgical knots and suturing wounds.
    d. Administering intravenous conscious sedation.

12. A study of nursing education with many implications for the contemporary nurse was *Nursing for the Future,* by Esther Lucille Brown, published in 1948. Brown recommended that:

    a. Educational programs for practical nursing be improved but that practical nurses not be licensed.

    b. The hospital environment foster the nurse's professional growth and free her to "nurse."

    c. Specialty hospitals be expanded and educational programs for nurse specialists be developed.

    d. Education for nurses remain hospital-based to provide the requisite clinical skills demanded by medical advances.

13. The 1997 AORN's Official Statement on the RN First Assistant acknowledged the importance of this nursing practice area in achieving optimal results for the patient. To provide this type of assistant at surgery, AORN recommended that the RN first assistant:

    a. Concurrently function as a scrub nurse.

    b. Obtain advanced preparation in a master's program.

    c. Have CNOR as a minimal certification.

    d. Be hired by a surgeon and be directly responsible to that surgeon.

14. The term *perioperative* encompasses

    a. Scrub nurses.

    b. Circulating nurses.

    c. RN first assistants.

    d. All of the above.

15. In the 1990s, the role of the RN first assistant

    a. Is primarily intraoperative.

    b. Is important in small hospitals without residents.

    c. Has expanded beyond the confines of the surgical suite.

    d. Is threatened by lack of nursing support.

■ Answer Key

1. b	6. d	11. c
2. a	7. b	12. b
3. d	8. a	13. c
4. b	9. d	14. d
5. c	10. b	15. c

REFERENCES

1. Wilbur CK: Revolutionary Medicine. Chester, Globe Pequot Press, 1980
2. Colp R, Keller MW: Textbook of Surgical Nursing. New York, Macmillan, 1927
3. Wilbur, p 1
4. Reverby S: A caring dilemma: Womanhood and nursing in historical perspective. Nurs Res 36:5–11, 1987
5. Ibid, p 6

6. Atkinson DT: Magic, Myth, and Medicine. New York, World Publishing, 1956
7. Nightingale F: Notes on Nursing. New York, Dover Publications, 1969 (Original work published 1859)
8. Keeling AF, Ramos MC: The role of nursing history in preparing nursing for the future. Nurs Health Care 16:30–33, 1995
9. Kitson AL: Johns Hopkins address: Does nursing have a future? Image 29:111–115, 1997
10. Kalisch PA, Kalisch BJ: The Advance of American Nursing. Boston, Little, Brown, 1978
11. Nightingale, p 71
12. Lynaugh J: Diary of a nurse. Nurs Res 40:254–255, 1991
13. Kalisch and Kalisch, pp 49–66
14. Sigerist HE: The Great Doctors. New York, WW Norton, 1933
15. Dannett SGL: Nobel Women of the North. New York, Thomas Yoseloff, 1959
16. Houck PW: A healing place. Civil War 9:40–43, May–June 1991
17. Ragge MM: Nursing and politics: A forgotten legacy. Nurs Res 36:26–30, 1986
18. Oates SB: A woman of valor—Clara Barton and the Civil War. Reflections 16–17, first quarter 1996
19. Ramage JA: I was there with Whitman at Armory Square. Civil War 9:8–9, May–June 1991
20. Kalisch and Kalisch, pp 216–220
21. Quandt E: Active service on the western front. Am J Nurs 18:454–455, 1918
22. Interviews with nurses and patients who served during World War I. Lebanon Veterans Hospital, 1955–1957
23. History of Nursing Museum, third floor, Pine Building, Pennsylvania Hospital, Philadelphia
24. Bledsoe, HW: American nurses for American men: A World War I diary. Nurs Health Care 18:11–14, 1997
25. Hanson KS: An analysis of the historical context of liberal education in nursing education from 1924–1939. J Prof Nurs 7:341–350, 1991
26. Kalisch and Kalisch, pp 471–478
27. Ibid, p 478
28. Ibid, p 483
29. Marks D: Social legislation: World War II posed new challenges for nursing. Am Nurse 28:20, 1996
30. Kalisch PA, Kalisch BJ: Nurses under fire: The World War II experiences of nurses on Bataan and Corregidor. Nurs Res 44:260–271, 1995
31. Stevens SY: Aviation pioneers: World War II air evacuation nurses. Image 26:95–98, 1994
32. Schwartz LS: Women and the Vietnam experience. Image 19:168–173, 1987
33. Scannell-Desch EA: The lived experience of women military nurses in Vietnam during the Vietnam War. Image 28:119–124, 1996
34. Van Devanter L: Home Before Morning. New York, Warner Books, 1983
35. Marshall K: In the Combat Zone. Boston, Little, Brown, 1987
36. Rogers WJ: Vietnam impressions by an orthopedic surgeon. AORN J 46:72–79, 1968
37. Some problems in grading our schools of nursing. Trained Nurse Hosp Rev 77:509, November, 1926
38. Kalisch and Kalisch, Advance of American Nursing, p 363
39. Ibid, p 478
40. Weeks CS: Textbook of Nursing, 2nd ed. New York, Appleton, 1897
41. Luce M: The duties of an operating room nurse. Am J Nurs 1:404, 1901
42. Fowler RS: The Operating Room and the Patient. Philadelphia, WB Saunders, 1918

43. VanSyckel J: The operating room technique at St Luke's Hospital, New York. Am J Nurs 10:635–638, 1910
44. Colp and Keller, p 291
45. Bertella M: Operating room routine: The training of students. Am J Nurs 24:377–380, 1924
46. Colp and Keller, p 14
47. Senn N: A Nurse's Guide for the Operating Room. Chicago, WT Keene, 1902
48. Weeks, p 199
49. Senn, p 13
50. Kalisch and Kalisch, Advance of American Nursing, p 183
51. Woodbury LC: Surgical nursing. Am J Nurs 13:688–693, 1903
52. DeLee JB: Obstetrics for Nurses, 3rd ed. Philadelphia, WB Saunders, 1909
53. Ibid, p 181
54. Weeks, p 245
55. Murphy EK: Evolving nursing care practices. Surg Services Management 1:15–17, 1995
56. Committee on Curriculum of the National League for Nursing Education: Nursing Schools of Today and Tomorrow. Final Report of the Committee on the Grading of Nursing Schools. New York, Committee on Grading of Nursing Schools, 1937
57. Stewart I: The Education of Nurses. New York, Macmillan, 1943
58. National League for Nursing Education: Nursing Education in Wartime (Complete Series of Fourteen Bulletins). New York, National League for Nursing Education, 1945
59. Taylor S, Worrall O: Principles of Surgery and Surgical Nursing. London, English Universities Press, 1961
60. LeMaitre G, Finnegan J: The Patient in Surgery, Philadelphia, WB Saunders, 1970
61. Ibid, pp 87–120
62. Moroney J: Surgery for Nurses. London, Churchill Livingstone, 1971
63. Pattersen P: Where will OR staff of the future come from? OR Manager 13:1, 1997
64. Brown EL: Nursing for the Future. New York, Russell Sage Foundation, 1948
65. Ibid, pp 57–72
66. Task force defines first assisting. AORN J 39:502–503, 1984
67. Survey shows state board position on first assistant. AORN J 37:428–436, 1984
68. Professional Nursing Law, Commonwealth of Pennsylvania. Act 151, 1974
69. Rules and Regulations of the State Board of Nurse Examiners for Registered Nurses, Commonwealth of Pennsylvania, 1983
70. Testimony of the Association of Operating Room Nurses on reimbursement for nonphysician providers before the Physician Payment Review Commission, Sept 13, 1990
71. Peirce AG: Re-examining Nightingale's vision: Clinical excellence and health services policy and research. Nurs Health Care 16:282–285, 1995

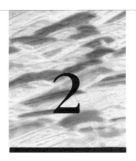

THE NURSE PRACTICE ACT
AND REGULATION
OF NURSING PRACTICE

JANE C. ROTHROCK

■

The practice of nursing for both registered nurses (RNs) and licensed practical nurses (LPNs) is enacted by state legislation, known as statutory law. The law is set forth in a nurse practice act, which must be approved by the state senate and house and signed by the governor. While nurse practice acts are unique to each state, they all have the underlying principle of the protection of the public through the regulation of nursing practice. In addition to the act, rules and regulations promulgated by the state board of nursing have the weight of law and clarify the implementation of the act. For example, the act requires that the RN have a current license to practice, and the rules and regulations spell out procedures and requirements for obtaining the license, including items such as required educational background and fees. Each RNFA should have a current copy of his or her state Nurse Practice Act. It is in reference to the act that first attempts are made to determine "what is nursing?" Each state's Nurse Practice Act contains a legal definition of nursing, delineating the minimum requirements for the safe and competent practice of nursing as regulated by law in that state. The enforcement of the act and the protection of the public from unqualified practitioners is delegated to boards of nursing located in each of the states.

◼ PURPOSE OF THE PRACTICE ACT

The purpose of statutory law and regulation of the health professions is to protect the consumer. By issuing nursing licenses, it is possible to control who practices nursing and to ensure that the practice meets approved standards. Thus, by limiting the practice of nursing to licensees and restricting impostors, substandard care is avoided. A trend among other health care personnel is to press for the rights of licensure so that their practice will be recognized, defined, and protected. It is necessary that RNFAs monitor this movement so that nursing practice is restricted to qualified personnel. Professional nurses have a responsibility to make sure that patients receive the best possible care, which involves more than performing tasks. It also includes assessment, diagnosing, planning, implementing, evaluating outcomes of care, and teaching, which must take into account the total family and the various resources available.

Early Licensure Efforts

The idea of licensing nurses began in England in 1867, when Henry Wentworth Ackland, a physician, made unsuccessful efforts to protect the public by recognizing qualified nurses. The banner was taken up by a nurse, Ethel Gordon Bedford Fenwick, but as early as the 1890s nurses were divided in their support of nursing licensure. Florence Nightingale was a strong opponent of licensure, because she was concerned that qualifications established for licensure would not give sufficient weight to moral characteristics. Because Nightingale fought to raise nursing to a respected profession rather than merely the work of servants and prostitutes, it is understandable that she would be protective. But this divisiveness in nursing resulted in the delay of licensing in England until 1919, long after the first nurse practice act was passed in New Zealand in 1901.[1]

In the United States, North Carolina passed its nurse practice act in 1903, followed shortly thereafter by New Jersey, New York, and Virginia. These acts included the major rights and requirements of nursing practice that remain relevant today. They specified the right to the title RN, required that graduates pass an examination, and provided a grandfather clause allowing those practicing to be licensed by waiver. The most impressive aspect of this success is that nurses managed to guide these acts through the legislative process at a time when women did not have the right to vote.[2] This demonstrates what can be accomplished when nurses work together. The cooperative, dedicated work of these early nurse leaders should be an example to all nurses.

Chaska divided the development of nursing legislation into three phases.[3] In the first phase, from 1903 to 1938, the focus was primarily on registration. From 1938 to 1971, as the profession developed, the emphasis was on defining the scope of practice. In the third phase, the profession struggled with the concepts of advanced practice and the expanded role of the nurse. As nursing moves toward the 21st century, issues of competence assessment, delegation, and new regulatory models are engaging the profession in dialogue and debate.

■ BOARDS OF NURSING

Each state or jurisdiction has its own board or boards; some have one board for RNs and another for LPNs. Boards are administered according to the statutes of the jurisdiction. Some nursing boards are under the jurisdiction of the education department; others are responsible to the commissioner of a bureau of professional regulation or licensure. The administrative organization has implications for the autonomy and independence of the board.

Board Composition

Appointment to the board varies in each state but usually requires senate approval; the appointment is made by the governor, commonly for a period of 4 to 6 years. In some states board members are elected. Most boards govern both RNs and LPNs and typically consist of RNs, LPNs, and consumers. In some states physicians serve on the nurse board. It is helpful to have a balanced board with members representing both practice and education as well as different regions of the state. All nurse members should be well prepared and active in professional nursing. The reasons for this will become apparent in the discussion of board functions.

National Council of State Boards of Nursing

At the 1978 convention of the American Nurses Association (ANA), the delegates voted to form the National Council of State Boards of Nursing (NCSBN), comprised of the member boards. Prior to that, representatives of state boards of nursing had met as a council within ANA. At the NCSBN annual meeting, two delegates from each member board vote on issues in the house of delegates meetings. The president and board of directors are elected and committees are elected or appointed as specified by the bylaws, mindful of the differing needs in each jurisdiction.

The purpose of the NCSBN is to provide an organization through which boards of nursing act and counsel together on matters of common interest and concern affecting the public health, safety, and welfare, including the development of licensing examinations in nursing. Decisions and recommendations are made by the delegate assembly and the board of directors. Member boards are grouped into geographic areas to discuss local issues, review the effects of national-level proposals on the region, share ideas, and prepare presentations to the delegate assembly that have national impact. The NCSBN performs policy analyses and promotes uniformity in relationship to the regulation of nursing practice throughout the states.

Licensing Examinations.   One of the most important services that the NCSBN provides for its member boards is preparing and delivering the National Council Licensing Examination for RNs (NCLEX-RN) and LPNs (NCLEX-PN). The board of directors solicits from each jurisdiction the names of nurses knowledgeable in specialty fields representing both nursing service and education. From these names the examination writers are selected. A professional testing service constructs the examination based on the test plan. Each examination includes a few trial items that are analyzed for reliability and difficulty level. As all states have the same required score for passing the examination, endorsement of licensure from one state to another is facilitated.

Purpose and Functions of State Boards

The purpose of state boards is to protect the public by supervising the implementation of the practice act(s): "The power of each state legislature to regulate practice through licensure laws is a result of the federal Constitution's delegation of the police power to the individual states under the 'state rights' provision of Article X of the U.S. Constitution."[4] The function of each board is based on the contents of the practice act. In general, those functions fall into three categories: licensure of the individual nurse, regulation of the educational programs that prepare nurses, and regulation of nursing practice.[5] Functions within this last category vary by jurisdiction but fall primarily into the areas of establishing standards for quality of practice and for quality of practice in specialized roles.

Nurse Practice Acts.   In 1980 the ANA updated its 1955 statement and published a document entitled "The Nursing Practice Act: Suggested State Legislation." Later, in 1982, the NCSBN published "The Model Nursing Practice Act." Both of these publications were based on extensive preparation, including the findings of committees and suggestions and comments from members. The NCSBN used the results of a research project to formulate its model act, which was approved by the house of delegates. In 1996, the ANA Model Practice Act was published in response to the changes that had occurred in the practice environment since the 1980 update. This model is reviewed annually to ensure incorporation of new legal decisions and state licensure laws.[6] Models provide guidelines for states rewriting their acts and provide a degree of consistency that facilitates interaction between states and reduces confusion for licensees.

Although nurse practice acts are similar in outline from state to state, they vary in detail, content, specificity, and length. All practice acts include a definition of nursing (which involves the scope of practice), and most include the organization of the state board, approval of nursing education programs, and conditions of licensure, including definition of violations and disciplinary actions. Other sections included by some states are definitions of advanced practice, expanded role, and entry level requirements.

The first task of the act is to define the practice of nursing. Most states have a flexible definition that allows nurses to practice in many varied settings, from critical care to preventive health care. Although necessary, this broad definition can be frustrating for the practicing nurse or RNFA who wants specific answers to questions of scope of practice. Some of these answers may be found in the rules and regulations or in specific statements made by the state board.

The ANA model act includes definitions of the RN, LPN, and advanced practice nurse. In its definition of nursing, the ANA notes that "nursing" means the performance of any acts for the health of the patient that require substantial specialized or general knowledge, judgment, and skill (both practice skills and cognitive skills) as defined in rules of the board of nursing. Although the model act does not specifically address unlicensed personnel, it does include provisions that would allow a board of nursing to develop standards for appropriate delegation. In 1995, the NCSBN published a paper on delegation, emphasizing and clarifying the responsibility of boards for the regulation of nursing, including nursing tasks performed by unlicensed health care workers. The NCSBN guideline clearly posited the responsibilities of the delegating nurse, who must individually assess the patient and the situation as well as the competence of the delegatee prior to delegation of any task, and must himself or herself be competent in the area of nursing relevant to the task to be delegated. It is important for RNFAs and their perioperative colleagues to understand that the functions of assessment, evaluation, and nursing judgment must not be delegated. The NCSBN goes on to offer the "five rights of delegation":

- the right task (one that is delegable for a *specific* patient)
- the right circumstances (consideration is given to the setting and the availability of adequate resources, including supervision)
- the right person (the right person is delegating to the right person)
- the right direction (task is described clearly, with limits and expectations)
- the right supervision (monitoring, evaluation, intervention, and feedback, as appropriate)[7]

The scope of practice decisions may be in the form of rules and regulations, statements of policy, or informed opinions. For example, in 1992, the Kentucky Board of Nursing issued an Advisory Opinion Statement entitled "Role of the Registered Nurse First Assistant."[8] In the Advisory Opinion, the board reviewed the definition of "registered nursing practice" in Kentucky. In light of that definition, it was the opinion of the board that the RNFA was within the scope of registered nursing practice. The board endorsed the 1984 AORN Official Statement on RN First Assistants (which was in effect at that time), and offered further opinions regarding the safe nursing practice for an RNFA. Rules and regulations, unlike an advisory opinion, must be promulgated, which entails publication in the official state bulletin, usually allowing a period during which the public has an opportunity to respond. If there is very limited opposition or no opposition, the decision bears the weight of statutory law; if violated, legal action can be taken against the licensee. A board of nursing's statement of policy or informed opinion may be used in case law. The only difference between the two is that the statement of policy is published in the state bulletin. However, depending on the statute, a waiting period for public comment is not always required. A licensee may perform an act defined as outside the scope of practice without legal repercussions, but if that nurse's practice is questioned, the licensee is subject to court hearing, where the opinion of the state board may be used by the prosecuting attorney.

Boards are frequently requested by nurses and administrators to issue scope of practice decisions; this is one of the most perplexing areas of board function. When making such a decision, the board must consider many factors, such as the difference between practice in large urban medical centers and in small rural hospitals, implications for quality improvement and risk management, and educational opportunities and levels of preparation and competence of nurses. Boards have moved away from generating lists of activities a nurse may or may not perform. The Nurse Practice Act defines basic parameters of legal practice for the professional nurse. The dynamic and evolving dimensions of nursing practice make it impossible, and undesirable, for the Nurse Practice Act to list specific activities; indeed, such an undertaking would impede and delay the growth of the discipline.[9] Instead, many boards, like the Pennsylvania Board of Nursing, have adopted a decision-making model (Chart 2–1).

Licensees should keep in mind that they should not undertake a task unless they believe that they can complete it safely—which presupposes knowledge of procedures necessary to deal with complications that may occur. This holds true in all situations except emergencies when life-saving measures are instituted. Because nursing is a profession, it carries with it certain responsibilities, including accountability and the use of sound judgment.

Organization of the board includes such considerations as membership and meetings. Three types of meetings are possible: open meetings where decisions are made, which are open to the public; work sessions where the preliminary work is done in preparation for meetings; and executive sessions, which are closed to the public and during which private concerns such as personnel matters are discussed.

The extent of the board's responsibility for educational matters is defined in the practice act. Some laws require supervision only of programs leading to licensure, which would include baccalaureate and associate degree programs as well as diploma programs. Other state boards are authorized to monitor RN/BSN completion programs and those programs offering a mas-

CHART 2–1

A Decision-Making Model for Determining RN/LPN Scope of Practice

1. **Describe the act being performed.**
2. **Is the act expressly permitted/prohibited by the PA Nurse Practice Act?**
   [This may be all the information you need to make your decision. If not, continue to the next step.]
3. **Does the act require you to have substantial specialized nursing knowledge, skill, and independent judgment?**
   [If you answer NO to this question, the act may be within the basic scope of practice for an RN or LPN.]
   [If you answer YES, it may be an act within the scope of practice of an RN only or for an advanced practice role (CRNP).]
4. **Is the act consistent with the scope of practice based upon at least one of the following factors?**
   a. Standards of Practice of a National Nursing Organization.
   b. Positive and conclusive data in nursing literature and research.
   c. Appropriately established policy and procedure of employing facility.
   [If you answer NO to this question, the act is *NOT* within your scope of practice.]
   [If the answer is YES, continue to the next step.]
5. **Do you personally possess the depth and breadth of knowledge to perform the act safely and effectively as demonstrated by knowledge acquired in a pre-licensure program, post-basic program, or continuing education program?**
   [If you answer NO, the act is *NOT* within your scope of practice.]
   [If you answer YES, maintain documented evidence and continue on.]
6. **Do you personally possess current clinical competence to perform the act safely?**
   [If you answer NO, the act is *NOT* within your current scope of practice unless competence is achieved.]
   [If you answer YES, continue on.]
7. **Is the performance of the act within the accepted "standard of care" which would be provided in similar circumstances by reasonable and prudent nurses who have similar training and experience?**
   [If you answer NO, the act is *NOT* within your scope of practice. Performance of the act may place both nurse and patient at risk.]
   [If you answer YES, continue on.]
8. **Are you prepared to accept the consequences of your action?**
   [If you answer NO, the act is *NOT* within your scope of practice.]
   [If you answer YES, then:]
   a. Perform the act—based upon valid order when necessary, and in accordance with appropriately established policies and procedures.
   b. Assume accountability for provision of safe care.

While nurse practice acts define the basic parameters of legal practice of nursing, nursing practice is dynamic and evolving. Thus, it is impossible for the acts to list all the specific duties a nurse may or may not perform. Instead, decision-making models such as this one have been adopted by some boards of nursing. Note that the nurse, in using such a decision-making tree to determine scope of practice, must consider the duty within circumstances that are consistent with the nurse's preparation, education, experience, and knowledge. (Source: Commonwealth of Pennsylvania, State Board of Nursing)

(continued)

CHART 2 – 1

A Decision-Making Model for Determining RN/LPN Scope of Practice *(continued)*

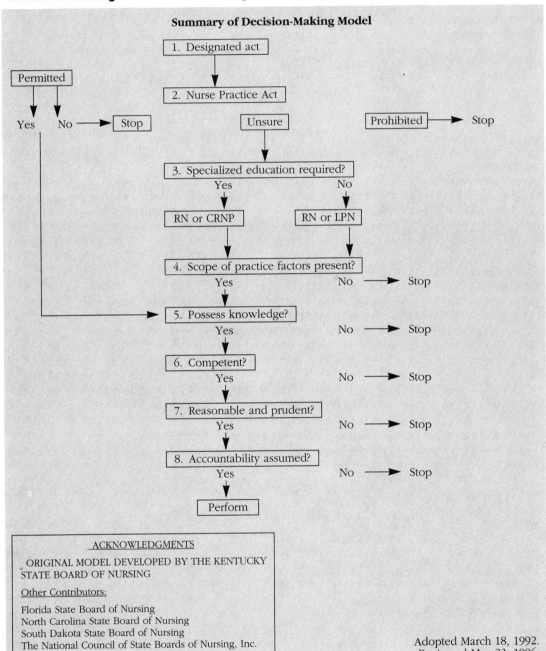

Summary of Decision-Making Model

1. Designated act

Permitted

2. Nurse Practice Act

Yes   No → Stop   Unsure   Prohibited → Stop

3. Specialized education required?

Yes   No

RN or CRNP   RN or LPN

4. Scope of practice factors present?

Yes   No → Stop

5. Possess knowledge?

Yes   No → Stop

6. Competent?

Yes   No → Stop

7. Reasonable and prudent?

Yes   No → Stop

8. Accountability assumed?

Yes   No → Stop

Perform

ACKNOWLEDGMENTS

ORIGINAL MODEL DEVELOPED BY THE KENTUCKY STATE BOARD OF NURSING

Other Contributors:

Florida State Board of Nursing
North Carolina State Board of Nursing
South Dakota State Board of Nursing
The National Council of State Boards of Nursing, Inc.

Adopted March 18, 1992.
Reviewed May 23, 1996.

ter's degree. The rules and regulations set forth standards for curriculum, faculty and administrators' qualifications, and student health and welfare policies. Educational institutions are visited on a regular basis.

Licensure.   The board's last major function is concerned with issuing and taking action against licensees. The general purpose of licensure laws is to protect the public from harm by ensuring that practitioners are qualified to "do good"; it seeks to ensure that only capable people, i.e., those licensed, perform activities that could potentially harm the recipient of such an activity or service.[10] Licensure laws commonly have provisions that include definitions, prohibition of unlicensed practice, minimum qualifications for licensure and, in the case of nursing, for curricula for schools that prepare nurses, as well as provisions for examination for licensure. The board in each state contracts with the NCSBN to administer the licensing examinations, issues licenses to successful candidates, and endorses licenses from nurses in other jurisdictions.

A license is a property right and cannot be taken without due process, which entitles the licensee to a hearing. The most frequent basis for action against a licensee is substance abuse. Many states have agreements that allow action against a license to be taken in one state based on action taken in another state. The NCSBN maintains a national disciplinary data bank so that action taken in each state is reported nationwide; however, not all jurisdictions avail themselves of this service.

Laws are being passed that facilitate action against licensees. Mandatory reporting laws require that if one licensee knows or strongly suspects that another licensee is breaking the law (for example, diverting controlled substances), then the first licensee must report the second licensee's behavior within a specified time or else face punishment by law. Another provision of law is that the state board may automatically suspend a license for a limited period pending formal action if it is deemed dangerous for the licensee to continue to practice. Mandatory reporting and automatic suspension laws usually include a clause that protects a person taking action in good faith.

Probation is sometimes used in conjunction with suspension; that is, the suspension is stayed for probation. The terms of probation for substance abuse may include drug screens, reports from treatment programs, and work evaluations. The advantage to probation is that should the licensee break the terms of probation, then the license can be suspended immediately without the need for a second hearing. The advantage to the licensee is that she or he may continue to practice in a safe and supervised manner, thus encouraging rehabilitation.

A suspended or revoked license may be reinstated. As mentioned before, suspensions frequently carry time limits; at the completion of this term, the licensee is usually requested to fulfill specific requirements to end the suspension. In cases of revocation, the plaintiff may at any time request reinstatement by board action. This frequently requires a formal hearing as the minimal condition for a decision.

As we approach a new century, multiple, complex changes continue to occur in systems for delivering health care. Technological advances, especially the advent of telehealth, pose questions related to patient safety, quality of service provision, and other legal, nursing, and economic issues. There is hardly an aspect of the health care system that has not experienced some fundamental change in the 1990s. Managed care, capitation, the move to an emphasis on home and long-term care in various delivery sites, and changes in both the utilization and requirements of health care providers have spurred intense discussion in the nursing community. Mergers and acquisitions have resulted in predictions that up to 50% of existing hospitals in the United States will close or merge, leaving four to six major, multistate delivery systems. Such changes may see nurses providing care by telephone and other electronic systems; case managers may oversee patients not in the boundaries of the state in which they are licensed. Thus, the profession has begun its dialogue about current (state-focused) regulatory models and their effectiveness in the predicted delivery systems of the future. The demands of the future, while daunting in some respects, afford RNFAs the opportunity to present solutions in designing a system that removes barriers to practice and contributes to quality improvement in the protection of the public.

Monitoring Boards of Nursing

Most state professional and occupational boards are monitored by the state's "sunset law." The purpose of this law is to ensure that only viable boards are continued, which is a reasonable requirement, as some boards do not even meet and some can rarely assemble a quorum to take action. Among boards, the nurse board usually has the highest number of licensees and many monitoring functions, so it conducts a large quantity of business.

Sunset Audit. The sunset audit involves investigation by an appointed group, usually supervised by a specified legislative senate or house committee. The committee reviews all aspects of function, including budget, number of cases investigated and completed, the consistency of minutes with actions, and the keeping of records. In addition to the internal audit, external professional groups and other licensees are invited to respond to questions regarding the operations of the board. Ideally, when the audit report is complete it is made available to the board for comment before being presented to the designated legislative committee at an open hearing. Testimony is heard and, based on all the findings, the practice act is revised as necessary. In revising the practice act, the responsible senate or house committee makes a recommendation that must be approved by both the senate and the house. If there is a difference of opinion, then a joint subcommittee is formed to negotiate agreement, and a date is set for final signature by the governor.

If the act is not acted on positively, then the board is disbanded. Many states include in their sunset laws a clause that creates a grace period for recreating or disbanding the board in an orderly way. This safeguard is the result of boards being disbanded because of a technical problem such as the legislature's not acting because of a heavy work schedule and then recessing. If the nurse board stopped functioning it would seriously affect licensees and the public. Among other things, no licenses could be issued or endorsed, no examinations could be given, and there would be no way to take action against licensees or to control practice.

Since the first sunset law was passed in Colorado in 1976, many states have accepted this procedure. As part of the process the acts are opened, thus creating an opportunity for special interest groups to submit recommendations for change. These recommendations must be carefully monitored so that the public is protected and the board can operate efficiently.

■ BEYOND THE GENERALIST

The movement toward advanced preparation or specialization in nursing, as in any other discipline, is initiated by forces such as new knowledge pertinent to the field, technological advances, and a response to public need or demand (consumerism). Since the early 1900s, consistent with rapid advances in technology and evolving professional and social demands, the practice of nursing has become more complex. Changes have resulted in new patterns of nursing, each with its own role and title. Specialization in nursing practice has seen a major proliferation over the last few decades, necessitating that nurses and nursing identify and refine scopes of practice, set professional practice standards, and certify practitioners in the specialty. This can certainly be construed as healthy growth within the profession; the great need and demand for nursing specialties and nurse specialists is a vital source of nursing's strength.

One danger of the increase in specialization, however, is the potential for lack of agreement about what constitutes each role, who should define the roles, and who should set and implement standards. Standards are authoritative statements used by the profession to describe the responsibilities for which its practitioners are accountable. They reflect the profession's values, priorities, and accountability to the public. To ameliorate confusion about the development of standards across specialties and to facilitate congruence in the organizing principles of all standards established by professional nursing associations, the ANA, through its Committee for Nursing Practice Standards and Guidelines, the Congress of Nursing Practice, ANA councils, and the specialty organizations, has led activity in the development of scopes and standards of nursing practice. These are periodically reviewed and revised after input from members of state nurses associations and specialty nursing organizations.

One requirement of a profession is that it be self-regulating. Nursing achieves this through the administrative authority vested in the nurse boards and through the definition of practice, ethical standards, certification of specialists, and criteria for accreditation developed by nursing organizations. The situation becomes more complex when one considers standards for advanced practice in the developing specialties. These standards may be implemented by government-supported agencies, such as state boards, or by professional organizations such as the ANA or, for perioperative nurses, the Association of Operating Room Nurses (AORN).

Nursing specialties originate and are recognized in many ways. Some of these include recognition by educational programs, state or national certification programs, specialty organizations, and councils such as those of the ANA. New specialties and the bodies that recognize them continue to change and proliferate. Styles, in an attempt to review, summarize, and analyze specialties in nursing, identified the following characteristics as indices of the maturity of a specialty:

practice: The practitioner is defined as a professional nurse; differentiation is recognized (though not necessarily through certification) between a generalist in a specialty area and a master's-prepared clinical nurse specialist or practitioner; definitions of functions and areas of responsibility exist; standards of practice are defined.

education: A baccalaureate degree in nursing is the prerequisite for entry into a specialty education program (or there is an intent to implement this standard); graduate level and continuing education in the specialty are available (or emerging); the specialty organization is accredited as a provider of continuing education.

research and development: Visible support and resources exist; the knowledge base for the specialty is identified, empirically based, and identifiable as advanced nursing knowledge; research symposia are conducted regularly.

credentialing: A rigorous program of certification in the specialty is available; a procedure (or plan) for recertification exists.

organization: Concerns and interests of the specialty are represented by an organized body; standards for practice are established; interests of the specialty are represented to nursing-at-large and to other groups as appropriate.

publications: Refereed journals are published; other mechanisms for regular communication are available.

relationship with other professions and disciplines: The specialty recognizes and undertakes joint ventures with the ANA (as the official organization-at-large); communication links and cooperative efforts with other specialty organizations are maintained.[11]

Pressure on state boards to recognize nurses in specialties is increasing, because recognition is needed for third-party reimbursement. As early as 1994, the Washington, DC–based Health Care Advisory Board noted a growing national trend to utilize RNFAs, citing such benefits as increased case load for the institution and improved surgeon and nurse satisfaction; they proposed establishment of RNFA services as a definitive, reimbursable nursing service as part of the solution to providing assistants at surgery.[12] In a survey on the RNFA perspective on health care reform, respondents indicated that their biggest concern regarding reform measures were (in rank order of response frequency) the potential for decreased use of RNFAs due to lack of recognition by employers and payers, inequity in reimbursement practices, and cost-cutting measures such as replacing a skilled RNFA with a less expensive assistant (sometimes referred to as "an extra pair of hands").[13] When asked about the single most important thing that must happen in health care reform efforts, RNFAs identified the achievement of reimbursement for their services. In a question asking participants to identify the most important things that should be accomplished during the years 1996–1999 to achieve a reformed health care delivery system, RNFA respondents agreed that any reform measure needed to include an emphasis on quality of care issues as well as adequate and fair reimbursement policies. RNFAs recognize that legitimacy for a specialty emanates in part from state and federal governmental or private third-party payers agreeing to reimburse certain "specialists." RNFAs in many states are partnering with the state nurses association (SNA) to introduce legislation for reimbursement of RNFAs. For example, RNFAs in Florida were successful in securing the passage of state legislation to support reimbursement of RNFAs through private insurers and Medicaid, and in getting Blue Cross and Blue Shield of Florida (BCBSF) to add an endorsement to its contracts:

> Surgical services rendered by a RNFA when acting as a surgical assistant when the assistance is medically necessary, may be covered services, subject to the applicable allowed amount. BCBSF's reimbursement level for surgical assistance provided by a RNFA is 20% of the physician's surgical allowance.[14]

In 1997, AORN developed a policy profile on reimbursement of RNFAs which discusses the role and credentials of RNFAs, federal legislation that AORN is supporting to obtain Medicare reimbursement, state RNFA reimbursement legislation, state service and provider laws, and model legislation for RNFAs to use when initiating efforts to make changes in a state's insurance code.[15] A 1997 survey conducted jointly by the AORN Specialty Assembly for RN First Assistants and *OR Manager* indicated that the largest single category of nonphysician assistant at surgery used in surveyed institutions was the RNFA.[16] However, the survey also indicated that only 40% of the institutions sought, or were able to obtain, reimbursement for this service.

At the federal level, however, most of the initiatives target advanced practitioners—certified nurse practitioners, clinical nurse specialists, certified nurse midwives, and nurse anesthetists. These advanced practice nurse categories emanate from definitions of "nonphysician providers" of Medicare services.

A significant change in the financing of health care services was the introduction of Medicare's prospective payment system. This major financing innovation had numerous implications for nursing payment systems in terms of cost of nursing services, efficient use of nursing resources, and support for expanded nursing roles. With a primary objective of minimizing costs, evolving payment systems continue to underscore the desirability of using midlevel practitioners whenever feasible; access to this level of provider has significant cost-saving implications. In 1997, direct Medicare reimbursement for nurse practitioners and clinical nurse specialists who serve as assistants at surgery was achieved as part of Public Law 105-33. As the groundwork for future health care reform is laid, RNFAs will need to continue identifying their cost-effectiveness (Charts 2–2 and 2–3), the value of their services (Chart 2–4), identify the nursing component of certain "physician services," and participate with the nursing profession in its analysis of the relationship of relative value scales for nursing services. The next phase of studies related to the role of the RNFA should focus on unique functions. Research findings on the nature of RNFAs' work will contribute to an understanding of the type, timing, and intensity of services provided to different patient groups and their families. Such studies will also facilitate the goal of assisting others to appreciate the knowledge and skills required by RNFAs to meet the complex needs of patients undergoing operative or other invasive interventions. Studies will then be needed to link those functions to outcomes (for the patient, family, cost of care). Finally, research is needed that compares practice patterns and

CHART 2–2
RNFA Cost-Effectiveness Analysis

CPT CODE	PROCEDURE	MD ASSIST 20%	RNFA ASSIST 16%	SAVINGS PER CASE	CASES PER YEAR	SAVINGS PER YEAR
Obstetrics-Gynecology						
58150	Total abdominal hysterectomy	$420.00	$336.00	$84.00	36	$3,024.00
56308	Laparoscopic-assisted vaginal hysterectomy	$500.00	$400.00	$100.00	36	$3,600.00
59514	Cesarean section	$500.00	$400.00	$100.00	36	$3,600.00
58260	Vaginal hysterectomy	$420.00	$336.00	$84.00	36	$3,024.00
Plastic/Reconstruction						
15755	Free flap (micro-vascular)	$1,142.00	$913.00	$228.00	36	$8,208.00
19318	Reduction mammo-plasty, bilateral	$754.00	$603.00	$151.00	36	$5,436.00
19316	Mastopexy	$600.00	$480.00	$120.00	36	$4,320.00
19367	Breast reconstruction with TRAM flap	$832.00	$666.00	$166.00	36	$5,976.00

C H A R T   2 – 2

RNFA Cost-Effectiveness Analysis *(continued)*

CPT CODE	PROCEDURE	MD ASSIST 20%	RNFA ASSIST 16%	SAVINGS PER CASE	CASES PER YEAR	SAVINGS PER YEAR
General						
56341	Laparoscopic chole-cystectomy with cholangiogram	$405.00	$324.00	$81.00	36	$2,916.00
44140	Colectomy, partial, with anastomosis	$378.00	$302.00	$76.00	36	$2,736.00
19240	Mastectomy, modified radical	$378.00	$302.00	$76.00	36	$2,736.00
60240	Thyroidectomy, total	$306.00	$245.00	$61.00	36	$2,196.00
Cardiovascular						
35301	Catroid endarterectomy	$521.00	$417.00	$104.00	36	$3,744.00
35583	Femoral-popliteal by-pass with in situ vein graft	$625.00	$500.00	$125.00	36	$4,500.00
33518/ 33533	Coronary artery bypass graft x 3 with IMA	$1,120.00	$896.00	$224.00	36	$8,064.00
35081	Abdominal aortic aneurysm repair	$1,000.00	$800.00	$200.00	36	$7,200.00
Neurological						
63075/ 22544	Anterior cervical fusion with bone graft	$760.00	$608.00	$152.00	36	$5,472.00
63030	Posterior laminotomy, one interspace, lumbar	$760.00	$608.00	$152.00	36	$5,472.00
Orthopedic						
27130	Total hip replacement	$780.00	$624.00	$156.00	36	$5,616.00
27447	Total knee replacement	$832.00	$666.00	$166.00	36	$5,976.00
27244	ORIF femoral fracture with plate and screws	$525.00	$420.00	$105.00	36	$3,780.00
27236	ORIF femoral fracture with prosthesis	$533.00	$426.00	$107.00	36	$3,852.00
23420	Repair of rotator cuff, shoulder	$476.00	$374.00	$93.00	36	$3,348.00
Total Savings						**$104,796.00**

Data such as these assist policy makers and legislators in recognizing the cost-effective nature of utilizing RNFAs. (Source: Rothrock JC: Where are we going, really? First Hand 11(2):2, 1996.)

CHART 2 – 3
RNFA Productivity Figures—Model

An RNFA employed by a cardiovascular surgery group providing assistance at sugery services, pre-admission workups, and some routine postoperative care:

1. Revenue generation:

Surgery assistance	(120 @ $850)	$102,000
Total Revenues		$102,000

2. Overhead reduction:

History and physicals	(120 @ $50)	6,000
Follow-up care—hospital	(120 @ $45)	5,400
Follow-up care—office	(210 @ $55)	11,550
Total Overhead Reduction		$22,950

3. Increased physician productivity:

Additional cases	(35 @ $5,750)	201,250
Additional consults	(40 @ $150)	6,000
Total Increased Physician Productivity		$ 207,250

Grand Total   **$332,200**

Note: Revenues are shown as net dollars. Figures represent annual amounts.

Models such as this one for a physician-employed RNFA elucidate contributions to productivity as an assistant at surgery and in the provision of preoperative and postoperative care. (Source: Rothrock JC: Managed care: Good, bad, or just ugly? First Hand 11(3):2, 1996.)

CHART 2 – 4
Practicing RNFA Contributions to Institutional Performance and Improvement

Top 10, ranked in order by frequency of response:
↓ Turnover time
↑ Consistency of service to surgeons
↑ Patient assessment/satisfaction
↑ Patient scheduling
↓ Lost time
↑ Surgeon productivity
↑ Nurse productivity via RNFA assistance to RN in room
↑ Staff resource (new and not-new staff)
↓ Operating time
↑ Internurse communication regarding patient/procedural requirements

In a 1995 study, hospital-employed RNFAs identified the ways they contributed to improving the employing institution's performance measures. (Source: Rothrock JC: Research results: Quantifying the RNFA's contributions. First Hand 10(3):3, 1995.)

outcomes of the RNFA with those of physicians and other nonphysician assistants at surgery.

ADVANCED PRACTICE ROLES

Definitions of advanced nursing practice should first be sought in a state's Nurse Practice Act. Many boards of nursing have, through statutes and administrative rules, recognized some level of advanced nursing practice. For example, nurse practitioners (NPs) are specifically regulated in numerous states. In other states, they function under a broad scope of practice with no specific title protection. In some states, both boards of nursing and boards of medicine regulate NPs. Thus, throughout the states, concepts and definitions of advanced nursing practice vary in interpretation and regulation.

In 1980, the ANA first published "Nursing: A Social Policy Statement." Part of this policy statement addressed the nature and scope of nursing practice and described important characteristics of specialization. An integral philosophic thrust of the policy statement originated in the belief that nursing, and the authority to practice as a nurse, is based on a social contract between society and the professions. Society grants the professions authority over their functions and autonomy in the conduct of their affairs. In return, the professions must uphold this public trust by acting responsibly and regulating themselves to ensure quality in performance of the profession. The 1980 document, however, did not use the term *advanced practice.*

As the nursing profession has matured, so has its body of knowledge and the needs and demands placed on it by the public. As complexity in required patient care services has grown, so has specialization in nursing. As early as 1957, an educational program for clinical nurse specialists was introduced, at Rutgers University. Shortly thereafter, other programs were developed, with many adding the functional role of teacher or administrator to the clinician role. A master of science in nursing (MSN), or a similarly titled degree, is awarded for successful completion of the program. The course content includes core courses (for example, research and theory) along with advanced pathophysiology and nursing science. Clinical nurse specialists function in hospitals and other health care agencies in line and staff positions in the roles of consultants, teachers, researchers, and supervisors, and they accept responsibility for patients requiring complex nursing care.

Some literature and demonstration projects in the early 1960s described the change in role and functions of the nurse as "extender" functions. More commonly referred to as "physician extenders," early role responsibilities focused on illness-oriented care and the assumption of patient care activities that formerly had been part of medical management. Although this was a natural evolution of nursing practice, nurse practitioner programs soon developed that incorporated a health focus. By the late 1960s and early 1970s, the term nurse practitioner was being used to designate a nurse who had completed a course of study, either institutional- or program-based, that prepared the nurse for expanded practice. But as nursing began to recognize the need to move these educational programs into the mainstream of education, recommendations were initiated to reserve the title "nurse practitioner" for nurses prepared at the master's level, in recognition of the specialized knowledge and skills required for autonomous practice.

By 1985, the NCSBN had adopted a position paper on advanced clinical nursing practice. Like the ANA, the NCSBN defined the educational preparation as at least a master's degree and recommended that boards of nursing regulate this advanced nursing practice through designation/recognition. Of all the approaches for regulating advanced nurse practice that the NCSBN could have suggested, designation/recognition was the least restrictive. This approach allowed boards of nursing to establish state-recognized credentials and authorize permission for a nurse to represent herself or himself with those credentials. Unfortunately, however, the resulting variability of titles, education, and scope of practice among jurisdictions created problems in credentialing, practice parameters, and geographic mobility for designated/recognized nurses in advanced practice.

In 1992 the NCSBN issued a draft position paper that recommended licensure of advanced nursing practice roles in the categories of nurse anesthetist, nurse midwife, nurse practitioner, and clinical nurse specialist. Advanced practice of nursing in these four categories is "based on knowledge and skills acquired in basic nursing education; licensure as a registered nurse; graduate degree and experience in the designated area of practice, which includes advanced nursing theory, substantial knowledge of physical and psychosocial assessment, appropriate interventions, and management of health care status."[17] The NCSBN position paper, amid a great deal of dissent in the nursing profession, was adopted in 1993. The debate regarding second licensure then moved to the states, where legislators, boards of nursing, and representatives of nursing organizations debated the extent to which a particular state would adopt the NCSBN model practice act. The ANA and many professional nursing organizations have opposed second licensure, maintaining that there should be one scope of nursing practice, only one license for registered nurses, and minimal statutory language about advanced practice, preferring that language regarding advanced practice be in rules and regulations.[18]

The RN First Assistant

Definitions and categories of advanced nursing practice do not include the specific title of "RN first assistant." While some RN first assistants have credentials as nurse practitioners or clinical nurse specialists, most do not. At one time, many states would not allow nurses to act as first assistants. In 1984, the AORN issued an official statement confirming that in the absence of a qualified physician, RNs with appropriate knowledge and skills were the best-qualified nonphysician personnel to act as first assistant. This position statement also described the definition, scope of practice, qualifications, preparation, and establishment of practice privileges. It was revised in 1993 to address the acceptance of the role by boards of nursing, to take a position on compensation for the RN who first assists, to focus on collaboration while removing the requirement for direct supervision by a surgeon, to recommend CNOR certification as a prerequisite to undergoing role preparation as an RNFA, and to recommend that education take place in institutions of higher education. In 1997, the official statement was again revised (the 1997 statement is presented in Appendix I) to recommend that programs that prepared RNFAs be in compliance with the AORN Recommended Education Standards for RN First Assistant Programs (these standards are presented in Appendix II).

Evolution of this role, and the increasing demand for it by both perioperative nurses and surgeons who value this patient care service, may be reviewed by examining the positions of the states and their boards of nursing. The February 1983 *AORN Journal* report of a first assistant survey listed each state's ruling on whether the RN may perform as first assistant: 17 states allowed RNs to act as first assistants, 14 did not, and 20 did not directly address the issue. In the January 1985 *AORN Journal*, the survey was updated, with 30 states allowing the RN to first assist, 9 clearly not allowing it, and 23 not giving a ruling interpretation. By 1990, only three states still did not permit the RN to first assist. By 1992, no state boards of nursing ruled that first assisting was outside the scope of nursing practice. There remain states where the board has chosen not to rule, however, and there is still active movement toward getting these states to issue opinions.

Many medical boards have a "right to delegate" clause under which the nurse has a broader scope of practice yet remains dependent on the physician. In nurse practice acts that are silent on the issue of first assisting, the inclusion in the act of some authority in accepting delegated medical acts or an "other acts" clause has been the basis for interpreting the act to permit first assisting because nothing in the act forbids it.[19] Most legal definitions of nursing are broad enough to permit a wide scope of practice. However, all RNs are clearly accountable for their actions and therefore are both legally and morally responsible for them.

INSTITUTIONAL LICENSURE AND EXPANDED PRACTICE

Institutional licensure, a process by which a state government regulates health institutions, has existed for many years. The focus has been on ensuring that health facilities have adequate standards to protect the consumer. For example, there must be sufficient footage around each patient's bed. A question raised repeatedly is whether institutional licensure should be extended to include personnel. This terminology is somewhat confusing, because licensure is usually defined as a process by which permission is granted by a governmental agency, whereas credentialing is a more inclusive term including accreditation, licensure, and certification. Where institutional licensure exists, it refers to a situation whereby the institution sets practice within the state government regulations. However, as the health care system continued to experience rapid change, policy makers began to suggest that the system for regulating health care providers also needed to change. In response to perceived problems, the Pew Health Professions Commission, established in 1989, created a Task Force on Health Care Workforce Regulation to explore how regulation protects the public's health. In December 1995, the task force published one of its reports, *Reforming Health Care Workforce Regulation: Policy Considerations for the 21st Century*. The report recommended changes such as standardizing regulatory terms and entry-to-practice requirements, removing barriers to full use of competent health professionals, ensuring practitioner competence, evaluating regulatory effectiveness, and understanding the organizational context of health professions regulation. The commission's report generated national debate around issues of licensure reform. Although the report did not use the term *institutional licensure,* nursing and other members of the health care community expressed concern over how barriers would be removed, what overlapping scopes of practice would be sanctioned and by whom, and how competence would be assessed and the results of such assessment used.

If job classification or the assignment of patient care functions is determined by an institution (an original concept in institutional licensure), a major drawback could be that systems may be developed by nonnurses who may interpret nursing care of patients in limited terms. Attention may be given only to physical tasks without understanding the nursing assessment, diagnosis, planning, and evaluation processes. The teaching and advocacy roles that nurses perceive as vital components in the nursing care of patients and families also may be omitted.

The first study of institutional licensure failed to show that the consumer was protected or that career mobility would not be inhibited.[20] In 1997, the Pew Health Professions Commission was reconstructed to build on recommendations issued in earlier reports. It will explore mechanisms by which the medical community can begin reducing the numbers of new physicians trained each year and determine new financing mechanisms for training health care professionals in nonhospital settings, such as in managed care. The commission will also examine federal policies, including financing of graduate medical education, and regulatory reforms at the state level. Such reform is intended to guarantee the competence and accountability of physicians, nurses, and other health professionals. The commission is expected to release specific recommendations in 1998.[21,22]

There are no simple solutions to questions of regulation or the roles of regulatory bodies in ensuring competence and accountability. Part of the answer lies with the institutions that employ nurses and other health professionals. Employment settings need to provide safe care for patients; they should incorporate standards of practice into their policies and evaluations. Health professions educators similarly need to incorporate standards into curricula and evaluate students by such standards, setting expectations for lifelong learning and professional accountability. Another part of the answer lies with individual nurses, who must accept the increased responsibility and accountability associated with being a professional, assess their own competence, recognize their legal and ethical obligations, engage in lifelong learning, and willingly participate in peer review. Yet another part lies with the professional organizations and the state nursing boards, which need to work together to establish standards for competence and to define models and mechanisms for competence demonstration for the protection of the public.[23] Underlying these suggestions is the need for nurses to work together to support each other.

■ RNFA INITIATIVES TO INFLUENCE PRACTICE

Nurses have the potential to affect not only nursing but the total health care delivery system through legislative action. This brings with it the need to act responsibly and in concert. Perhaps the most difficult part is setting up an information network. An immediate resource is the vice president for nursing, who should have copies of the state's Nurse Practice Act and rules and regulations. The health care facility probably subscribes to the official state bulletin, which provides regular reports on the activities of the boards of nursing, medicine, health, welfare, and education. Nursing organizations such as ANA and AORN have publications that include legislative information; the RN first assistant must belong to the organizations to receive their mailings. In 1992, AORN supported the formation of specialty assemblies; the Specialty Assembly for RN First Assistants is an important resource when establishing an information network. Some state councils of operating room nurses have task forces or other subcommittees that monitor and respond to issues affecting the practice of RNFAs. A newsletter for RN first assistants, *First Hand,* is another information resource; information about this newsletter and other current practice and policy information about RNFAs can be accessed on the Internet at www.rnfa-firsthand.com.[24] In 1997, the AORN's board of directors approved the National Legislative Committee's (and its 52 state coordinators') recommendation that reimbursement for RNFAs be the association's number one legislative priority. AORN is developing a legislative and government relations program, with a major focus being RNFA reimbursement. Information regarding AORN's activities and the Specialty Assembly for RNFAs can be accessed on the Internet at www.aorn.org.

State boards operate under the sunshine act, and meetings are open to the public. RNFAs should set up a roster to send representatives to meetings. Another source of information is related to the professional nurse role as consumer advocate. Contacting local health agencies allows the RNFA to determine health care needs in specific geographic areas. Patients are another excellent source of information about needed services.

Once an information and resource base has been identified, the RNFA should start working with state representatives and senators in both the work district and area of residence. Useful strategies include building a working relationship with them before it becomes necessary to solicit their legislative support; becoming familiar with how they have voted on health issues; offering to assist with elections by making phone calls or volunteering in campaigns; and, if there is pertinent legislation in the state house or senate, informing legislators of how it would affect health care. The RNFA should know the legislative staff who frequently brief legislators on pending legislation.

It is easy to complain about the "system," but in a democracy the individuals are the system, which makes complaining rather futile. The RNFA should be a productive professional by knowing the issues, developing ways to be heard, and then acting in an effective way to improve the health care delivery system and nursing. As contemporary trends in health care continue to evolve, RNFAs must remain at the forefront of patient advocacy, making known the essential attributes of their nursing services as they work to promote quality patient care. In visible leadership roles, RNFAs will need to closely monitor and influence health policy initiatives at both the state and federal levels, as most policy issues today are being implemented simultaneously at both levels of government.

■ CONCLUSION

The dramatic revolution in systems for delivering and financing health care have created new and significant challenges for RNFAs and for the regulation of nursing practice. The primary function of professional regulation is to protect the public; this is accomplished by establishing and enforcing standards of practice. Nurse practice acts are statutes passed by state legislatures. They define what constitutes nursing. Scopes of practice have evolved to reflect changes in health care delivery systems, advances in technology, and innovations in contemporary nursing practice. The state nurse practice acts also make provisions for creating state boards of nursing. As administrators of the nurse practice acts, state boards of nursing promulgate rules and regulations. It is this board that handles specific concerns regarding nursing practice and makes rules to more specifically implement and enforce the state's Nurse Practice Act. States have similar statutes that define the practice of medicine. RNFAs should review both the Medical Practice Act and their state's Nurse Practice Act, as well as all relevant guidelines, qualifications, or other documents the board may have developed regarding the RNFA. Regardless of how the role is defined by the board, the RNFA must have the proper education and skill competence to perform the nursing behaviors required of first assistants.

The AORN Official Statement on RN First Assistants requires preparation for role assumption through the completion of a formal education program, which takes place in an institution approved by the appropriate regional accrediting body for higher education and awards a degree or certificate upon successful program completion. Many state boards of nursing have adopted the AORN position in their decision that RNs may first assist as part of the scope of nursing practice. Once the RN first assistant is clear about the position and opinions of the board of nursing and has obtained the requisite education for role assumption, clear institutional policies and credentialing mechanisms must be put in place to ensure that the nurse who acts as first assistant is qualified to do so. That is the topic of the next chapter.

Review Questions

Use the following list of terms to identify the definitions in questions 1–12:

a. Attorney general opinion
b. Constitutional law
c. Law
d. Legal
e. License and licensure
f. Personal liability
g. Policies
h. Rules and regulations
i. Scope of practice
j. Standard of care
k. Standards
l. Statutes

1. _____: criteria of measuring and conformity to established practice

2. _____: branch of law dealing with organization and function of government

3. _____: guidelines within which employees of an institution must operate

4. _____: opinion of the attorney general; opinion is not law, but is given credence should litigation arise on the issue discussed in an opinion

5. _____: legislative enactments; acts of legislature declaring, commanding, or prohibiting something

6. _____: the sum total of human-made rules and regulations by which society is governed in a formally and legally binding manner

7. _____: permission granted by the state to conduct a certain activity that the state board regulates and controls

8. _____: clear and concise statements mandating or prohibiting certain activities

9. _____: each person is responsible for his or her own acts

10. _____: that area of practice legally considered to fall within the expertise of the registered nurse

11. _____: permitted or authorized by law

12. _____: the professional is expected to exercise that degree of care that other reasonably prudent professionals would exercise under similar situations

Select the best response to the following questions.

13. Nurses may look to several sources of law to determine their scope of practice. These include:
    a. The state's Nurse Practice Act.
    b. Rules and regulations.
    c. Attorney general opinions.
    d. All of the above.

14. The state's power and authority to regulate through licensure are primarily directed toward:
    a. Allowing for disciplinary action of licensees.
    b. Establishing a testing process to determine licensee competence.
    c. Protecting the public's health, welfare, and safety.
    d. Preventing encroachment on nursing practice.

15. The organization that has as its purpose to provide a mechanism through which boards of nursing act and counsel together is the
    a. National League for Nursing.
    b. National Council of State Boards of Nursing.
    c. American Nurses Association.
    d. Association of Nurse Attorneys.

16. Many nurse practice acts include a definition of nursing similar to which of the following?
    a. Nursing is the responsibility for knowing the law, practicing within legal boundaries, being accountable for judgments, and maintaining competency in its art and science.
    b. Nursing is the performance of selected acts requiring additional education and preparation.
    c. Nursing is an independent practice that does not require the supervision of a physician.
    d. Nursing is the diagnosis and treatment of human responses to actual or potential health problems.

17. When a state board of nursing gives an opinion regarding a practice issue (such as determining that the RN first assistant may harvest veins), then

    a. All RN first assistants may engage in the practice.

    b. Institutions must include this in their job descriptions for RN first assistants.

    c. Institutions may decide whether the function is acceptable as part of the job description.

    d. The RN first assistant may legitimately bill the patient for the service.

Consider the following situation and then mark T (true) or F (false) for the questions posed.

Rachael Hutting is a perioperative nurse with 4 years of experience in an operating room. She has her CNOR and is going to a nearby university to obtain her BSN. Rachael has a friend, Brittany, who is an RN first assistant. Brittany attended a college course that required 340 hours of study and supervised clinical practice in first assisting. Rachael also wants to first assist. She believes that her 4 years of experience and her CNOR have prepared her to take on this function. In determining whether Rachael is within the scope of nursing practice to first assist at surgery, the following are proper courses of action:

18. _____ Rachael should see whether other perioperative nurses in her AORN chapter are first assisting without having educational preparation.

19. _____ Rachael should write to AORN and request the *RN First Assistant Guide to Practice.*

20. _____ Rachael should write to the state board of nursing, requesting any guidelines, opinions, or rules or regulations about the RN first assistant.

21. _____ If the state board of nursing responds to Rachael that it has chosen not to address this issue, then Rachael cannot pursue her goal of first assisting at surgery.

22. _____ On reading her state's Nurse Practice Act, Rachael notes a provision for "delegated medical acts." She correctly realizes that this means first assisting is within her scope of practice.

23. _____ In reviewing the AORN Official Statement on RN First Assistants, Rachael finds a definition stating that "the RNFA practices perioperative nursing and must have acquired the necessary specific knowledge, skills, and judgment."

24. _____ Rachael's state board of nursing has determined that first assisting at surgery is within the scope of nursing practice. Therefore, she no longer needs to concern herself with the AORN Official Statement.

25. _____ Rachael's state board of nursing has determined that first assisting at surgery is within the scope of nursing practice. Therefore, Rachael has the right to demand that her employing institution allow her to first assist, because it is law.

◼ Answer Key

1. k
2. b
3. g
4. a
5. l
6. c
7. e
8. h
9. f
10. i
11. d
12. j
13. d
14. c
15. b
16. d
17. c
18. F (Although Rachael may be interested in this information, it does not obviate her responsibility for conforming to her state Nurse Practice Act. That is the first source of authority. Rachael should also be guided by information from her specialty nursing association (AORN) and institutional guidelines. A nurse cannot assume that a practice is permissible simply because another nurse performs it.)
19. T (This was previously referred to as the *RN First Assistant Practice Resource Manual*. It was revised and expanded in 1997 and renamed the *RN First Assistant Guide to Practice*.)
20. T
21. F (If the state board is silent on the issue, this does not mean that it is not permissible.)
22. F (Provisions for "delegated medical acts" may be found in the Nurse Practice Act or the Medical Practice Act. However, scope of practice varies, depending on patient populations, practice environment, institutional policy, the state Nurse Practice Act, and standard-setting bodies such as AORN. Rachael cannot disregard any of these.)
23. T
24. F (Nurse practice acts of each state set bounds of practice for nurses licensed under those statutes and serve as a standard of practice. However, standards of practice from specialty nursing associations such as AORN can be used as guidelines for nursing practice. The AORN official position statement should not be ignored.)
25. F (Institutions have the right and responsibility to determine their own policies and procedures. An institution is not required to make provision for the role of RN first assistant simply because it has been determined by the board of nursing to be within the scope of nursing practice.)

REFERENCES

1. Sheets V: Public Protection or Professional Self-Preservation? Chicago, National Council of State Boards of Nursing, 1996

2. Catalano JT: Contemporary Professional Nursing. Philadelphia, FA Davis Co, 1996
3. Chaska NL: The Nursing Profession: A Time to Speak. New York, McGraw-Hill, 1983, pp 613–614
4. Snyder M, LaBar C: Issues in Professional Nursing Practice. Nursing: Legal Authority for Practice. Washington, DC, American Nurses' Association, 1984, p 2
5. Dalton JA, Speakman M, Duffey M, Carlson J: The evolution of a profession: Where do boards of nursing fit in? Profess Nurs, 10:319–324, 1994
6. American Nurses Association: Model Practice Act. Washington, DC, American Nurses Association, 1996
7. National Council of State Boards of Nursing: Delegation: Concepts and Decision-Making Process, Chicago, National Council of State Boards of Nursing, 1995
8. Kentucky Board of Nursing: Advisory Opinion Statement: Role of the Registered Nurse First Assistant. Louisville, Kentucky Board of Nursing, 1993
9. Pennsylvania State Board of Nursing: *Newsletter.* Harrisburg, Pa, 1995, pp 5–6
10. Hall JK: Nursing Ethics and Law. Philadelphia, WB Saunders, 1996
11. Styles MM: On Specialization in Nursing: Toward a New Empowerment. Kansas City, Mo, American Nurses Foundation, 1989
12. Health Care Advisory Board: Nurse Issue Tracking: Hospitals Benefit by Using Registered Nurse First Assistants (RNFAs) to Assist in Surgery. Washington, DC, Health Care Advisory Board, 1994
13. Rothrock JC: The RNFA perspective on health care reform: Survey results, First Hand 10(1): 2–3, 1995
14. Rothrock JC: Blue Cross/Blue Shield of Florida endorsement of RNFAs. First Hand 12(1): 4, 1997
15. Romig CL: AORN Policy Profile: Reimbursement of RNFAs. Denver, Association of Operating Room Nurses, 1997
16. Patterson P: Who's first assisting? OR Manager 13:1, 1997
17. National Council of State Boards of Nursing: Position Paper on the Licensure of Advanced Nursing Practice. Revised draft. Chicago, National Council of State Boards of Nursing, Aug 13, 1992
18. Cronenwett LR: Molding the future of advanced practice nursing. Nurs Outlook 43:112–118, 1995
19. Murphy EK: When is the RN first assistant practicing within the scope of nursing? AORN J 40:256–260, 1984
20. Ibid, pp 111–112
21. Recognizing Continuing Oversupply of MDs, National Commission Revived to Recommend New Financing Strategies for Training Physicians, San Francisco, Center for Health Professions, 1997
22. Health Professions Licensure Reform, San Francisco, Health Policy Tracking Service, 1997
23. National Council of State Boards of Nursing: Assuring Competence: A Regulatory Responsibility, Chicago, National Council of State Boards of Nursing, 1996
24. *First Hand*, c/o QuestRN, Inc, PO Box 20, Wallingford, Pa 19086

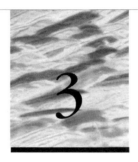

INSTITUTIONAL CREDENTIALING
OF THE RN FIRST ASSISTANT

NANCY B. DAVIS

■

As we approach the new millennium, there is little debate regarding the commonness of using RN first assistants or the effectiveness of such providers of patient care services. A 1997 study by the Association of Operating Room Nurses (AORN) RN First Assistant Specialty Assembly and the journal *OR Manager* indicated that the RNFA was the largest single category of nonphysician assistant at surgery used in responding hospitals.[1] Through either rulings or opinions of boards of nursing, states have determined that the practice of an RN as an assistant in surgery is either within the scope of nursing or permissible under a portion of the practice act that addresses delegated medical functions. There are no states that consider first assisting outside of the scope of practice of the registered nurse. Some states have published sets of guidelines for RNs acting in this capacity and specified the content of policies and procedures to be in place in institutions that utilize RNFAs.[2] Nonetheless, most states expect that the functions outlined in policies and procedures will be performed only after practice privileges have been granted by a credentialing committee established by the institution. Clear definitions of the role of the RNFA must be established within institutional policy; policies should be explicit with regard to the knowledge and skills that an RNFA should possess. Institutional practice privileges can limit activities associated with practice as a RNFA, but they cannot expand the RNFA's practice beyond the legal parameters established by a state's Nurse Practice Act and the board's interpretation of the act.

◼ CREDENTIALING AND PRACTICE PRIVILEGES

Each institution establishes its own guidelines for credentialing. Although there are no national standards for credentialing RNFAs per se, there are resources available for the institution to use in establishing a credentialing policy. The AORN's Official Statement on RN First Assistants (reprinted in Appendix I)[3] addresses the need to establish practice privileges in the institution where the RNFA is practicing. The position of the American College of Surgeons (ACS) regarding qualifications of the first assistant in the operating room is that "practice privileges of those acting as first assistant should be based on verified credentials reviewed and approved by the hospital credentialing committee."[4] Such requirements are part of the institution's duty toward its patients—ensuring that those persons who provide patient care services are qualified to do so. While credentialing and the granting of practice privileges is a legal process that is part of the institution's bylaws and approved by the board of the institution, the rationale for credentialing is to ensure quality patient care.[5] Practice privileges also meet the American Nurses Association (ANA) requirement that the nursing profession provide methods of identifying and recognizing nurses with specialized skills and experience.

Thus, the right to perform certain activities within an institution is a privilege granted through a credentialing process. This process determines whether the individual is qualified to perform the activities for which the application is being made. This verification is essential for both employees and nonemployees of the institution, although it is possible that the institution's credentialing process will differ for employees and nonemployees. In both instances the credentialing process aims to ensure that established and accepted legal and professional standards for the nurse functioning in the role of first assistant are met. By verifying that the professional nurse is competent to function in the role of first assistant, the institution ensures that patients will receive quality care and minimizes the liability exposure of itself and of its staff.[6]

It is important not to confuse the credentialing process with institutional licensure. The term "institutional licensure" has been discussed for several years without being widely accepted or implemented. This system would allow the institution to determine "who can do what" within the institution. Scope of practice would not be determined by professional standards or by legal action. Competency would be determined by standards set within each institution, and variations potentially could have a negative effect on the quality of patient care. Professional associations such as the ANA are opposed to the system of institutional licensure, for obvious reasons.

History of Hospital Credentialing

The hospital credentialing process was instituted for the purpose of granting hospital privileges to physicians. This process became necessary as increasing numbers of physicians began using hospitals. In the early 1900s there was a growing acceptance of hospitals as centers for treating patients with acute illnesses and for performing surgical interventions. More and more physicians wanted to use the hospital facility as a "workshop." Hospitals were eager for physicians to admit their patients, especially those patients able to pay the hospital for their care. Because physicians determined which patients were to be admitted, they were powerful in influencing how hospitals were managed and controlled.

Physicians who had obtained hospital privileges soon controlled the "credentialing process." Often, other physicians were not granted hospital privileges and were unable to use the hospital for their patients. In 1907 a survey of New York physicians in the Bronx and in Manhattan found that only 10% had hospital privileges. Those physicians who were excluded began establishing their own hospitals, and increasing competition forced hospitals to open their staff privileges to qualified physicians. By 1933, 75% of all physicians had some type of hospital privileges.[7]

Initially, the authority in hospitals passed from trustees to physicians because of financial reasons. In the 1930s and 1940s, however, hospital administrators began challenging physicians' authority over hospitals. Administrators assumed more authority, reflecting the increasing complexity of the hospital's internal organization and its relationship with outside agencies.

There are other reasons for increased control of hospitals by governing boards and administrators. Hospitals have a moral, ethical, and legal responsibility for overseeing the care that patients receive. Because they are legally responsible for physician competence, health care institutions cannot simply rubber-stamp medical staff recommendations regarding staff privileges. Licenses convey the right to practice; hospital privileges provide the opportunity.

Nonphysician Providers

In recent years, nonphysician providers of patient care, such as nurse practitioners, physician assistants, and RN first assistants, have successfully increased their efforts to obtain hospital practice privileges. Although economic independence is certainly a factor in this movement, a major force is the opportunity for professional autonomy. Opposition has come primarily from physicians concerned about the fragmentation of patient care and the competition for health care dollars. Antitrust actions have been initiated by nonphysicians who were denied hospital privileges. In 1982 Tennessee Federal Trade Commission testimony, it was asserted that "access to an essential facility—the hospital—by nonphysician providers in appropriate circumstances may lead to substantial consumer benefits. Both new consumer options and competitive pressures on practitioners already in the market (leading to lower cost and improvements in quality) have potentials for providing important improvements in consumer welfare in the health care field."[8]

Since 1982, health care has undergone profound changes, requiring the health professions to redefine their responsibilities in order to respond more quickly and effectively to the needs of consumers. The regulation of these professions, which has as its intended effect protection of the public, has come under scrutiny. Health care workforce regulation is performed by each individual state; there are more than 100 health occupations or professions in the 50 states. Regulatory systems, aimed at standardizing levels of care, originated with early efforts by surgeons in an era when there were few health professions.

◼ THE JOINT COMMISSION ON ACCREDITATION OF HEALTHCARE ORGANIZATIONS

In 1918 the ACS established the Hospital Standardization Program to standardize hospital care so that a minimum level of care could be ensured. In 1951 other organizations were asked to participate, and the Joint Commission on Accreditation of Hospitals (Joint Commission) was formed. Initially, the participating organizations were the American College of Physicians, the American Medical Association, the American Hospital Association, and the Canadian Medical Association. The Canadian Medical Association withdrew in 1959 to form its own organization. In 1979, the American Dental Association was granted Joint Commission membership. As accreditation by Joint Commission extended to organizations other than hospitals, its name was changed to the Joint Commission on Accreditation of Healthcare Organizations.

The Joint Commission accreditation process is voluntarily accepted by health care organizations. Reimbursement by third-party payers often requires Joint Commission approval of the institution. This economic determinant increases the use of the accrediting process. Additional benefits to the accredited institution include enhancement of community confidence in the facility; recruitment of medical staff; provision of educational tools to improve care, services, and programs; and partial or complete fulfillment of state and federal requirements for licensure and certification.

To assist facilities seeking accreditation, the Joint Commission publishes the *Comprehensive Accreditation Manual for Hospitals*, which identifies the standards to be met by the institution, specifies the characteristics of each standard, and describes the measures that the institution must implement to meet the standard. Credentialing procedures for RNFAs who apply for practice privileges within the institution must comply with the Joint Commission requirements.

CREDENTIALING MECHANISMS

Institutions have credentialing mechanisms for granting or denying practice privileges. These mechanisms are based on standards that ensure the accountability and competence of the individual in performing activities within the institution. Criteria established by the institution for the credentialing process must be substantially related to the position and/or function of the applicant. There must also exist an appellate process if an applicant is denied privileges. In 1981, the Joint Commission revised its standards to reflect, among other changes in health care, the broadened scope of practice of various providers of patient care services. This change established mechanisms to monitor the provider's preparation and competence to perform the functions identified in the application for practice privileges.[9]

In the 1997 *Manual*, the Joint Commission standards address the need for the institution's governing body to approve the following:

- the medical staff
- the mechanism used to review credentials and to delineate individual clinical privileges
- recommendations of individuals for medical staff membership
- recommendations for delineated clinical privileges for each eligible individual
- the organization of the quality assessment and improvement activities of the medical staff as well as the mechanism used to conduct, evaluate, and revise such activities
- the mechanism by which membership on the medical staff may be terminated
- the mechanism for fair-hearing procedures[10]

The governing body usually bases its approval on recommendations from the medical staff executive committee.

The Joint Commission also posits that the medical staff is responsible for monitoring and evaluating the clinical performance of individuals with privileges and that there must be mechanisms to ensure that each practitioner provides only those services in which he or she has been determined to be competent. Clinical privileges are based on the individual's license, experience, competence, ability, and judgment. When an individual is being considered for reappointment to the medical staff, or when an individual's clinical privileges are being renewed or revised, information regarding the individual's professional performance, judgment, and clinical and technical skills must be assessed.[11] The Joint Commission fully expects that when an individual has performance problems that cannot be improved, modifications (or other appropriate action) in clinical privileges will be made.

RN First Assistants Employed by the Institution

Perioperative nursing in many institutions includes first assistant functions and nursing behaviors. Additional formal education and experience are necessary for nurses who act as first assistants. The AORN Official Statement on RN First Assistants clearly states that "the RN first assistant practices perioperative nursing and must have acquired the necessary knowledge, skills, and judgment specific to clinical practice."[12] The AORN standards for RNFA education programs specify that this education be obtained by the perioperative nurse through matriculation in an educational program for RN first assistants in a college or university, which includes a semester of didactic instruction and a semester of clinical internship, awards college credits, and grants a degree or certificate upon program completion.[13] Many such programs are available in the United States. Specific information regarding program prerequisites, length, and curricular content may be obtained from the *Specialty Course Directory,* available from AORN. Beginning in January 1998, all applicants for the certification examination for RN first assistants (CRNFA) must have completed a formal RNFA program, as described in the AORN's education standards. In 1997, the Certification Board for Perioperative Nursing (CBPN, formerly the National Certification Board: Perioperative Nursing, Inc.) implemented a process for RNFA programs to apply for acceptance by CBPN; the list of acceptable programs is sent to CRNFA examination candidates.

Joint Commission standards require a process or processes designed to ensure that all individuals who provide patient care services, but who are not subject to the medical staff privilege delineation process, are competent to provide such services. Competence is the primary consideration in assigning responsibilities to nursing staff. Nursing care standards determine the scope of responsibility based on educational preparation, any applicable licensing laws or regulations, and assessment of current competence. Determination of competence includes an objective assessment of the nurse's performance in delivering patient care services. As early as 1985, the National Council of State Boards of Nursing (NCSBN) had developed a position statement on continued competence; in 1991, the NCSBN published a framework for measuring competence from both an empirical and a standard-setting perspective. In 1993, the NCSBN advanced the responsibility for the individual licensee in self-assessment of competence and limiting practice accordingly. By 1996, the NCSBN had adopted the following definition of competence: "Competence is the application of knowledge and the interpersonal, decision-making, and psychomotor skills expected for the nurse's practice role, within the context of public health, welfare, and safety."[14] This action, and the accompanying standards for competence developed by the NCSBN, evolved in part from the challenge faced by health care professionals in attaining, maintaining, and advancing their professional competence in the face of accelerating technological and scientific developments. Additionally, the 1995 report of the Pew Health Profession's Commission's Task Force on Health Care Workforce regulation clearly articulated several recommendations regarding competence.[15] RNFAs should collaboratively participate in processes that examine issues of competence assessment and work to include these in policies and procedures for credentialing and recredentialing.

Employee credentialing by the institution is a mechanism that can be used for meeting these requirements. This mechanism provides a method for ensuring that the nurse is competent to function in the first assistant role. Not only does this affect the quality of patient care, it also gives the RNFA recognition for the additional education and clinical expertise needed to function in this role.

The AORN perioperative nursing credentialing model describes a credentialing process that can be used by an institution.[16] This model is directed toward the credentialing of nurses practicing in the operating room. Specific criteria regarding the employee or new employee are verified by the institution. Files maintained on each employee, updated annually, should contain documentation of the following information:

- educational qualification (i.e., diplomas, degrees, certificate of completion of RN first assistant program)
- licensure (verify original and copy for file)
- peer evaluation (references, letters of recommendation)
- certification (i.e., CNOR, CRNFA)
- evidence of continuing education and in-service education
- verification of orientation
- job description and skill list
- performance appraisal and documentation of competence
- professional development activities (i.e., professional association activity, research, publications) (see Figure 3–1)

Institutions in which first assisting is an expanded perioperative nursing role need to develop a job description specific to first assisting that identifies the qualifications, responsibilities, and functions for the position. The institution may wish to use the job description for the staff nurse position in the operating room that relates to the scrub position and develop a separate job description for first assisting as a supplement. Perioperative nursing staff may function in various roles, such as scrubbing, circulating, or first assisting. A sample job description is shown in Chart 3–1.

A skills list is used in conjunction with the job description. The list is based on the knowledge required to actualize the role and on the employee's ability to perform the specific tasks required. A skills list is maintained on each employee; often this will be the employee's responsibility. The skills may be incorporated into a checklist system or a gradation system, ranging from 1, "not performed,"

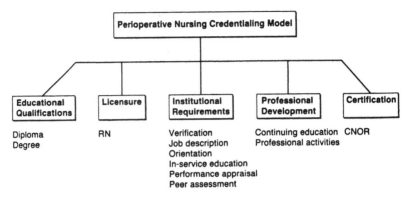

FIGURE 3–1

AORN's perioperative nursing credentialing model. (Source: AORN J 43(1), 1986.[16] Copyright © AORN, Inc., Denver, Colo. All rights reserved.)

to 5, "able to teach." The skills list for the professional nurse acting as a first assistant must address behaviors specific to that role. The behaviors might be classified in terms of suturing, handling tissue, providing exposure, using instruments, and achieving hemostasis. Documentation of the numbers and types of operative procedures in which the nurse has assisted is suggested. The skills list is useful for evaluating the nurse's performance and for providing evidence of continued competence. A sample skills checklist is shown in Chart 3–2.

RN First Assistants Not Employed by the Institution

RNs not employed by an institution but who wish to function as first assistants within that institution must have practice privileges. Application for privileges is usually made through the medical staff, as an affiliate member. Nonphysicians are considered "limited" health care practitioners, in contrast to physicians. Practice privileges are based on the legal scope of the applicant's professional practice and on the need for the services that the individual desires to provide within the institution.

In some institutions, nurses are considered "dependent" practitioners. When functioning as a first assistant, the nurse is under the supervision of the surgeon and is therefore "dependent." The nurse's practice privileges usually require a professional association and collaboration with a specific surgeon or group of surgeons. According to the ANA's *Guidelines for Appointment of Nurses for Individual Practice Privileges in Health Care Organizations*, this is a Type B appointment: "The appointee collaborates with physicians in implementing medical therapies in specified areas."[17] (See Chart 3–3 for more details on the ANA guidelines.)

(text continues on page 61)

C H A R T   3 – 1

Millard Fillmore Hospitals Job Description

JOB TITLE: RN First Assistant   **APPROVED BY:**
DEPARTMENT: Operating Room   **DATE:**
REPORTS TO: (TITLE)   Nursing Director
                                Surgical Services

MAIN FUNCTION: Under the direct supervision and direction of the operating surgeon functions during the assisting phase of the role until the conclusion of the operative procedure. Does not function concurrently as a scrub nurse.

DUTIES AND RESPONSIBILITIES:
1. Performs preoperative patient assessment and teaching.
2. Recognizes safety hazards and initiates appropriate corrective action.
3. Applies principles of asepsis and infection control skillfully.
4. Applies knowledge of surgical anatomy, physiology, and operative technique relative to operative procedures wherein the RN first assistant assists.
5. Performs positioning, prepping, and draping of the patient.
6. Provides hemostasis by clamping blood vessels, coagulating bleeding points, ligating vessels, and by other means as directed by the surgeon.
7. Provides exposure through appropriate use of instruments, retractors, suctioning, and sponging techniques.
8. Handles tissue as directed by the surgeon during the operative procedure.
9. Performs wound closure as directed by the surgeon; sutures the peritoneum, fascia, subcutaneous tissue, and skin.
10. Applies surgical dressings.
11. Assists with transfer of the patient from the operating room.
12. Performs postoperative patient evaluation and teaching.
13. Practices within limitations of preparation and experience.
14. Maintains continuing education relative to practice.

EDUCATION REQUIRED: (minimal formal education or its equivalent required to perform the job):
1. Graduate of approved school of nursing—RN
2. Completion of approved course in RN first assisting

MINIMUM TIME TO LEARN JOB:
The minimum time required to learn job is 3–6 months; relative to opportunity for experience.

SPECIAL REQUIREMENTS (registration, license, certification) OR OTHER HIRING SPECIFICATIONS (courses, studies, special skills needed or prior experience desired):
1. Licensed as a Registered Nurse in the State of New York
2. CPR certification
3. CNOR certification
4. Minimum 5 years diversified perioperative nursing experience; both scrubbing and circulating proficiency

C H A R T   3 – 2

RN First Assistant Skills List

RN FIRST ASSISTANT NAME: _____

EVALUATOR: _____

DATE: _____ YEARS PERIOPERATIVE EXPERIENCE: _____

YEARS RN FIRST ASSISTANT: _____

**Key		*1	2	3	4	5
A.	1. Identifies normal/abnormal anatomy.					
	2. Participates in clinical decision making.					
	3. Modifies techniques based on findings.					
	4. Anticipates steps in surgical procedure.					
B.	1. Interviews patient and family preoperatively and assesses patient's needs.					
	2. Implements and evaluates care plan.					
	3. Implements revised care plan based on patient's outcomes.					
C.	1. Communicates relevant data to team members (physical findings, lab data, x-rays).					
	2. Discusses radiological/surgical procedures to be implemented during surgery.					
	3. Discusses unusual techniques/instruments required based on data collected.					
D.	1. Assists team members as needed.					
	2. Collaborates with surgical team members to plan perioperative patient care plan.					
	3. Analyzes critical situations and implements appropriate action.					
E.	1. Reports safety hazards and variances in aseptic technique.					
	2. Relates changes in patient's condition.					
	3. Demonstrates CPR technique.					
	4. Reports concerns to appropriate members.					
	5. Prioritizes calmly and efficiently in stressful or emergency situations.					
F.	1. Provides appropriate retraction.					
	2. Demonstrates proper handling of tissue.					
	3. Uses appropriate suctioning techniques.					
	4. Demonstrates manual dexterity in the use of surgical instruments.					

(continued)

CHART 3-2

RN First Assistant Skills List *(continued)*

**Key	*1	2	3	4	5
5. Provides hemostasis using:					
electrosurgery					
bipolar cautery					
clamps					
pressure/sponging					
collagens					
bone wax					
other (state)					
6. Demonstrates suturing skills:					
tying techniques					
ligating vessels					
wound closing					
approximation					
subcuticular closure					
skin closure					
staples					
securing drains					
7. Demonstrates appropriate use of instruments.					
G. 1. Reviews postoperative orders with surgeon and team members.					
2. Reports patient's status to PACU/OPU/ICU personnel.					
3. Participates in patient's and family's education and discharge planning.					

As defined by Patricia Benner in "Novice to Expert," the Dreyfus Model, pages 21–32.

The Dreyfus Model (page 21) distinguishes between the level of skilled performance that can be achieved through principles and theory learned in the classroom and the context-dependent judgments and skills that can be acquired only in real situations.

STAGE 1.   *NOVICE*
- has no experience of the situations in which he or she is expected to perform.
- is *given* context-free *rules* to guide actions to different *attributes*.
- is unfamiliar with goals and tools of patient care.

STAGE 2.   *ADVANCED BEGINNER*
- *demonstrates* marginally acceptable performance and has coped with enough real situations to note the recurring "aspects of the situation."
- *formulates guidelines* (rather than rules) that dictate actions in terms of attributes and aspects.

(continued)

STAGE 3.   *COMPETENT*
- begins to see his or her actions in terms of *long-range goals or plans* of which he or she is *consciously aware.*
- *establishes a prospective and a plan* based on considerable *conscious*, abstract, analytic contemplation of the problem and *helps to achieve efficiency and organization* (characteristic of this skill level).
- *begins to see* his or her actions in terms of long-range goals or plans of which she or he is consciously aware.
- *has a feeling of mastery* and has the *ability to cope with and manage the many contingencies* of clinical nursing.
- lacks speed and flexibility of the proficient nurse and does not base conclusions on salient points of the whole picture.

STAGE 4.   *PROFICIENT*
- *perceives situations as a whole guided by maxims,* rather than in terms of aspects and attributes. Maxims reflect *nuances* of situations and provide directions as to what must be taken into consideration. *Perception is the key.* Practice is not "thought out" but "presents itself" based on experience and recent events.
- has a *holistic* undertaking of situations which improves decision making.

STAGE 5.   *EXPERT*
- *possesses multifaceted knowledge with concrete referents* that cannot be put into abstract principles or explicit guidelines, but rather is based on an intuitive grasp of the situation. No longer relies on analytic principles (rules, guidelines, maxims) to connect his or her understanding of the situation, but zeros in on the accurate region of the problem without wasteful consideration of a large range of unfruitful alternative diagnoses and solutions.
- *operates from a deep understanding of the total situation. The vision of "what is possible"* is one of the characteristics that separate competent from proficient and expert performance.
- *possesses an intuitive and holistic overview.*
- *implements rapid decision making.*

RN FIRST ASSISTANT NAME: _____

EVALUATOR: _____

DATE: _____

EXPLANATION OF CATEGORIES A, B, C, etc.

**Key	**Performance Evaluation**	**Criteria Met**
A.	Demonstrates knowledge base of procedures to which he or she is assigned.	_____
B.	Assesses, plans, implements, and evaluates patients' needs and needs of the surgical team.	_____
C.	Communicates relevant data to team members.	_____
D.	Demonstrates qualities of a team member.	_____
E.	Practices continuous surveillance as related to safety hazards, aseptic technique, and changes in patient's condition, and initiates appropriate action.	_____
F.	Demonstrates assisting skills.	_____
G.	Assists in planning the postoperative care and education of the patient and in the education of the family/others.	_____

Forence T. Wilson, R.N., CNOR, RNFA   Division: Nursing Department of Surgery

The Arlington Hospital   Formulated: August, 1991

Arlington, Virginia   Revised: May, 1992

CHART 3-3

ANA Guidelines for Privileges

The ANA believes that nurses (external to organized nursing services) should have the opportunity, through the mechanism of nursing appointments, to gain access to the consumer in health care organizations for the purpose of providing continuity of care in an accountable systematic manner. The nurse appointment is a method of putting into operation the belief that all persons have the right to health care that is accessible, continuing, and comprehensive.

Because of the diversity of the various types of nursing practice, the nurse should apply for a specific type of appointment, one that is within the nurse's limits of competence and meets the consumer's and family's needs. The type(s) of appointment(s) requested may not encompass all the nurse's professional competencies but will reflect the desired area of practice of the nurse in the health care organization to which she applies.

Types of Appointments

The following are examples of types of appointments.

Type A. The appointee gives support to the consumer and family through the health care organization by:
1. providing data to nurses and other health care providers
2. participating in the planning for discharges with the health care team, including the consumer and family
3. maintaining contact with the consumer and family.

Type B. The appointee collaborates with physicians in implementing medical therapies in specified areas.

Type C. The appointee administers direct consumer nursing intervention by:
1. collecting data for nursing intervention, e.g., health history, physical examination, limited laboratory work
2. identifying and providing a specific part of the nursing intervention.

Type D. The appointee provides consultation in a collaborative relationship that allows the appointee to be active in planning part or all of the nursing intervention (nursing order) in conjunction with the staff of the department of nursing services.

In general, there are two kinds of application for nursing services exclusively, as reflected in Types A, C, and D of the preceding examples; the other is for applicants interested in performing designated activities, as in Type B.

(Source: American Nurses Association: Guidelines for Appointment of Nurses for Individual Practice Privileges in Health Care Organizations, Kansas City, Mo., American Nurses Association, 1978, pp 1–2. Reprinted with permission.)

Although credentialing is done through the medical staff, the nursing department is also involved in the process. Standards for nursing care within the institution are the responsibility of the nursing department, and first assisting by RNs is considered a perioperative nursing role.

It is usually necessary for the applicant to provide the credentialing committee with information that might include a description of the role of the

RNFA, the legal interpretation and constraints of the practice in the involved state, historical information, national trends, acceptance, and support from professional associations (i.e., AORN, ANA, ACS), as well as educational and certification credentials. This documentation should be gathered and submitted before applying for practice privileges. In institutions where there has not been an RNFA applicant for practice privileges previously, the nurse applying for privileges should remember that change occurs slowly and requires planning, patience, and persistence.

The application process begins with submission of the application form and requisite information to the appropriate committee; this will most likely be the operating room committee or surgical committee, if the medical staff is structured by services. From this committee, the application is usually sent to the executive committee of the medical staff and then to the governing body for the final decision.

Before applying for practice privileges, the nurse should review the institutional policies that apply to practicing within that health care setting. If the institution does not have a policy related to RNFAs or nonphysician assistants, such a policy should be developed and approved before the official application process can begin. Chart 3–4 lists the policy of a medical center in Boise, Idaho.

Institutional policies that govern the role of the RNFA should cover activities that may be performed, qualifications required, and the mechanism for supervision by the surgeon. The nursing department, medical staff, and administration must be jointly involved in developing policies. AORN's Official Statement on RN First Assistants can provide general guidance to an institution in developing a policy that is specific to the institution.

When the RNFA applies for institutional practice privileges, it is important to provide the information required by the Joint Commission. The 1997 standards specify that criteria for all applicants for medical staff privileges or delineated clinical privileges should include at least the following:

- evidence of current licensure
- relevant training and experience
- current competence (usually verified through references and peer recommendations)
- health status[18]

Information regarding the RNFA's licensure, specific educational preparation, experience, and current competence will be verified by the institution. Additional information, such as current professional liability insurance, likely will be requested. Medical staff bylaws or policies will also require provision of:

- information related to involvement in professional liability actions
- information related to any challenges (previously successful or currently pending) to licensure or registration or voluntary relinquishment of licensure or registration

CHART 3-4

Associated Health Care Professional Policy: Nonphysician First Assistant, St. Luke's Regional Medical Center

Purpose

The purpose of the nonphysician first assistant is to assist the surgeon/employer in those specific procedures that have been identified by the surgeon/employer, and that the nonphysician first assistant has demonstrated the knowledge, experience, and skill to perform as assistant for those procedures. The OR/Surgical Supervisory Committee grants privileges to the nonphysician first assistant.

Qualifications

A. Current Idaho registered nurse license or physician assistant registered with the Board of Medicine.

B. Three years of experience as a registered nurse in the operating room with demonstrated knowledge and skill in those procedures for which requesting privileges as a first assistant or evidence of graduation from a physician assistant program with curriculum that includes courses in surgical procedures which have prepared the physician assistant to function in this role.

C. Credentials approved by OR/Surgical Supervisory Committee through the following procedure:

1. Employing surgeon submits letter to the OR/Surgical Supervisory Committee requesting privileges for nonphysician first assistant and a copy of liability insurance coverage for nonphysician first assistant.

2. Applicant completes application for nonphysician first assistant privileges, including three current letters of references who can attest to the applicant's clinical skills and ability to perform procedures for which requesting privileges.

3. Submit completed application for nonphysician first assistant to the Medical Staff office, which will verify licensure or registration, insurance coverage, educational preparation, and references.

4. The Director of the Operating Room will orient the applicant to the operating room and complete a skills checklist of knowledge and skills requested by the applicant.

5. The OR/Surgical Supervisory Committee will review the application and recommendations. If all are satisfactory, the applicant will be appointed to Associate Health Care professional status for a 1-year period. Privileges are limited to the operating room.

6. Annual review of privileges will include recommendation by the Director of the Operating Room that the performance meets accepted standards. The Medical Staff office will verify continuation of insurance coverage, current licensure or certification, and continuing education.

7. Renewal of privileges will be granted by the OR/Surgical Supervisory Committee.

D. For privileges for the nonphysician first assistant to function outside the operating room, request must be made by the employing surgeon and reviewed by the OR/Surgical Supervisory Committee.

Date Reviewed: May 1990
(Source: Rules and Regulations, Article XVI, Associated Health Care Professional. Courtesy of St. Luke's Regional Medical Center, Boise, Idaho.)

■ any limitation, reduction, or loss of privileges at another institution (voluntary or involuntary)

The institution is concerned with both legal constraints to practice and evidence of competence in relation to the activities or services that are to be provided by the applicant. Chart 3–5 provides a sample application for medical affiliate staff privileges.

AORN's Official Statement on RN First Assistants provides additional information regarding the credentialing process. It calls for a mechanism for the following:

■ assessing individual qualifications for practice
■ assessing continuing proficiency
■ evaluating performance annually
■ assessing compliance with relevant institutional and departmental policies
■ defining lines of accountability
■ retrieving documentation of participation as first assistant
■ establishing a system for peer review[19]

The ACS's Qualifications of the First Assistant in the Operating Room address applying for practice privileges by surgeon assistants and physician assistants. The criteria outlined could be applied to RNFAs applying for practice privileges, and include the following:

■ outline of qualifications and credentials
■ request to "assist in a surgeon's practice including assisting at the operating table"
■ identity of the surgeon responsible for the applicant's performance
■ requirement that the qualifications be reviewed and approved by the hospital (institutional) board[20]

When an application for practice privileges is submitted, the institution usually requests specific information related to first assistant activities. The request may be for information in the form of a narrative description of the RNFA's role, or for a checklist. The RNFA may apply for privileges in all surgical specialties or in a specific surgical area or areas, such as cardiovascular, orthopedics, and so on. The privileges will be granted only in those specialty areas designated by the applicant. Examples of activities to include on the application are:

■ providing preoperative assessment of the patient and preoperative education of the patient, family, and significant others
■ assisting with patient positioning, prepping, and draping
■ providing exposure by suctioning, sponging, and retracting
■ providing hemostasis by applying hemostatic clamps or clips, coagulating bleeding points, and ligating bleeding vessels
■ suturing

CHART 3 – 5

Application—Associated Health Care Professional

APPLICANT'S NAME: _____
(Please type, for legibility)

[ ] CRNA
[ ] Dental Assistant
[ ] Nonphysician First Assistant
[ ] Nurse Practitioner
[ ] Physician Assistant
[ ] Private Scrub
[ ] Other (specify)

NAME IN FULL: _____   DATE: _____
　　　　　　　　FIRST　　　　　　　MIDDLE　　　　　　LAST

EMPLOYER: _____

EMPLOYER'S OFFICE ADDRESS: _____   TELEPHONE: _____

RESIDENCE ADDRESS: _____   TELEPHONE: _____

DATE OF BIRTH: _____   SOCIAL SECURITY NUMBER: _____

POSITION/DUTIES: _____

EDUCATION: _____
　　　　　　　College or University　　　　Address　　　City/State/Zip　　　Degree　　　Date

EDUCATION: _____
　　　　　　　College or University　　　　Address　　　City/State/Zip　　　Degree　　　Date

PROFESSIONAL EDUCATION: _____

EXPERIENCE:
Hospital: _____
　　　　　　　　　　Dates: From/To

Position: _____
Address　　　　　　City　　　　　　State　　　　　　Zip

Hospital: _____
　　　　　　　　　　Dates: From/To

Position: _____
Address　　　　　　City　　　　　　State　　　　　　Zip

Have your clinical privileges ever been voluntarily or involuntarily suspended, diminished, revoked, refused, relinquished, or limited at any hospital or other health care facility? Yes _____ No _____. If yes, explain on a separate page.

Have you ever withdrawn your application for appointment, reappointment, and clinical privileges or resigned before a decision was made by a hospital's or health care facility's governing board? Yes _____ No _____. If yes, explain on a separate page.

Have you ever been the subject of disciplinary proceedings or investigations at any hospital or health care facility? Yes _____ No _____. If yes, explain on a separate page.

(continued)

C H A R T 3 – 5

Application—Associated Health Care Professional *(continued)*

Current Licensure/Certification (Attach Copy)

State: _____   Number: _____   Expiration Date: _____
Registration State Board of Medicine/Dentistry   Date: _____
Registration State Board of Nursing   Date: _____

Has your license or certificate to practice in any jurisdiction ever been suspended, revoked, or not re-newed? Yes _____ No _____. If yes, please explain in detail on separate sheet.

Membership in Professional Organizations:

_____

Continuing Education: (last 5 years)
1. _____   2. _____

   _____   _____

HEALTH ASSESSMENT
Have you ever abused or been addicted to drugs and/or alcohol?   No _____ Yes _____
Have you ever been hospitalized for drug and/or alcohol related problems?   No _____ Yes _____
If your answer is "yes" to any of the above questions/ please explain fully on an additional page.

Have you ever been a defendent in a felony criminal matter?   No _____ Yes _____

If "yes," what was the nature of the allegation(s)?

_____

_____

If "yes", what was the finding:
    Guilty ( )   Pending Trial or Appeal ( )
    Not Guilty ( )   Other: _____( )

Personal References: Medical references who are able to attest to your current competence at performing the privileges you request

NAME	COMPLETE ADDRESS: (Street, City, State, Zip)	PHONE
1.		
2.		
3.		

List below the nature and scope of those privileges you are requesting as an associated health care pro-fessional:

_____

_____

_____

In making application to associated health care professional status of St. Luke's Regional Medical Center, I agree to abide by the bylaws, rules, and regulations of the medical staff, as well as the bylaws and poli-cies of the hospital which pertain to me.

(continued)

CHART 3 – 5

Application—Associated Health Care Professional *(continued)*

I attest that I am physically and mentally capable of accepting appointment to associated health care professional status and any privileges granted to me. I fully understand that any significant misstatement in or omissions from this application constitutes cause for summary dismissal from the staff.

APPLICANT'S SIGNATURE: _____ Date: _____

****PLEASE ATTACH CERTIFICATE OF LIABILITY INSURANCE****

RELEASE OF LIABILITY:

I release from any liability all individuals and organizations who provide information to St. Luke's Regional Medical Center in good faith and without malice concerning the applicant's professional qualifications, clinical competence, mental and emotional stability, physical health, ethics, character, and other qualifications for medical staff appointment and clinical privileges, including otherwise privileged or confidential information.

I authorize all listed references included in my application to release any and all information as requested by the Medical Staff Office of St. Luke's Regional Medical Center, Boise, Idaho 83712

APPLICANT'S NAME: (please print)   _____ Date: _____

APPLICANT'S SIGNATURE: _____ Date: _____

NOTE: It is the responsibility of the applicant to keep the hospital informed and current regarding changes in address, status, continuing education, teaching appointments, licenses, etc.

DEPARTMENT CHAIRMAN: _____ Date: _____

CREDENTIALS COMMITTEE CHAIRMAN: _____ Date: _____

ADMINISTRATION: _____ Date: _____

APPROVED: EXECUTIVE COMMITTEE: Date: _____

APPROVED: BOARD OF DIRECTORS: Date: _____

(Source: St. Luke's Regional Medical Center, Boise, Idaho.)

■ performing postoperative activities, which may include removing sutures, chest tubes, drains, or pacing wires; performing postoperative evaluation; and providing discharge instructions

It may be necessary to identify specific operative procedures in which the RNFA will be assisting as either first or second assistant. This is not desirable, for it requires constant revision and is limiting in emergency and on-call situations. It is important to state that intraoperative activities will be performed in collaboration with the operating surgeon and to delineate the nature of the surgeon's supervisory functions.

Privileges may be granted on a temporary basis, providing an opportunity to evaluate the RNFA's competence. The provisional period required after the initial appointment to the medical staff can vary from 3 months to 2 years. At the end of this provisional period, the institution decides either to continue, expand, or curtail the RNFA's practice privileges. All appointments and reappointments, as well as renewal or revision of clinical privileges, are made for a period not longer than 2 years.

Reappointment or renewal of practice privileges will be determined in relation to competence. Information concerning professional performance, clinical judgment and decision making, interpersonal skills, and clinical or technical skills will be requested during the reappointment process. Peer recommendations are part of the basis for reappointment; these, as well as documentation of continuing education activities, should be prepared. Also required are recommendations from the department or major clinical service where the RNFA functions.

For applicants who are denied clinical privileges or who receive adverse decisions, the Joint Commission requires that institutions offer a mechanism for appropriate action, including a fair hearing and an appeal process. Sex, race, creed, and national origin are not bases for decisions on granting or denying appointment or clinical privileges. The institution must abide by antitrust laws that prohibit restraint of trade or attempts to monopolize by excluding certain providers from access to the institution. The bylaws of the medical staff must define the criteria for admission to or denial of medical staff privileges within the institution. Decisions or recommendations cannot be made on the basis of competitive considerations.[21] The RNFA who is denied staff privileges may find it necessary to seek legal advice or counsel prior to appealing the institution's decision.

Applying for Privileges as an RN First Assistant Intern

The importance of educational preparation for assisting at surgery is well documented. In its Official Statement on RN First Assistants, AORN clearly states that "the RN first assistant practices perioperative nursing and must have acquired the necessary knowledge, skills, and judgment specific to clinical practice . . . through completion of an RNFA program that meets the AORN Recommended Education Standards for RN First Assistant Programs."[22] The AORN Recommended Education Standards for RN First Assistant Programs further clarify the nature of the didactic and supervised clinical learning required to develop the cognitive, psychomotor, and affective behaviors necessary to role assumption as an RNFA.

The 1990s have seen a significant interest in and institutional need for nurses to act as first assistants. Although it may seem expedient to assign a perioperative nurse who is available to assist, this practice is not advisable. If an injury occurs because a nurse who has not received adequate instruction and is not acting pursuant to an institutional policy assumes the role of a first assistant, the consequences to the nurse and to the institution can be severe.[6,23]

Educational programs for RN first assistants require a clinical internship, during which the nurse builds on a knowledge base acquired through classroom instruction. The internship is supervised by faculty or a surgeon and an experienced RNFA. These internships require acquisition of a depth and breadth of clinical skills. For example, in one collegiate program for RNFAs, interns average 250 hours during their internship.[24] To engage in such internship activities, the RN first assistant student may need to apply for privileges as an RN first assistant intern. The delineation of privileges may vary from institution to institution and is often based on the clinical requirements of the educational program. A sample application for RNFA internship privileges is shown in Chart 3–6.

CHART 3 – 6
Application for RNFA Internship Privileges

I _____
request permission to practice as an RN First Assistant intern at Millard Fillmore Hospitals. The anticipated time frame for my clinical internship activities will be from:

_____   to   _____.

Attached you will find verification of:

1. Enrollment in an approved RN first assistant course requiring a clinical internship experience
2. Goals and objectives for the internship
3. Clinical activities associated with the internship
4. CNOR status
5. RN licensure
6. Malpractice insurance

_____
Signature of Applicant   Date

Privileges   Granted _____
                    Denied _____   Date _____
_____

(Source: Millard Fillmore Hospitals, Buffalo, NY.)

CONCLUSION

A credentialing process provides a system in the institution for identifying and validating the individual RNFA's knowledge and skill. This is important as a competency assessment and quality improvement mechanism. With credentialing, the institution has a method for evaluating each RNFA and assigning specific aspects of patient care based on the RNFA's qualifications, ensuring patient safety and contributing to quality of care, increased productivity, and efficiency.

A credentialing system can also be used for identifying the educational needs of individual staff members. The RNFA's individual professional growth can be enhanced with such a system. Viewed in this framework, a credentialing system benefits the RNFA, the institution, and the patient.

Review Questions

1. A surgeon tells an RNFA to execute a medical order they both know is not part of the RNFA's practice privileges. The patient is injured and sues the RNFA. In terms of the RNFA's liability,
    a. The surgeon's verbal assurance to the RNFA will provide adequate protection from legal liability to the patient.
    b. The Nurse Practice Act addresses the function; therefore, no one can sue the RNFA.
    c. The hospital may hold the RNFA liable for performing a function for which she or he was not granted practice privileges.
    d. The "borrowed servant" law absolves the RNFA from responsibility.

2. Because most nurse practice acts either permit the nurse to function as assistant in surgery or are silent on it,
    a. Most hospitals must also permit it.
    b. Clear definitions of the role still need to be established in the institution.
    c. Surgeons may determine the role functions by the "captain of the ship" doctrine.
    d. A nurse who functions as an RNFA could not be sued for wrongful conduct.

3. While employed as an RNFA at a hospital with a job description for the role, and credentialed by the institution to perform the role, RNFA Hutt negligently injures a patient. Which of the following conclusions (if any) would apply?
    a. If the injured patient sues and collects damages from the hospital, RNFA Hutt cannot also be held liable.
    b. RNFA Hutt cannot be held liable under any circumstances, because the hospital, by virtue of the job description and credentialing mechanism, has agreed to assume all liability.

    c. Both RNFA Hutt and the hospital can be held liable for the negligence.

    d. None of the conclusions apply.

4. The law will absolve RNFAs from liability:

    a. If they are employed by a hospital with a credentialing mechanism for RNFAs, even if the nurse practice act is silent on scope of practice for RNFAs.

    b. If they can show they were carrying out a surgeon's orders.

    c. In both of the above instances.

    d. In neither of the above instances.

5. A surgeon may safely assume that:

    a. Any perioperative nurse on staff is competent to carry out first assisting functions.

    b. Some surgical maneuvers cannot be delegated to an RNFA no matter what the circumstances.

    c. A CRNFA carries his or her own liability insurance.

    d. As long as the RNFA has practice privileges, she or he is competent to carry out any assigned assisting duties.

6. A perioperative patient care coordinator directs an RNFA intern to assist at major abdominal surgery even though the intern has only assisted at minor procedures in the past. As a result of the intern's lack of competence, the patient is injured. On what basis could the RNFA intern be held liable?

    a. For not discussing with the coordinator his or her limitations prior to assisting at the surgery.

    b. For not carrying student liability insurance.

    c. Both of the above.

    d. Neither of the above.

7. Credentialing processes

    a. Place the burden of liability on the RNFA.

    b. Attempt to decrease institutional liability.

    c. Are required by the AORN and ANA.

    d. Are part of the institution's duty toward patients.

8. If the perioperative credentialing model is used as a guideline, files maintained would contain annual documentation of:

    a. Changes in the Nurse Practice Act.

    b. A review by the risk manager of liability claims.

    c. Performance appraisal and documentation of competence.

    d. Current membership in the AORN RNFA Specialty Assembly.

9. When an institution develops a job description for the RNFA, such a description should:

    a. Be separate from descriptions of staff nursing positions.

    b. Not be part of nonphysician credentialing.

     c. Require a master's degree (or evidence of a degree in progress).

     d. Be specific to assisting functions and responsibilities.

10. Joint Commission standards require

     a. A process that ensures that all individuals who provide patient care services are qualified to do so.

     b. That only medical staff appointments are subject to competence review and privilege granting/renewal.

     c. Additional education and experience for nurses who request privileges as first assistants.

     d. Advanced certification as an RNFA or physician assistant for any nonphysician provider of assistant at surgery services.

Indicate whether each of the following statements is true (T) or false (F):

11. _____ The rights to perform certain activities within an institution are privileges granted through a credentialing process.

12. _____ The Joint Commission requires that credentialing processes be the same for institutional employees and nonemployees.

13. _____ By verifying that an applicant is competent to function as a first assistant, the institution ensures that patients will receive quality care.

14. _____ Credentialing by an institution as an RNFA is the same as being given institutional licensure as an RNFA.

15. _____ Competence is the only requirement in determining assignment of an RNFA to a patient procedure.

16. _____ A skills list should be used in conjunction with a job description as evidence of the RNFA's continued competence.

17. _____ If an RNFA is granted "limited" privileges, it means that his or her competence is not yet at a level deserving "full" privileges.

18. _____ When applying for institutional practice privileges, the RNFA should be prepared to provide information on formal educational preparation and/or experience.

19. _____ It is a violation of the RNFA's privacy to be queried regarding any professional liability actions.

20. _____ It is important that institutions have mechanisms for retrieving documentation of the RNFA's participation in surgical procedures as a first assistant.

Answer Key

    1. c
    2. b
    3. c
    4. d

5. b
6. a
7. d
8. c
9. d
10. a
11. T
12. F (Credentialing processes are often different for employees and nonemployees.)
13. T
14. F (Institutional licensure would allow an institution to determine "who can do what" without regard to professional standards. Credentialing processes, on the other hand, rely on many professional standards to ensure competence and appropriate scope of practice delineations.)
15. F (Competence is important in assignment, but there must be an institutional position description that clearly identifies what is permissible.)
16. T
17. F ("Limited" privileges usually refer to the RNFA's nonphysician status, not to competence.)
18. T
19. F (This is permissible and relates to the institution's duty to provide quality care by competent professionals.)
20. T

REFERENCES

1. Patterson P: Who's first assisting? ORs turn to non-MDs but reimbursement lags. OR Manager 13(9):1, 1997
2. Delaware Board of Nursing: Registered Nurse Surgical First Assistant Position Statement. Dover, Del, July 2, 1987
3. Association of Operating Room Nurses: AORN Official Statement on RN First Assistants. Adopted 4/2/98, House of Delegates, Orlando, Fla.
4. American College of Surgeons: Qualifications of the first assistant in the operating room. AORN J 32:1012, 1980
5. LoCicero J: Credentialing, decredentialing, and recredentialing. Paper presented at the American College of Surgeons Symposium X, Chicago, May 12, 1997
6. Patterson P: Who's first assisting? Personnel used as FAs: Are they qualified? OR Manager 13(9):19, 1997
7. Starr P: The Social Transformation of American Medicine. New York, Basic Books, 1982, pp 162, 167.
8. The question of hospital privileges for allied health professionals. QRB 19:18, 1984
9. Moss RW: Privileging essential to APN autonomy. Am Nurse 25(10):7, 1993
10. Joint Commission on Accreditation of Healthcare Organizations: Comprehensive Accreditation Manual for Hospitals. Chicago, Joint Commission on Accreditation of Healthcare Organizations, 1996
11. VanderVeer JB: How my practice profile almost got me fired. Med Econ 74(16):111–117, 1997
12. Association of Operating Room Nurses: Official Statement
13. Association of Operating Room Nurses: AORN Recommended Education Standards for RN First Assistant Programs. In: AORN Standards, Recommended Practices and Guidelines. Denver, Colo., Association of Operating Room Nurses, 1997, pp 37, 39

14. National Council of State Boards of Nursing Continued Competence Subcommittee: Report at the 1996 NCSBN Annual Meeting, Baltimore, Aug 6–10, 1996
15. Seifert PC: Health care work force regulation in Canada and the United States: The Ontario Regulated Health Professions Act of 1991 and the Pew Commission recommendations. Conference Proceedings: The 1997 World Conference of Operating Room Nurses—X. Toronto, Canada, 1997, pp 65–78
16. Association of Operating Room Nurses: Perioperative nursing credentialing model. AORN J 43:262–264, 1986
17. American Nurses Association: Guidelines for Appointment of Nurses for Individual Practice Privileges in Health Care Organizations. Kansas City, Mo, American Nurses Association, 1978
18. Joint Commission on Accreditation of Healthcare Organizations: 1997
19. Association of Operating Room Nurses: Official Statement
20. American College of Surgeons, p 1012
21. Scott PE: Legal considerations. In: Care of the Surgical Patient, Vol II. New York, Scientific American—American College of Surgeons, 1991, pp X3-1–X3-12
22. Association of Operating Room Nurses: Official Statement.
23. Murphy EK: OR nursing law. AORN J 45:140–142, 1987
24. RN First Assistant Program, Delaware County Community College, Media, Pa, 1997

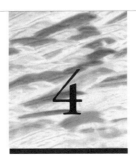

INFECTION CONTROL

CECIL A. KING

■

Asepsis means the absence of germs, infection, and septic matter. For RNFAs and their perioperative colleagues, aseptic technique is the foundation of infection control. Components of surgical asepsis include rigorous environmental control, processing supplies and equipment, selecting and evaluating barrier materials, surgical hand scrubbing, patient skin preparation, preparing and maintaining a sterile field, and continuous monitoring of both the patient and the perioperative environment.

▨ NURSING ROLE IN THE DEVELOPMENT OF ASEPSIS

"Every day sanitary knowledge, or the knowledge of nursing, or in other words, of how to put the constitution in such a state as that it will have no disease, or that it can recover from disease, takes a higher place."[1] Florence Nightingale, in her *Notes on Nursing,* was the first to connect sanitary science to preventing mortality associated with disease. Her work to improve sanitary conditions during the Crimean War reduced the mortality rate from 42% to 2%. Nightingale firmly established nursing's role in infection control by being the first nurse to validate the relationship of sanitary science to medical institutions through outcome measurement, data collection, and analysis. Her belief that nurses could intervene to prevent infection continues to influence the nursing process and nurses' roles in infection prevention to this day.[2]

In 1989, William H. Welch, William S. Halsted, a surgeon, and Sir William Osler established Johns Hopkins University in Baltimore to train doctors and nurses. A graduate of Bellevue training school, Isabel Hampton Robb was chosen to head what would become known as the department of surgical nursing. Robb worked with Halsted to develop operating room nursing, which was identified as an area of specialization and became nursing's first specialty.[3] This was an era of carbolic acid hand rinses; surgical masks and sterile gowns were not worn. Because of the severe dermatosis experienced by Robb when using carbolic acid, Halsted contracted with the Goodyear Company to develop surgical rubber gloves. Eventually this led to the wearing of sterile surgical gloves, and it serves as an early example of collaborative practice between a nurse and a surgeon in advancing surgical asepsis.

During this era, the Boston Training School added a lecture on bacteriology, and in 1891 student nurses were responsible for cleaning and sterilizing instruments for Saturday surgeries. By 1896, student nurses were assisting with Saturday surgery. The early 1900s saw the start of perioperative nursing. In 1901, Martha Luce of Boston described the responsibilities of an operating room nurse, which required knowledge of the principles of asepsis, careful attention to details, and much forethought in planning and preparing the operative theater. Since the days of Nightingale, nursing has contributed to the advance of surgical asepsis and the prevention of postoperative surgical site infections (SSIs).

Perioperative nursing is the first recognized nursing specialty, and nurses no doubt have functioned as first assistants throughout time. RNFAs have an important role to play in incorporating their nursing actions into indicator criteria and surveillance programs in an effort to identify predictive outcomes for surgical patients as part of facilitywide continuous improvement to promote quality outcomes and decrease SSIs.

■ EPIDEMIOLOGY OF SURGICAL SITE INFECTIONS

The Centers for Disease Control and Prevention (CDC) have dropped the term *wound* from the modified definitions of surgical site infection. The term *incisional* SSI refers to infections that involve only the incision. *Superficial incisional* SSI infections are those involving the skin and subcutaneous tissue. *Deep incisional* SSI involves deep soft tissue, fascia, and muscle. *Organ/space* SSI involves any part of the anatomy other than the incision.

Of the plethora of known bacterial organisms, only a small number are actually pathogenic and cause infection.

The first line of defense in protection from infection is the skin, which is violated during operative and other invasive procedures. There are two major sources of potential contamination during surgery that may transmit pathogens to the patient. *Endogenous* sources are bacterial organisms commonly found on the skin (e.g., *Staphylococcus aureus* and *S. epidermidis*) and in the gut (e.g., *Escherichia coli*). *Exogenous* sources are those organisms found on objects outside the patient (e.g., bioburden). Factors that influence the development of SSIs are the source of colonization, the microbial agent involved, the route of transmission, the susceptibility of the patient, and the environment. Surgical asepsis is designed to restrict contamination by microorganisms in the environment and on equipment that comes in contact with the patient.

Pathogenicity of Bacteria

Once pathogens attach to their host cell surface receptors, they demonstrate their virulence through various cellular mechanisms. Toxin production is one mechanism of pathogenicity. Diphtheria, tetanus, and botulism are caused by microbes that rely on toxin production for their infectious property. Protective cellular outer capsules prevent *Staphylococcus, Streptococcus, Neisseria,* and *Hemophilus* from being ingested by phagocytic leukocytes, contributing to their pathogenicity. A chief immune system defense is the humoral response, whereby antibodies coat the capsule, render it to complement fixation, and prepare it for sequestration by the spleen (Figure 4–1). Any patient who is asplenic, age-extreme (the elderly or the infant), or has an impaired immune system, such as in immunosuppression, has an increased vulnerability to encapsulated organisms.

Some organisms are viable outside a host. Such microbes survive phagocytic ingestion and remain viable within the presence of antibodies in complement. These organisms are intracellular and can survive and multiply for years within the phagocyte, surfacing later under ideal conditions to result in clinical infection (e.g., tuberculosis bacillus and pathogenic fungi). Other organisms, such as viruses (e.g., human immunodeficiency virus, rickettsiae, and chlamydia) live within the cell and use the patient's metabolic elements (e.g., DNA or RNA) for their survival and reproduction. These obligate cellular parasites can resurface repeatedly, causing recurrent clinical infection (e.g., herpesvirus).

Although some organisms possess high degrees of innate virulence and have no difficulty overcoming the patient's defense mechanisms, other, less virulent microbes, those usually implicated in SSIs, rely on suppression of the patient's normal immune system. Burns, trauma, and surgery violate the skin's barrier, allowing low-virulence organisms, such as *Staphylococcus epidermidis* and *S. aureus,* to contaminate the surgical wound, resulting in SSI. The very antibiotics used to prevent postoperative SSI can contribute to weakening the normal immune response. Additionally, radiation and chemotherapy suppress the phagocytes and lymphocytes or damage the mucosal barriers of the bowel. Various disease states can result in poor nutrition and organ dysfunction, leaving the patient with little resistance to infection. It is important for the RNFA to understand that the event that allows organisms to penetrate the vulnerable interior of the patient is modern surgical technology.

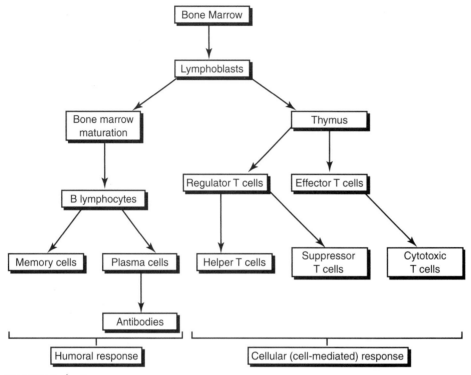

FIGURE 4–1

There are three primary immune system defenses: the phagocytic response, the humoral (or antibody) response, and the cellular response. The phagocytic response (not pictured) involves the granulocytes and macrophages, which engulf and digest invading agents. The humoral response, sometimes referred to as the antibody response, begins with lymphocytes, which can transform themselves into plasma cells that manufacture antibodies. The cellular response also involves lymphocytes, which can also turn into special cytotoxic T-cells that attack the pathogen. (Source: Smeltzer SC, Bare, BG: Brunner and Suddarth's Textbook of Medical-Surgical Nursing. Philadelphia, Lippincott-Raven, 1996, p 1367, Figure 48–2.)

▓ BACTERIAL MICROORGANISMS OF PERIOPERATIVE IMPORTANCE

In the past two decades, postoperative SSI surveillance has revealed that the most common organisms isolated from clean, clean-contaminated, and contaminated surgical sites are *Staphylococcus aureus,* coagulase-negative staphylococci, enterococci, *Pseudomonas,* and *Staphylococcus epidermidis.* The type and virulence of an organism play a pivotal role in the likelihood of infection.

Staphylococci

Staphylococci are gram-positive, non-spore-forming microbes that form in clumps and are pyogenic. *S. aureus* is involved in about 20% of SSIs.[4] *S. epidermidis,* once considered nonthreatening, is becoming more resistant; in 80% of cases the strain is methicillin resistant, and resistance has been identified to cephalosporins and vancomycin. *S. epidermidis* has become more common as the causative agent in clean wound infections, especially during implant surgery (prosthetic joints, valves, and other invasive medical devices).

Staphylococci are ubiquitous in the hospital environment; infected and colonized patients are the most important sources. Transmission occurs primarily via the hands of health care workers, which can become contaminated through contact with the colonized or infected body site. Health care workers can become colonized and serve as reservoirs and disseminators; carriage of *S. aureus* is most common in the anterior nares, but other sites, such as the hands, axilla, perineum, oropharynx, and nasopharynx, may be involved. Staphyloccal infections are commonly characterized by odorless, red, tender wounds with a creamy exudate. Septicemia and deep organ involvement can occur, but most often after local SSIs. The degree of virulence depends on the specific extracellular enzymes and toxin production by the causative agent. Toxin-producing strains of *Staphylococcus* can cause toxic shock syndrome under certain conditions (e.g., nasal and vaginal packing). Staphylococcal organisms are resistant to destruction by heat and chemical disinfectants. Their ability to survive under adverse conditions makes the use of barrier materials critical during operative procedures.

Streptococci

Streptococci are gram-positive cocci, non-spore-forming and pyogenic. Surgical patients may be colonized with Group B streptococci; the most common sites are the vaginal mucosa, the male urethral meatus, the throat, and the rectum. Streptococci are spread by hand-to-hand contact, aerosolized droplets, or as dust-borne bacteria. Pathogenically they infect a wound in association with other organisms. They are usually implicated in SSIs following cesarean birth or gynecologic procedures or in systemic infection in immunocompromised patients. Streptococci are commonly present in lower gastrointestinal surgery, in diffuse cellulitis, and in vascular stasis ulcers and gangrene in diabetic patients. Group A streptococci may cause cutaneous infections, while Group B streptococci can cause significant infections in neonates. *Streptococcus pneumoniae* has become the most common pathogen in nearly all studies of hospitalized adults with community-acquired pneumonia, and has increasingly become resistant to penicillin (PRSP).[5]

Enteric Bacilli

The enteric bacilli are gram-negative, non-spore-forming, aerobic organisms endogenous to the gastrointestinal tract. Types include *Escherichia coli, Proteus mirabilis, Klebsiella,* and *Enterobacter.* When enteric bacilli are the causative agent in SSIs, it is often as a result of autoinfection by endogenous flora. The wound is usually necrotic and purulent. These infections are frequently seen following bowel surgery without a prep, with ruptured appendix, and with diverticulitis presenting as a diffuse peritonitis. The enteric bacilli can also cause infection following instrumentation of the gastrointestinal tract and septicemia in the necrotic tissue of burn patients. Enteric bacilli can be destroyed by heat and chemical methods of sterilization, but in the last few years they have become a formidable nosocomial infectious agent, as they have developed resistance to vancomycin.

Pseudomonas

The *Pseudomonas* organism is gram-negative and non-spore-forming. *Pseudomonas* is found in the environment in water, soil, and decomposing organic matter. It is often a secondary organism in SSI; its presence is detected by a characteristic bluish green discharge with an acrid, musty odor. *Pseudomonas* can also cause pneumonia and can be fatal in the respirator-dependent patient. It is susceptible to routine sterilization techniques but may emerge in SSIs during prolonged use of broad-spectrum antibiotics.

Clostridia

The clostridia are anaerobic, gram-positive, spore-forming organisms. Important species include *C. tetani, C. welchii,* and *C. sordelli.* These organisms are common in the soil and the intestinal tract, where the spores can remain viable for years. In their pathogenic form, they are the causative agent in tetanus and gas gangrene. They are also implicated in deep necrotic wounds associated with trauma. Because they are spore-forming, they are resistant to routine disinfectants and some sterilization methods.

Multiple-Antibiotic-Resistant Organisms

Infectious diseases, once thought to be eliminated as a public health threat, remain the leading cause of death worldwide and are among the leading causes of illness and death in the United States. Over the past 40 years a number of factors, such as the overuse and indiscriminate use of antibiotics, have resulted in multiple-antibiotic-resistant organisms (MAROs), often referred to as "superbugs." Bacteria become resistant to antibiotics in at least three ways. The most common is through conjugation: genetic material related to resistance on the outside of organisms is shared among related and unrelated bacteria. This can occur, for example, by shaking a bag of urine, which disrupts the cell walls of organisms, allowing their resistant genetic material to be transmitted to other bacteria in the urine bag. Mutations involve a change in the organism's response to exposure to antibiotics, inducing resistance. In transduction, viruses that contain genetic material that make them resistant attack bacteria; genetic material is transmitted to the bacteria, making them also resistant.[6] This is an emerging global problem of antimicrobial resistance which has multiple aspects and involves multiple pathogens.[7]

Methicillin-resistant *S. aureus* (MRSA), vancomycin-resistant *Enterococcus* (VRE), and multiple-drug-resistant tuberculosis (MDR-TB) are three strains of infectious microbes of significance to the RNFA. In 1997, a vancomycin-resistant strain of *S. aureus* (VISA—vancomycin-intermediate-resistant *S. aureus*) was announced by researchers in Japan; within months, researchers in the United States had documented two cases of resistance to the drug, considered the last uniformly effective antibiotic against this microbe for serious infections.[8]

Methicillin-resistant *S. aureus* has been implicated as a prevalent nosocomial infection in many health care facilities. The majority of such infections have been in patients with extensive burns and surgical wounds. The term MRSA is misleading, because this strain of *S. aureus* is also resistant to oxacillin, nafcillin, and cephalosporin antibiotics. Ten to 15% of all nosocomial infections are attributable to MRSA. Colonized or infected patients are the major sources of infection. Most often MRSA is spread from one patient to another by the hands of health care providers (e.g., while changing dressings or during tracheal suctioning). MRSA, which remains viable on the hands for many hours, is then carried to subsequent patients. Hand washing remains the most effective measure to prevent transmission of MRSA. The sites in or excretions of patients colonized with MRSA most often are the anterior nares, sputum, surgical or burn wounds, decubitus ulcers, perineum, rectum, and tracheostomies or gastrostomies.

Extended hospital stays and the use of broad-spectrum antibiotics add to the risk of MRSA infection. The highest risk is in patients in ICUs, infants, the elderly, those with suppressed immune systems, and those in burn units. Patients with open wounds or invasive devices (e.g., gastrostomy tubes, indwelling catheters) are much more likely to acquire MRSA. Although patients can transmit MRSA to health care providers, such transmission is rare. MRSA infections in health care providers usually manifest as cellulitis, impetigo, or conjunctivitis. Health care providers can become colonized, MRSA-present without infection, at rates of 2% to 6% in the anterior nares, and thereby become a source of MRSA infections among patients. The current antibiotic of choice for MRSA infection is vancomycin, but the emergence of VISA compounds treatment dilemmas. Vancomycin must be given parenterally and carries the risks of tissue irritation or necrosis if it extravasates, red neck syndrome, ototoxicity, and nephrotoxicity. MRSA is an attendant-borne (e.g., spread through health care provider hands or equipment) organism and requires body substance isolation and contact isolation measures to prevent transmission within the facility to other patients.[9]

With the emergence of VISA, the CDC issued interim guidelines to assist health care facilities in preventing and preparing for possible breakouts. These guidelines include detecting *Staphylococcus* with reduced vancomycin susceptibility via laboratory determination, then immediately contacting infection control experts to conduct an epidemiological investigation. RNFAs should be aware that guidelines suggest patient isolation in a private room, use of contact isolation, and limiting the numbers of health care workers who have access to the colonized or infected patient.[10]

Because vancomycin has been aggressively used to treat MRSA since the 1970s, the stage was set for resistance to vancomycin to occur. This is especially true during prolonged empirical use or inappropriate use of broad-spectrum antibiotics. What has emerged, in addition to VISA, is vancomycin-resistant *Enterococcus* (VRE), which is second to MRSA as the most common pathogen of nosocomial infections. With the ability of pathogenic bacteria to achieve inherent resistance to various antibiotics, enterococci account for 12% of all nosocomial infections. Enterococci are normal flora of the gastrointestinal tract, oral cavity, vagina, hepatobiliary tree, soft tissue sites (such as those used for intravenous access), and decubitus ulcers. Patients at greatest risk for VRE are also those at greatest risk for MRSA. Those particularly threatened by VRE are patients whose defenses have been bypassed by invasive medical devices or compromised by aggressive surgery, and those whose normal flora has been altered by antibiotic therapy. There has been an alarming 20-fold increase in VRE infections in the past eight years. Standard precautions and body substance isolation methods remain the most effective ways to prevent colonization of patients with VRE and MRSA. Patients acquiring VRE will need an infectious disease consult and careful planning to combine various antibiotics to resolve the infection. RNFAs should pay careful attention to recommending appropriate disinfectants to assistive personnel during environmental sanitation. VRE survives for long periods of time on clothing and objects; however, the organisms are susceptible to disinfection by quaternary ammonium compounds, phenols, and alcohol.[11]

■ NON-ANTIBIOTIC-RELATED RISK FACTORS FOR SSI

Four independent risk factors have been identified as highly predictive for subsequent SSI. These are the surgical wound class, American Society of Anesthesiologists (ASA) physical status, duration of surgery, and results of intraoperative cultures. The ASA physical status classification is a standardized numerical determination used to assess patients preoperatively. The ASA classification takes into consideration a variety of patient factors that are directly related to patient risk of developing SSI. These factors are age, nutritional status, the presence of systemic diseases, and projected mortality. Table 4–l lists possible risk factors for postoperative SSIs. The most critical factors in preventing SSIs are sound clinical judgment, proper operative technique, and the general health of the patient. During clean surgical procedures there is a generally low infection rate (<3%), which is expected due to airborne exogenous microorganisms.

Table 4–1 also lists other factors sometimes considered, without convincing evidence, to influence the development of SSI.

Preoperative Stay

There is a strong correlation between the duration of preoperative hospitalization and the development of SSI. The rate of infection can double with each week that a patient is hospitalized before surgery. Virtually every patient will be colonized with an infective bacterium within two weeks of admission to an ICU. These infections often involve a resistant nosocomial organism. The current trend toward same-day admissions and ambulatory surgery may be decreasing the rate of SSIs. However, failure to report and subsequent loss to postoperative follow-up in this population is problematic; therefore it is only speculated that current trends toward ambulatory surgery are decreasing the rate of nosocomial SSIs.

T A B L E   4 – 1 . RISK FACTORS FOR POSTOPERATIVE SSI

Patient Factors	Operative Factors
Age	Emergency/elective
Sex	Hair removal technique
Premorbid illness	Service
ASA classification	Surgeon
Immunocompromising diseases	Site of surgery
Diabetes mellitus	Procedure related
Cancer	Perioperative antibiotics
HIV/AIDS	Duration of surgery
Nutritional status	Drains
Presence of other infections	Packing
Duration of preoperative stay	Primary or secondary closure
Chemotherapy	Drapes
Radiation therapy	Irrigation
	Gloves

(Source: Adapted from Garibaldi RA, Cushing D, Lerer T: Risk factors for postoperative infection. Am J Med 91(suppl 3B):38-1595, 1991.)

Preoperative Shave

Preoperative shaving is associated with a significantly higher rate of SSIs. As early as 1971, researchers proposed using a depilatory agent for hair removal, based on findings of a 0.6% infection rate with depilatories, in contrast to a 5.6% infection rate with razor preparations before surgery. In 1973, another study reported the lowest infection rate in patients who had not been shaved. The investigators proposed the alternative method of using hair clippers, which yielded a 1.7% infection rate, in patients who needed hair removed at the operative site.

In 1991, a randomized, prospective study of 200 patients indicated that hair clipping in the immediate preoperative period was a viable alternative to shaving, especially when cost and patient comfort were considered. Thus, research findings indicate that, if it is necessary to remove hair at the operative site, RNFAs should recommend it be done just prior to surgery, with clippers (or a razor, if required by the surgeon).

Length of Operation

With each hour of surgery, the chance of infection almost doubles. As early as 1982, reports indicated that an increased duration of surgery was associated with a decreased effect of antibiotic prophylaxis (when indicated) in preventing infection. These findings relate to the pharmacokinetics of the antibiotic prophylaxis used as well as the increased bacterial wound contamination that occurs in lengthy, complicated procedures. Other studies have supported the association between increased infection rates and lengthy surgical procedures. Even in clean procedures, there is a doubling effect for every hour of surgery. These studies support the current practice of repeating the dosage of prophylactic antibiotics, when indicated, in procedures exceeding two to three hours.

Abdominal Drains

Numerous clinical and experimental studies have demonstrated the risks associated with the use of prophylactic drains in abdominal surgery. On the basis of these studies, the prophylactic use of abdominal drains should be done cautiously by RNFAs; they may actually enhance SSI rates.[12]

Preoperative Showering

Bathing or showering with an antiseptic agent on the evening before surgery decreases the rate of SSI. For same-day admission patients, the RNFA may wish to suggest that the patient shower or bathe just before leaving home.[12]

Skin Preparation

The RNFA should select a patient preoperative skin preparation agent that is broad spectrum, fast-acting, nonirritating, and designed for frequent use. It is difficult to conduct clinical trials to ascertain the optimal agent for skin preparation because of the multitude of perioperative variables and the ethical issues surrounding enrolling patients in such clinical trials. The vast majority of clinical studies evaluating various skin preparations were conducted during the 1980s. An integrative review of the literature on the effectiveness of preoperative skin preparatory agents found chlorhexidine to reduce the incidence of postoperative infections. Using either 70% isopropyl alcohol or iodophor-in-alcohol solution for one minute before applying antimicrobial-impregnated plastic adhesive drapes appears to greatly reduce the colony count of endogenous flora at the incisional site. An isopropyl alcohol skin preparation in conjunction with an iodophor-impregnated plastic adhesive drape appeared to be the most effective skin preparation in reducing the risk of endogenous contamination of the surgical site. When using alcohol or alcohol-based solutions, RNFAs must exercise caution because of its flammability.

Presence of Infections

The presence of any active infection at the time of elective surgery significantly influences the development of subsequent SSI. These infections occur, in order of frequency, in the urinary tract, skin, and respiratory tract. Antibiotic prophylaxis in this patient population does not decrease the incidence of SSI. However, preoperative treatment (>24 hours preoperatively) has been shown to reduce SSI rates significantly. Therefore, RNFAs should recommend postponing elective surgery in patients presenting with an underlying concurrent infection to optimize wound healing and decrease the risk of SSI.[12]

■ SURVEILLANCE SYSTEMS

In the past, detecting and following SSI rates was less complicated because patients remained in the hospital longer postoperatively. Today's trend toward ambulatory surgery has made tracking SSI rates more complicated; more of the RNFA's patients are seen postoperatively outside the facility where the surgery was performed. RNFAs are challenged by such trends to develop a comprehensive outcome measurement system to track variances in this population. In a study of outpatient surgical patients to determine if postoperative telephone interviews, in addition to physician surveys, were adequate in detecting SSI, it was concluded that telephone follow-up was inefficient in the detection of SSI. Using clinical pathways and case management methods may enhance the RNFA's ability to measure important outcomes, including the rate of SSI.[13] This may mean conducting postoperative assessments in the patient's home, the clinic, or the physician's office to enhance SSI surveillance.

Controversy surrounds what is considered an acceptable SSI rate based on the categories of wound classification. As early as 1985, infection control literature emphasized the importance of identifying patients at high risk of developing SSI in each category of surgical procedure to increase the efficiency of routine SSI surveillance and control. Analyzing ten possible risk factors by stepwise multiple logistic regression, researchers developed a model containing four risk factors—abdominal operations, operations lasting longer than two hours, contaminated or dirty/infected operations according to traditional wound classification, and patients having three or more diagnoses. Utilizing this model, levels of developing SSI were identified in each of the categories of wound classification. The infection rates by wound classification were found to be clean (2.9%), clean-contaminated (3.9%), contaminated (8.5%) and dirty/infected (12.6%). Wound class is a moderately effective predictor of SSI risk; however, the ASA score is at least as good as the traditional wound classification system. A number of studies have reported declines in the incidence of SSIs when information on SSI rates is reported back to the practitioner involved in the operation. Such feedback is an essential component of an effective infection control program.

Another factor that affects wound healing is the normal stress response. During times of stress and anxiety, the stress response results in the release of cortisol, which is an immunosuppressor. Cortisol's direct immunosuppressive effect results in a decrease in T-cells and decreased lymphocyte response. The RNFA can dramatically reduce the assault of the stress response by providing preoperative teaching and comforting measures to decrease patient anxiety and thereby decrease the stress response.[14] Perhaps more than any other member of the surgical team, the nurse is sensitive to promoting an optimal psychological state, which contributes to positive postoperative outcomes.

Various alternative therapies are beginning to demonstrate improved patient outcomes when they are employed during the perioperative experience. Therapeutic touch and music therapy are only two of many alternative therapies being explored to improve postoperative outcomes.

Health and Economic Impact of SSI

SSIs may add from 7.4 to 10.1 days to hospitalization, and each year approximately 325,000 patients develop SSIs, at an additional cost of $2,700 per patient.[15] These SSIs account for 25% of nosocomial infections.[16] These figures do not reflect the increased morbidity and delay in return to normal activities of daily living for the patient or the strain imposed on the patient's family. This information supports the cost savings in preventing SSI through appropriate aseptic technique in conjunction with appropriate perioperative antibiotic prophylaxis.

STANDARDS OF PERIOPERATIVE ANTIBIOTIC PROPHYLAXIS

A consensus paper, "Quality Standard for Antimicrobial Prophylaxis in Surgical Procedures," addresses recommended standards to establish more uniform and reliable administration of prophylactic antibiotics during those procedures where their value has been demonstrated.[17] The standards are intended to provide a mechanism that will facilitate administration of antibiotics during procedures judged to be beneficial to the patient and to help facilities formulate policies for implementation of standards. The outcome should be a reduction in the rates of SSIs with a limit on the amount of antibiotic agents used where they are not likely to benefit the patient. Unnecessary antibiotic use favors the emergence of resistant organisms. All patients for whom prophylactic antibiotics are recommended should receive them. The agents given should be appropriate to the surgical procedure and should be given only for a 24-hour period or less.

Antibiotic Agent

In general, the agent chosen should be effective against the pathogens most often recovered from infections occurring after a specific procedure and the endogenous flora of the operative site. Cefazolin is recommended for operations on the distal ileum, appendix, or colon. The advanced generation agents have not been proved to be more effective than cefazolin, cefoxitin, or cefotetan. Regimens of ampicillin, amoxicillin, or vancomycin combined with gentamicin, known to be active against enterococci, are recommended for prophylaxis of endocarditis when a patient with certain cardiac lesions undergoes genitourinary or gastrointestinal tract operations. Vancomycin can be given instead of cefazolin to patients allergic to cephalosporin or in settings where MRSA is prevalent.[17]

Specific Factors

Timing. Laboratory studies have demonstrated that for an antibiotic to be effective in preventing SSI, it should be initiated 120 minutes before the incision is made. Pharmacokinetic data indicate the desirability of administration as close to the time of incision as possible (i.e., at the time of anesthesia induction). Postoperative administration is not recommended, nor is administering the first dose

T A B L E   4 – 2 .   PROCEDURAL GUIDELINES FOR THE ADMINISTRATION OF PARENTERAL ANTIBIOTIC PROPHYLAXIS

Parenteral Antibiotics Indicated
Procedures on the head and neck that involve the oropharynx
Abdominal and lower extremity vascular surgery
Craniotomy
Orthopedic hardware insertion
Cardiac surgery with median sternotomy
Hysterectomy
Primary cesarean section or prolonged rupture of membranes
Implantation of permanent prosthetic device

Parenteral Antibiotics Optional
Breast operations
Hernia operations
Clean procedures in high-risk settings (e.g., MRSA)
Low-risk gastric and biliary operations

after the incision. Cesarean section is a specific exception (Table 4–2). When indicated, additional intraoperative doses of an antibiotic should be given at intervals of one or two times during the half-life of the drug to maintain adequate blood levels throughout the procedure. Antibiotic prophylaxis in the absence of contamination or infection is not warranted beyond 24 hours postoperatively.[17]

Dose.   The prophylactic dose should never be smaller than the standard therapeutic dose. It is more reasonable to use a high dose (such as 1–2 grams of cefazolin, cefoxitin, or cefotetan for adults, 30–40 mg/kg for children).[17]

Procedures.   The standards developed and set forth in the consensus report[17] are procedure-specific and categorized to reflect the strength and quality of evidence supporting their use perioperatively. Table 4–2 summarizes the use of prophylactic antibiotics for specific procedures. The first category, *parenteral antibiotics indicated,* is supported by good evidence from at least one properly randomized, controlled, clinical trial. *Parenteral antibiotics optional* indicates that there is moderate to poor evidence; antibiotic use is recommended based on the opinions of respected authorities and their clinical experience. For minimally invasive procedures, there is poor evidence to support the use of antibiotic prophylaxis. However, pending further studies, it seems safest to apply the standards that would be used for the same procedure done via a traditional approach. There is moderate empirical evidence to support antibiotic prophylaxis during urologic procedures. It seems prudent to treat bacteriuria before performing any urinary tract procedures. For procedures involving newborns (<30 days old), there is moderate empirical evidence to support antibiotic prophylaxis as beneficial; however, it is common practice for pediatric surgeons to administer broad-spectrum antibiotics prophylactically.

Standards can be incorporated into routine procedures by either the anesthesia provider or the perioperative nurse (i.e., circulating nurse). It might be helpful to develop preprinted standing orders for antibiotic prophylaxis for all operations in which prophylaxis is deemed appropriate. These standing order forms should be developed by a joint committee of surgeons, anesthesia providers, and nurses, with participation of the institution's operating room, pharmacy and therapeutics, and infection control personnel. They should include recommendations about the usual drug choices (including a reminder about the need for anaerobic coverage in cases involving the colon).

The implementation and continued monitoring of a standard of perioperative antibiotic prophylaxis is an ideal quality improvement project that the RNFA can assume an active part in. Reviewing SSI rates in conjunction with the use of antibiotic prophylaxis with infection control and quality improvement committees can provide the RNFA with another means of evaluating outcomes and improving care through collaborative practice.

POSTOPERATIVE INDICATORS OF SSI

The incubation period for SSI is 3 to 8 days postoperatively. In patients who are not immunocompromised, infection usually presents with the cardinal signs of inflammation: redness, heat, pain, and swelling. The clinical sign of fever, which is 38 °C (100.4 °F) or higher, occurs after the normal postoperative temperature elevation has resolved. The white blood cell count is usually elevated, and the presence of an infection is confirmed by cultures of the surgical site.[18] Gram stain for preliminary identification of the organism assists with identification and appropriate treatment based on the offending organism. Culture with sensitivities will guide the choice of treatment. Chest x-ray, aspiration of potentially infected fluid, or ultrasonography or computed tomography (CT) of the operative site may be required to make a definitive diagnosis and determine the most appropriate treatment.

Determining the existence of SSI and appropriate treatment in immunocompromised, elderly, major trauma, chronic premorbid disease, and endorgan failure patients is often not as straightforward; consultation with an infection disease specialist may be required. Empirical antibiotic therapy may be indicated before microbiological confirmation of SSI.

TREATMENT OF SSI

Due to the vast array of antibiotic treatments available, the RNFA will need to be familiar with the various chemotherapeutics available and the risk involved with each treatment to best educate patients during the treatment of

SSI. Adequate and appropriate patient teaching must be tailored to the patient and emphasize the need for the patient to continue the prescribed antibiotic for the duration of therapy to resolve the infection and avert the possible development of antibiotic-resistant infection.

The RNFA must keep in mind that antibiotic therapy cannot replace wound drainage when an abscess or hematoma is present. Nor can antibiotics replace surgical debridement of devitalized or necrotic tissue, especially in the presence of anaerobic bacteria. Surgical wounds needing debridement may have to be sequentially debrided before it can be determined what viable tissue remains. This is especially challenging to the RNFA and distressing for the patient. The need for further surgery may be accompanied by anxieties and fears during the subsequent procedures. This patient population needs a great deal of support from the RNFA during the recovery period.

Antibiotics usually fail when a prosthetic implant has become infected early in the postoperative phase. Postoperative irrigation of infected wounds with antibiotic solution has not been shown to be more beneficial than simple mechanical debridement. In fact, continuous antibiotic irrigation has been shown to allow resistant organisms to enter the wound and proliferate. The routine use of pulsatile lavage is contraindicated; irrigation under pressure may actually predispose to systemic infection through dissemination of infectious agents into the peripheral circulation.

The antibiotic chosen to treat SSI must be able to penetrate the area involved. The physician determines the antibiotic of choice based on the area of involvement and confirmed by microbiological assay. The goal is to provide the least toxic, most cost-effective narrow-spectrum coverage to prevent damage to the patient's protective flora. These kinds of complex decisions warrant consultation with an infectious disease specialist.

■ IMPLICATIONS FOR THE RNFA

A complete understanding of the pathogenicity of infectious diseases is the foundation for the nursing diagnosis of *High Risk for Infection related to surgical intervention*. Once the skin is violated, the patient is exposed to potential infectious agents from endogenous and exogenous sources. To achieve the outcome standard—a patient free from signs and symptoms of infection—the RNFA actions focus on aseptic technique and methods known to reduce the risk of contamination during the operation.[19] Measuring variances in any given patient population is a means of outcomes management that can enhance patient care by identifying those variances that are unavoidable (e.g., premorbid disease) and those variances that may contribute to SSI (e.g., use of disposable versus reusable instrumentation). Collaboration with infection control practitioners in tracking SSI can greatly enhance improved practice through outcomes management.

Transmission Risk of Bloodborne and Microbiological Infections

The RNFA is at greatest risk during surgery to exposure from blood and body fluids. Of primary concern to the RNFA is the exposure to bloodborne pathogens such as hepatitis B virus (HBV) and hepatitis C virus (HCV). The risk of acquiring HBV from a puncture with a hollow-bore needle in RNFAs not vaccinated against HBV is 30%, in striking contrast to the 0.3% risk of acquiring HIV. Between 6% and 30% of nonimmunized health care providers exposed to HBV through a needle stick, who do not receive postexposure prophylaxis, develop HBV infection.[20]

There are primarily three types of exposure that may occur: from RNFA to patient, from patient to patient, and from patient to RNFA (occupational exposure). These types of exposure apply to both bloodborne and microbial pathogens, but bloodborne pathogens pose the greatest risk to the RNFA. The greater risk to the patient is the acquisition of bacterial infections from the RNFA, equipment, or instrumentation. Such attendant-borne transmission is of special concern with MARO (e.g., MRSA, VRE). The most frequent attendant carrier of bacterial infections is the health care provider's hands. Hand washing remains the bulwark of transmission prevention. The hands should be washed between contacts with patients and after glove removal, each and every time. The majority of endemic outbreaks of MARO have been directly correlated with lax hand washing among health care providers. The risk of acquiring MARO infection by the RNFA is slight. Bioburden on instrumentation is perhaps the greatest source of concern to the RNFA, and applying sound aseptic technique and sterilization methods will eliminate the risk of transmission to patients.

Airborne Pathogens. *Mycobacterium tuberculosis* (TB) has resurged as a significant public health problem in North America.[21] Those at highest risk for TB are the homeless, those infected with HIV, intravenous drug users, and immigrants from areas with endogenously high rates of TB (e.g., Asia). TB is airborne, with particles of 0.05 micron in size, remains suspended in the room air on dust particles, and is therefore highly contagious in confined areas with poor ventilation. Persons infected with TB easily dispel the TB particles into the air during coughing, sneezing, or talking. This has been further complicated by the emergence of multiple-drug-resistant tuberculous strains. Ventilator control and mask barriers (airborne isolation) provide the most effective means of reducing the risk of TB transmission. However, the role of disinfection cannot be ignored in nosocomial transmission. In 1997, two cases of transmission of TB via a contaminated bronchoscope were documented.[22] The Association for Professionals in Infection Control and Epidemiology (APIC) recommends precleaning followed by immersion in a 2% glutaraldehyde solution at 20 °C for at least 20 minutes.[23] A particulate respirator is to be worn by health care providers who come in contact with patients infected with TB. The patient needs to be in an isolation room with negative-pressure air flow and 15 air exchanges per minute. The negative pressure prevents air exhaled by the patient from passing into public areas. During transport, the patient wears a high-efficiency particulate mask (i.e., filter particles up to 0.5 micron in size). Patients with TB are to be considered infectious until they have been on chemotherapy long enough to have two acid-fast bacillus-negative cultures on three consecutive days.

Hepatitis A to G.   Viral hepatitis has evolved over the past 20 years from infectious hepatitis (hepatitis A virus) and serum hepatitis (hepatitis B virus) into six strains of viral hepatitis. Hepatitis refers to the acute inflammatory disease of the liver caused by the virus. The degree of inflammation and necrosis depends on the individual's direct or immune response to the virus. There are four strains of hepatitis virus of primary concern to the RNFA because they are bloodborne viral pathogens: HBV, HCV, HDV, and HGV. Hepatitis A virus and hepatitis E virus are enteric viruses spread by fecal–oral routes (i.e., via feces), saliva, contaminated water, and household and sexual contacts) (Table 4–3). HBV vaccination is strongly recommended for RNFAs, and standard precautions continue to be the most effective way to prevent occupational acquisition of bloodborne hepatitis viruses. These precautions include appropriate hand washing, the use of barrier methods to prevent contact with blood and body fluids, and techniques and devices to reduce the risk of percutaneous injury. (See Chapter 10 for a discussion of blunt needles and other strategies for use by RNFAs during suturing.) No vaccines against HCV are currently available, nor are there recommendations for postexposure prophylaxis.[24] The CDC's postexposure recommendations for HBV depend on the HBsAg status of the source of the exposure as well as the immunization status of the person exposed.

Herpesvirus.   The herpes simplex viruses (HSVs) became of concern to perioperative personnel during the same decade as HIV. HSVs cause a relapsing mucocutaneous viral infection. A thorough perioperative assessment can detect patients infected with HSV. HSV is divided into two types. Type I has a propensity for causing infection on the face and lips; type II generally causes genital infection. Crossover between sites can occur. While acyclovir can control clinical symptoms and suppress relapses, there is no cure for HSV. Although nosocomial transmission of HSV is rare, RNFAs can contract HSV infection on the hands in the form of herpetic whitlow if they have direct contact with a patient's oral, vaginal, or cutaneous lesions or virus-containing secretions. With the use of standard precautions and an intact glove barrier, the risk of occupational acquisition approaches zero.

Acquired Immunodeficiency Syndrome.   Perhaps the viral bloodborne pathogen of greatest concern to perioperative personnel is HIV, the

T A B L E 4 – 3 . VIRAL HEPATITIS A–G

	Hepatitis A Virus (HAV)	Hepatitis B Virus (HBV)
Etiologic agent	Single-stranded ribonucleic acid (RNA) virus; virus of the entero-virus group (replicates in liver)	Double-stranded deoxyribonucleicacid hepadnavirus
Transmission	Fecal-oral route; spread by feces, saliva, contaminated water, household and sexual contacts; parenterally (rare)	Percutaneous/permucosal exposure to blood; sexual contact; HBV can survive on surfaces for 1 wk and lead to unknown exposures
Infectious period	Highest concentration of virus in stool during 2 wk before onset of symptoms; ends 1 wk after symptoms subside	From before symptoms occur; may be lifelong if individual becomes chronic carrier
Prevention	Vaccine recommended for children and those traveling to areas where HAV is endemic	Vaccine. Standard precautions; control of blood, blood products, skin-piercing instruments; good personal hygiene
Postexposure treatment	Postexposure immune globulin within 2 wk of exposure	Vaccine and HBV immune globulin therapy for postexposure; interferon alpha-2b for chronic state
Risk factors	Close personal contact; handling feces and contaminated articles; eating raw shellfish; working with animals imported from endemic areas. At risk are health care providers, patients with multiple blood transfusions and dialysis, homosexually active males, morticians, intravenous drug users	Health care providers, patients with multiple blood transfusions and dialy-sis, homosexually active males, morti-cians, intravenous drug users
Course of disease	Acute, self-limiting; rarely fulminant; chronic form not known	HBV may be acute with insidious onset; may become chronic; may progress to cirrhosis or end-stage liver disease

	Hepatitis C Virus (HCV)	Hepatitis D Virus (HDV)
Etiologic agent	Single-stranded RNA virus; little specific information available	Defective, incomplete single-stranded RNA virus that is dependent on HBV for replication
Transmission	Parenteral/percutaneous/permu-cosal exposure to blood and blood products; sexual, personal contact suspected; possible fecal–oral route	Appears as a coinfection or superinfec-tion with HBV; transmitted same as HBV
Infectious period	Before onset of symptoms; may persist for lifetime if individual becomes a carrier	Not known
Prevention	No vaccine. Standard precautions; control of blood, blood products, skin-piercing instruments; good personal hygiene	Same as HBV

(continued)

T A B L E   4 – 3 .   VIRAL HEPATITIS A–G (continued)

	Hepatitis C Virus (HCV)	Hepatitis D Virus (HDV)
Postexposure treatment	Standard immunoglobulin for postexposure; interferon alpha-2b for chronic HCV	Same as HBV (interferon alpha-2b trials are underway)
Risk Factors	Same as HBV	Same as HBV
Course of disease	Insidious onset; 40%–60% become chronic carriers; 20% of acute HCV cases may progress to cirrhosis	Acute onset; may resolve without sequelae; may lead to serious fulminant hepatitis; more likely leads to chronic HDV and liver failure

	Hepatitis E Virus (HEV)	Hepatitis G Virus (HGV)
Etiologic agent	Undeveloped, single-stranded RNA virus	Hepatitis G virus, although causal association remains to be confirmed
Transmission	Fecal–oral route; spread via feces and contaminated water	Bloodborne; transfusion recipients, intravenous drug users; frequent coinfection with HCV; ?other
Infectious period	Not known	Not known
Prevention	No vaccine. Standard precautions	No vaccine. Standard precautions. Confirmation of disease association, determination of routes of transmission, and development of serologic screening assays are necessary before prevention measures can be considered
Postexposure treatment	No postexposure prophylaxis available	No vaccine. Pending further knowledge of HGV
Risk factors	Often seen after natural disaster in developing countries	Transfusion recipients, intravenous drug users; ?other
Course of disease	Acute process; 99% of patients recover uneventfully	0.3% of acute viral hepatitis; estimated 900–2,000 infections/yr, most may be asymptomatic; chronic infection develops in 90%–100% of infected persons; chronic disease state may be rare or not occur

(Source: Adapted from Lisanti P, Talotta D: An overview of viral hepatitis. AORN J 59(5):1000–1001, 1994.)

causative agent of acquired immunodeficiency syndrome (AIDS). HIV is an RNA retrovirus that destroys the CD4+ and T-helper lymphocytes of the immune system, resulting in progressive impairment of the immune response that leaves the person defenseless against numerous opportunistic infections. The most common of these opportunistic infections are Kaposi's sarcoma and *Pneumocystis carinii* pneumonia. HIV, like HBV, HCV, and HDV, is a bloodborne pathogen transmitted by parenteral (blood-to-blood) contact, sexual contact, and perinatally (mother to baby) contact. Like the hepatitis viruses, HIV has been isolated in many body fluids known to pose an occupational risk to health care providers. The risk of transmission of HIV during a percutaneous exposure (e.g., needle stick with a hollow-bore needle) is about 0.3%, significantly less than that of HBV or HVC.

There is concern that exposure to patients infected with HIV, their body fluids, and organs during surgery might transmit HIV through a suture needle or scalpel injury. Current studies estimating positive exposure from a needle stick are based on hollow-bore needles (hypodermic needles) and not on the volume of blood or body fluid transmitted during percutaneous injury with a suture needle. Although the transmission risk has been compared to that of HBV, there is a significant difference in actual risk. A drop of blood or saliva of a patient infected with HBV contains a large number of viral particles per milliliter of blood. Although HBV can be contracted from a needle stick, this is less likely with HIV. A small volume of blood from a person infected with HIV does not contain enough viral particles to be considered infectious. It would appear that to contract HIV, one would need either a large inoculum exposure (e.g., blood transfusion or 0.001 milliliters of blood) or repeated sexual contact. The acquisition of HIV is perhaps even more complex than what may occur during an occupational exposure to contaminated blood or body fluids.

Laboratory studies indicate that HIV has a difficult time entering the CD4+ lymphocyte unless the lymphocyte is activated by recurrent antigenic stimulation. This is proposed to be a reason why the major risk groups for HIV infection continue to be homosexual and bisexual men, intravenous drug users, sexual partners of intravenous drug users, and newborns of infected mothers. Clinical evidence supports antiretroviral therapy with zidovudine (AZT) during pregnancy to prevent HIV infection in newborns of HIV-infected mothers.[24] In prospective studies of persons sustaining percutaneous exposures to HIV-infected blood (hollow-bore-needle sticks), the incidence of seroconversion appears to be less than 0.5%.[25]

Based on retrospective and prospective studies, HBV and HCV continue to be the greatest risk to RNFAs and their perioperative colleagues. The CDC emphasizes standard precautions as the most effective means of preventing occupational exposure to bloodborne pathogens. CDC recommendations for postexposure prophylaxis are based on a two-drug regimen, AZT and 3TC, given for four weeks, and a protease inhibitor when exposure is very risky (both a deep injury with a hollow-bore needle that had been in an artery or vein and a patient with end-stage AIDS, for example), and treatment is started as soon as possible (within hours).[25]

Creutzfeldt-Jakob Disease.   Creutzfeldt-Jakob disease (CJD) is a fatal neurodegenerative disorder. The actual route of transmission is unknown. The CJD organism is difficult to eradicate and is therefore of special concern to the RNFA. CJD is a spongiform viral encephalopathy and is closely linked to bovine spongiform encephalopathy ("mad cow disease"). The CJD virus is a "slow virus" that causes insidious and rapid progression to neurological degeneration and death. It usually does not manifest until the person is in the late fifties or early sixties, with an incubation period of 1 to 4 decades. Both sexes are affected equally. Genetic predisposition is seen as an autosomal dominate gene. Libyan Jewish immigrants to Israel and Tunisian and Algerian immigrants to France have a higher incidence. CJD has also been reported in inbred Czechoslovakians and in certain areas of Chile.[26]

Nosocomial infection has been documented in a patient who received a human dura mater graft, and clusters of infections have been noted in Great Britain, attributed to iatrogenic inoculation during dental surgery, corneal grafting, and stereotaxic EEG depth electrodes previously used on a patient with CJD. The viral particles of spongiform encephalopathies are viable under a variety of physical and chemical conditions. The CJD virus is resistant to heat, formalin, freezing, autolysis, drying, ionizing radiation, ultraviolet light, and some organic solvents. Tissues and fluids of infectious patients are known to transmit CJD, with the highest infectious titers in the central nervous system tissues, including the CSF and optic tissues; transmission has also been attributed to contaminated human growth hormone. The highest risk for acquiring CJD is through direct inoculation with the infectious agent. Standard precautions are but one means of preventing transmission. Table 4–4 summarizes recommendations for handling instrumentation and equipment used for CJD patients by the Committee on Health Care Issues of the American Neurologic Association. Because biopsy is the only means of accurate diagnosis, with subsequent culture growth of the CJD organism, these recommendations should be carefully considered when performing surgical interventions on patients suspected to be infected with CJD.

T A B L E 4 – 4. MANAGEMENT OF INSTRUMENTS AND EQUIPMENT IN CREUTZFELDT-JAKOB DISEASE

1. Use as many disposable items as possible.
2. Implement standard precautions when coming in contact with blood, body fluids, and CNS tissue.
3. Wash hands thoroughly with soap and water or detergent after contact with patient when contact does not involve handling blood, percutaneous fluid, or body tissues.
4. Irrigate percutaneous exposure to blood, CSF, and tissue immediately with 0.5% sodium hypochlorite (household bleach).
5. Label all specimens sent as biohazard.
6. Sterilize all potentially contaminated materials in a gravity displacement autoclave at 132 °C for a least 1h before discarding, handling, or reprocessing. Preferred to autoclave contaminated materials in a prevacuum autoclave at 134–138 °C for 18 min.
7. Immerse all reusable equipment having contact with the patient in 1 N sodium hydroxide for 1 h at room temperature. Alternative method is to use 5% sodium hypochlorite (full-strength household bleach) for 2 h. Full-strength bleach will damage instruments. The extended time ensures deactivation of CJD agent.
8. Autoclave all instruments before they are handled for reprocessing.
9. Disinfect all OR surfaces with 5% sodium hypochlorite.
10. Bag and label all linens and disposables as biohazard.

(Source: Adapted from Bailes BK: Creutzfeldt-Jakob disease. AORN J 52(5):982, 1990.)

▰ STANDARD PRECAUTIONS

Standard precautions synthesize the major features of universal precautions and body substance isolation precautions, recognizing the potential of all body fluids, secretions, and excretions to transmit pathogens. The revised guidelines also address specific clinical syndromes that are highly suspicious for infection and identify appropriate transmission-based precautions to use on an empirical, temporary basis until a definitive diagnosis can be made. Transmission-based and empiric precautions are to be used in addition to Standard Precautions. The new recommendations have two tiers. *Standard precautions* are implemented for all patients regardless of diagnosis or infection status. *Transmission-based precautions* are implemented for patients known or suspected to be infected or colonized with "epidemiologically important" pathogens transmitted by the airborne, droplet, or contact routes.[27]

Standard precautions (Table 4–5) apply to all patients regardless of diagnosis or presumed infection and are to be used for anticipated contact with blood, all body fluids, secretions, excretions (regardless of whether they con-

T A B L E 4 – 5 . STANDARD PRECAUTIONS

Standard Precautions incorporate universal blood and body fluid precautions and body substance isolation measures.

- **Apply to all patients** regardless of diagnosis.
- To be used for:
  - **Blood**
  - **All body fluids,** secretions, excretions; regardless of whether there is visible blood.
  - **Nonintact skin**
  - **Mucous membranes**

1. **Wash hands** before and after contact with potentially infectious material (blood, body fluids, secretions, excretions, and contaminated items) *even if you are wearing gloves.*
2. **Wear gloves** any time there is likely chance of exposure to potentially infectious materials.
3. **Use personal protective equipment.** Wear fluid-repellent gowns, protective eyewear, and masks when there are likely to be splashes or sprays of potentially infectious material.
4. **Avoid recapping needles.** Use a neutral zone for placing sharps. No two people should touch the same sharp at the same time.
5. **Clean blood spills.** Use gloves and personal protective equipment. Confine spill and clean with a hospital-grade disinfectant.
6. **Patient placement.** Place patients who may contaminate the environment in private/isolation rooms.
7. **Handle used, contaminated patient care equipment/articles carefully.** Limit traffic in the OR to essential personnel.

TABLE 4-6. TRANSMISSION-BASED PRECAUTIONS (BODY SUBSTANCE ISOLATION)

Transmission-based precautions: For known or suspected infection/colonization with epidemiologically important pathogens transmitted by the airborne, droplet, or contact routes.

Airborne precautions apply to those infections spread through the air, such as TB, varicella, disseminated zoster and rubeola. Negative-pressure isolation room. Wear respiratory protection (high-efficiency particulate air [HEPA] filter respirator or N95 respirator when in close contact with patient [in isolation room or OR]. Patient wears HEPA mask for transport. Note that surgical masks filter *expired* air. Respirators filter *inspired* air.

Droplet precautions apply to those infections spread by large particle droplets containing the infectious agent. Infections include rubella, diphtheria, mumps, pertussis, influenza, and adenovirus. Private rooms and negative pressure are not required. These epidemiologically important pathogens can infect via the conjunctivae, nares, mucosa, or mouth. Wear a surgical mask when coming within 3 ft of the patient.

Contact precautions apply to pathogens spread by direct contact (skin to skin) and indirect contact (touch) with a contaminated object (e.g., instruments, needle, dressing, or bed). Wear gloves and isolation gown when entering the infected patient's environment. Conditions requiring contact precautions include (1) gastrointestinal, respiratory, skin, or wound infections colonized with MARO; (2) *Clostridium difficile*, respiratory syncytial virus, hepatitis A in incontinent patients; (3) highly contagious skin diseases such as impetigo, scabies, pediculosis, varicella, and zoster (disseminated in any patient and localized in immunocompromised patients).

When transferring a patient with virulent pathogens:

- The patient wears appropriate barriers (e.g., mask) and knows how to help prevent the spread of pathogens.
- The transporter has implemented necessary precautions (e.g., uses personal protective equipment).
- The staff in the receiving unit have been notified and understand the necessary precautions.

Keep in mind that under the new guidelines, some pathogens and conditions fall into two categories because the organisms are transmitted in more than one way. For example, varicella and zoster can spread through both airborne and contact routes.

---

tain visible blood), nonintact skin, and mucous membranes. Transmission-based precautions (Table 4–6) are additional precautions for patients with known or suspected infection with highly transmissible pathogens. These precautions address the three routes of known transmission—airborne, droplet, and contact transmission. Empiric precautions (Table 4–7) are transmission-based precautions to be used in undiagnosed patients with certain clinical syndromes and conditions.

Contact transmission is the most frequent route of transmission of nosocomial infections and can be divided into two categories: direct contact and indirect contact. Direct-contact transmission involves actual surface contact

TABLE 4–7. EMPIRIC ISOLATION PRECAUTIONS

Clinical Syndrome/Condition	Potential Pathogens	Empiric Precautions
Diarrhea, acute, with likely	Enteric pathogens	Contact
infectious cause	*Clostridium difficile*	Contact
Meningitis	*Neisseria meningitidis*	Droplet
Rash or exanthems, generalized, etiology unknown		
Petechiae/ecchymosis with fever	*Neisseria meningitidis*	Droplet
Vesicular rash	Varicella virus	Airborne and contact
Maculopapular with coryza and fever	Rubeola virus	Airborne
Respiratory infections		
Cough/fever/upper lobe infiltrate in HIV-negative patient at low risk for HIV infection	*Mycobacterium tuberculosis*	Airborne
Cough/fever/pulmonary infiltrate in any lung location in HIV-infected patient at high risk for HIV infection	*Mycobacterium tuberculosis*	Airborne
Paroxysmal/severe persistent cough during periods of pertussis activity	*Bordetella pertussis*	Droplet
Bronchiolitis and croup in infants and young children	*Respiratory syncytial or parainfluenza virus*	Contact
Risk of MARO		
History of infection/colonization with MARO	Resistant bacteria	Contact
Skin, wound, or urinary tract infection in those with recent hospital or nursing home stay	Resistant bacteria	Contact
Skin or wound infection		
Abscess or draining wound that cannnot be covered	*S. aureus,* Group A streptococcus	Contact

(Adapted from Centers for Disease Control and Prevention. "Recommendations for isolation precautions in hospitals," 1997, Atlanta, GA)

with the infected patient to transfer pathogens, such as occurs during direct patient care activities. Indirect contact involves contact with a contaminated intermediate object, such as instruments, contaminated hands, and dressings.

Droplet transmission occurs when droplets are generated by the patient, primarily during coughing, sneezing, talking, suctioning, and bronchoscopy. Transmission occurs when the droplet is propelled a short distance and is deposited on the conjunctiva, nasal mucosa, or mouth. Droplets do not remain suspended in the air, so special air handling is not required. These droplets are larger than 5 microns in size.[27]

Airborne transmission occurs when droplet nuclei of 5 microns or smaller remain suspended in the air for long periods of time. Because of the small size of these droplets, they can remain suspended on dust particles. These pathogens can be carried widely by air currents and require special air handling ventilation (negative-pressure rooms). *Mycobacterium tuberculosis*, rubeola, and varicella viruses are considered airborne pathogens.

Under the new guidelines, some infections and conditions fall into two categories because the pathogens can be transmitted in more than one way. For example, varicella (chickenpox) and zoster can spread through both the airborne and contact routes. A complete understanding of transmission-based precautions, implemented in conjunction with standard precautions, can avert the potential for cross-contamination infection in both surgical patients and RNFAs.

■ SUMMARY

The RNFA plays a significant role in preventing postoperative SSIs by focusing on sound infection control practices and surgical asepsis as the most appropriate means of infection prevention. Antibiotics should never replace infection control practices. Familiarity with standards and recommended practices, with current text and journal readings, and with guidelines promulgated by external agencies is essential to the safe care of the surgical patient. The expected patient outcome, freedom from infection, is only as tenable as the knowledge base and competent practice of the RNFA and other surgical team members.

■ Review Questions

1. The term incisional *surgical site infection* (SSI) refers to infection involving
   a. Only the incision.
   b. The incision and subcutaneous tissue.
   c. The incision and fascia.
   d. The skin and subcutaneous tissue.

2. The most common organisms isolated from SSIs are
   a. *S. aureus* and *Klebsiella*.
   b. *S. aureus, Staphylococcus,* and *Enterococcus*.
   c. *S. aureus, Staphylococcus, Enterococcus,* and *Pseudomonas*.
   d. *Staphylococcus* and *Pseudomonas*.

3. Skin provides the first line of defense. Opening the skin, either surgically or traumatically, potentiates
   a. Immunoincompetency.
   b. Infection.

   c. The need for antibiotic therapy.

   d. A slower rate of wound healing.

4. Methicillin-resistant *S. aureus* is a strain of *S. aureus* resistant to
   a. Methicillin and oxacillin.
   b. Methicillin, oxacillin, and nafcillin.
   c. Methicillin, oxacillin, nafcillin, and vancomycin.
   d. Methicillin, oxacillin, nafcillin, and cephalosporins.

5. Multiple-antibiotic-resistant organisms (MAROs) are most often transmitted by
   a. The hands of health care providers.
   b. Food handlers.
   c. Personal hygiene items belonging to the patient.
   d. Eating utensils.

6. Surgical wound class, ASA classification, duration of surgery, and results of intraoperative cultures are all highly predictive of
   a. Subsequent pneumonia in cancer patients.
   b. Subsequent deep venous thrombosis.
   c. Subsequent SSI.
   d. Subsequent return to activities of daily living.

7. When enteric bacilli are the causative agent in SSI, it is more often a result of
   a. Endogenous flora.
   b. Airborne exogenous microorganisms.
   c. Exogenous factors such as a compromised immune system.
   d. Endogenous factors such as poor environmental sanitation.

8. A pathogenic microorganism that relies on toxin production is
   a. *Staphylococcus.*
   b. *Streptococcus.*
   c. *Corynebacterium diptheriae.*
   d. *Rickettsia.*

9. An acceptable SSI rate for clean, elective procedures is
   a. 5%.
   b. 3%.
   c. 10%.
   d. 2%.

10. The RNFA can have a direct effect on the stress response by
    a. Administering prophylactic antibiotics 60 minutes before incision.
    b. Providing preoperative teaching and comfort measures to decrease anxiety.
    c. Conducting a postoperative assessment in the PACU.
    d. Discussing the prognosis of other patients undergoing the same procedure.

11. Prophylactic antibiotics are usually not indicated in
    a. Clean procedures.
    b. Clean-contaminated procedures.
    c. Contaminated procedures.
    d. Procedures involving the nasopharynx.

12. For prophylactic antibiotics to have optimum effect, they should be initiated
    a. 60 minutes before the incision.
    b. At the same time as the incision.
    c. 120 minutes before the incision.
    d. 160 minutes before the incision.

13. Unless the patient has an allergy to it, the antibiotic of choice for systemic prophylaxis is
    a. Ampicillin.
    b. Gentamicin.
    c. Cefazolin.
    d. Vancomycin.

14. The most frequent route of transmission of hepatitis B virus is
    a. Fecal–oral.
    b. Body fluids.
    c. Percutaneous.
    d. Perinatal.

15. The hepatitis virus most often implicated in posttransfusion hepatitis is
    a. Hepatitis A.
    b. Hepatitis B.
    c. Hepatitis G.
    d. Hepatitis C.

16. An important transmission precaution for herpes viruses is
    a. Anti-HDV immunization.
    b. Wearing gloves.
    c. Immune globulin.
    d. Acyclovir.

17. Following exposure to hepatitis B virus, the RNFA should receive
    a. Immune serum globulin.
    b. Hepatitis A vaccination.
    c. Acyclovir.
    d. AZT.

18. Standard precautions apply to
    a. Blood only.
    b. Only body fluids with visible blood.
    c. Blood and excretions.
    d. All body fluids, secretions, and excretions.

19. Airborne precautions require the use of
    a. A negative-pressure room.
    b. A negative-pressure room and surgical mask.
    c. A negative-pressure room and an HEPA filter respirator.
    d. Gloves and gown for contact with the patient.
20. Contact precautions apply to epidemiologically important pathogens transmitted by
    a. Droplets.
    b. Direct and indirect contact.
    c. Excretions only.
    d. Secretions only.

Answer Key

1. a	6. c	11. a	16. b
2. c	7. a	12. c	17. a
3. b	8. c	13. c	18. d
4. d	9. b	14. c	19. c
5. a	10. b	15. d	20. b

REFERENCES

1. Nightingale F: Notes on Nursing: What It Is, and What It Is Not. London, Harrison, 1859
2. Donahue MP: Nursing, the Finest Art. St Louis, CV Mosby, 1985, pp 360–364
3. Groah LK: Perioperative Nursing, 3rd ed. Stamford, Conn, Appleton & Lange, 1996, pp 121–136
4. Infection experts ready protocols as superbug looms. OR Manager 13(8):1, 1997
5. Capriotti T: Emerging antibiotic resistance among community-acquired and nosocomial bacterial pathogens. Medsurg Nurs 6:296–298, 1997
6. Mathias JM: OR has role in controlling "superbugs." OR Manager 11(5):25–26, 1995
7. Schwartz B, Bell DM, Hughes JM: Preventing the emergence of antimicrobial resistance. JAMA 278(11):944–945, 1997
8. Stephenson J: Worry grows as antibiotic-resistant bacteria continue to gain ground. JAMA 278(23):2049–2050, 1997
9. Ronk LL: Surgical patients with multiantibiotic-resistant bacteria. AORN J 61:1023–1033, 1995
10. Staph with lower vancomycin resistance in US. OR Manager 13(10):7, 1997
11. VRE is everywhere. OR Manager 13(8):32, 1997
12. Nichols RL: Surgical wound infection. Am J Med 91(suppl 3B): 3B-54S, 1991
13. Mathias JM: Clinical pathway leads to infection control changes. OR Manager 13(8):23, 1997
14. Morse JM: Responding to threats to integrity of self. Adv Nurs Sci 19(4):21–36, 1997
15. Reporting of infection rates stirring debate. OR Manager 13(7):24–25, 1997

16. Wheelock SM, Lookinland S: Effect of surgical hand scrub time on subsequent bacterial growth. AORN J 65:1087–1098, 1997
17. Dellinger PE, Gross PA, Barret TL, Krause PJ, Martone WJ, McGowan JE, Sweet RL, Wenzel, RP: Quality standard for antimicrobial prophylaxis in surgical procedures (consensus paper). Infect Control Hosp Epidemiol 180–188, 1994
18. Litwack K: Practical points in the evaluation of postoperative fever. J Perianesth Nurs 12(4):100–104, 1997
19. Association of Operating Room Nurses: Patient outcomes: Standards of perioperative care. In: Standards, Guidelines and Recommended Practices. Denver, Colo, AORN Publications, 1998, pp 141–152
20. CDC Draft guideline for infection control in health care personnel. Fed Reg 62(173):47276–47314, 1997
21. Agerton T, Valaway S, Gore B, Pozsik C, Plikaytis B, Woodley C, Onorato I: Transmission of a highly drug-resistant strain (strain W1) of *Mycobacterium tuberculosis*. JAMA 278:1073–1077, 1997
22. Mathias JM: New APIC guideline on disinfection, sterilization. OR Manager 13(1):9, 1997
23. Recommendations for follow-up of health care workers after occupational exposure to hepatitis C virus. JAMA 278:1056–1057, 1997
24. Ungvarski PJ: Update on HIV infection. Am J Nurs 97:44–52, 1997
25. HCV greatest bloodborne threat, expert says. OR Manager 13(6):26, 1997
26. Bailes BK:Creutzfeldt-Jakob disease. AORN J 52(5):976–985, 1990
27. Garner JS: Guidelines for isolation precautions in hospitals. Infect Control Hosp Epidemiol 17:53–80,1996

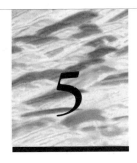

THE DIAGNOSTIC PROCESS

JANE C. ROTHROCK

■

The diagnostic process involves recognizing, identifying, localizing, and evaluating information provided by and about the patient. The history and physical examination begin the diagnostic process; they are the foci around which diagnosis and subsequent treatment revolve. The RN first assistant most often will target the history on a specific patient complaint. The patient complaint guides the physical examination; it is the symptom(s) or concern(s) that have induced the patient to seek care or advice. The history of the present illness expands on the chief complaint, providing a full chronological description of how the symptom developed, what is related to it, how the patient feels about it, and how it has affected the patient's life and functional ability. The data obtained from the history and physical examination are grouped and analyzed. The RNFA confirms or validates a tentative diagnosis regarding the body structures and processes most likely involved and collaborates in reviewing the results of the diagnostic tests and studies that follow.

The RN first assistant's commitment to focusing on the individual patient as a whole requires that assessment cover physical parameters, self-care behaviors, health promotion, spiritual development and beliefs, culture and values, family and social roles, and developmental tasks. Holistic health, part of the rich history of the nursing profession, focuses both on curing (alleviating physical signs and symptoms) and healing (integration of the mind, body, and spirit).[1,2] Both subjective data—what the patient says during the history—and objective data—what the RNFA observes by inspecting, palpating, percussing, and auscultating during the physical examination—form the initial patient database.

EVALUATION FOR NONEMERGENCY SURGERY

Preoperative assessment of the patient scheduled for nonemergency surgery begins with the history and physical examination. Both of these assessments focus on the patient's presenting complaint while at the same time screening for risk factors and any related patient problems. It has been suggested that, diagnostically, the history is three times more productive than the physical examination and 11 times more effective than routine laboratory tests; when the history is combined with the physical examination, it is diagnostic in 75% to 90% of patients.[3] Once the history and physical examination are completed, a tentative diagnosis is established and appropriate screening and diagnostic tests are performed to confirm the diagnosis. Any concomitant risk factors or conditions are stabilized or corrected; this will determine whether surgery is delayed or whether the patient's operative risk is acceptable.

OBTAINING THE HISTORY

Obtaining the patient's history may be the initiation of the relationship between the RN first assistant and the patient. Each patient is a unique individual, and the purpose of the history is to learn about the patient as the nurse–patient relationship is established. The organization of the data derived from the patient's history may reflect both a nursing model and a medical model. The RNFA relies on a medical model when working collaboratively with a surgeon in the diagnosis and treatment of disease; a nursing model is used with the medical model to focus assessment on core nursing problems. A nursing model commonly includes the clinical use of nursing diagnoses. Nursing diagnoses were introduced to aid the profession in developing a standard language that would assist in describing nursing phenomena and contribute to nursing knowledge by identifying areas for clinical research.[4] A common foundation of knowledge about the patient facilitates collaboration between the RNFA, the patient, the surgeon, and the rest of the health care team.

A health history has several components, each with a specific purpose. The history's components are fairly widely accepted: chief complaint, present illness/problem, past medical history, current health status, family history, social/experiential history, and systems review. This chronological and detailed structure elicits information about a wide range of variables that may affect the patient's health status. Chart 5–1 presents these components for an adult patient.

Before conducting a patient history, the RN first assistant should quickly review the patient's medical record. This review yields a snapshot of the patient, providing demographic and other information. By knowing the patient's name and some background information, the RNFA is able to set a tone of courtesy, interest, and helpfulness. The environment for the interview should

(text continues on page 111)

CHART 5–1
Comprehensive History: Adult Patient

DATE OF HISTORY _____

Identifying Data, including age, sex, race, place of birth, marital status, occupation, and religion.

SOURCE OF REFERRAL, if any, and the purpose of it.

SOURCE OF HISTORY, such as the patient, a relative, a friend, the patient's medical record, or a referral letter.

RELIABILITY, if relevant. For example, "The patient is consistently clear about her symptoms but vague about when they began."

CHIEF COMPLAINTS, when possible in the patient's own words. "My stomach hurts and I feel awful." Sometimes patients have no overt complaints; ascertain their goals instead. "I have come for my regular checkup" or "I've been admitted for a thorough evaluation of my heart."

PRESENT ILLNESS. This section is a clear chronological account of the problems for which the patient is seeking care. The data come from the patient but the organization is yours. The narrative should include the onset of the problem, the setting in which it developed, its manifestations, and any treatments. The principal symptoms should be described in terms of (1) location, (2) quality, (3) quantity or severity, (4) timing (i.e., onset, duration, and frequency), (5) the setting in which they occur, (6) factors that have aggravated or relieved them, and (7) associated manifestations. Also note significant negatives (the absence of certain symptoms that will aid in differential diagnosis).

A present illness should also include patients' responses to their own symptoms and incapacities. What does the patient think has caused the problem? What are the underlying worries that have led to seeking professional attention? ("I think I may have appendicitis.") And why is that a worry? ("My Uncle Charlie died of a ruptured appendix.") Further, what effects has the illness had on the patient's life? This question is especially important in understanding a patient with chronic illness. "What can't you do now that you could do before? How has the backache, shortness of breath, or whatever, affected your ability to work? Your life at home? Your social activities? Your role as a parent? Your role as a husband, or wife? The way you feel about yourself as a man, or a woman?"

PAST HISTORY

General State of Health as the patient perceives it.

Childhood Illnesses, such as measles, rubella, mumps, whooping cough, chickenpox, rheumatic fever, scarlet fever, polio.

Adult Illnesses

Psychiatric Illnesses

(continued)

CHART 5-1

Comprehensive History: Adult Patient (continued)

Accidents and Injuries

Operations

Hospitalizations not already described.

CURRENT HEALTH STATUS. Although some of the variables grouped under this heading have past as well as current components, they may all affect current health.

Current Medications, including home remedies, nonprescription drugs, vitamin/mineral supplements, and medicines borrowed from family or friends. Ask about doses and frequency of use. You may need to ask patients to bring you all their medicines and show you what they take.

Allergies

Tobacco, including the type (smoked, e.g., cigarettes, or smokeless, e.g., chewing tobacco or snuff), amount, and duration of use, e.g., cigarettes, a pack a day for 12 years.

Alcohol, Drugs, and Related Substances.

Diet, including usual daily intake and any dietary restrictions or supplements. Ask about coffee, tea, cola drinks, and other caffeine-containing beverages.

Screening Tests appropriate to the patient, such as tuberculin tests, Pap smears, mammograms, stools for occult blood, and cholesterol tests, together with the results and the dates they were last performed.

Immunizations, such as tetanus, pertussis, diphtheria, polio, measles, rubella, mumps, influenza, hepatitis B, *Hemophilus influenzae* type b, and pneumococcal vaccine.

Sleep Patterns, including times that the person goes to bed and awakens, daytime naps, and any difficulties in falling asleep or staying asleep.

Exercise and Leisure Activities

Environmental Hazards, including those in the home, school, and workplace.

Use of Safety Measures, such as seat belts, smoke detectors, and other devices related to specific hazards.

CHART 5 - 1

Comprehensive History: Adult Patient (continued)

FAMILY HISTORY

The age and health, or age and cause of death, of each immediate family member (i.e., parents, siblings, spouse, and children). Data on grandparents or grandchildren may also be useful.

The occurrence within the family of any of the following conditions: diabetes, heart disease, hypercholesterolemia, high blood pressure, stroke, kidney disease, tuberculosis, cancer, arthritis, anemia, allergies, asthma, headaches, epilepsy, mental illness, alcoholism, drug addiction, and symptoms like those of the patient.

PSYCHOSOCIAL HISTORY. This is an outline or narrative description that captures the important and relevant information about the patient as a person.

Home Situation and Significant Others. "Who lives at home with you? Tell me a little about them, and about your friends." "Who helps you when you are sick, or need assistance?"

Daily Life, from the time of arising to bedtime. "What is a typical day like? What do you do first? Next?"

Important Experiences, including upbringing, schooling, military service, job history, financial situation, marriage, recreation, retirement.

Religious Beliefs relevant to perceptions of health, illness, and treatment.

The Patient's Outlook on the present and on the future.

REVIEW OF SYSTEMS

General. Usual weight, recent weight change, any clothes that fit tighter or looser than before. Weakness, fatigue, fever.

Skin. Rashes, lumps, sores, itching, dryness, color change, changes in hair or nails.

Head. Headache, head injury.

Eyes. Vision, glasses or contact lenses, last eye examination, pain, redness, excessive tearing, double vision, blurred vision, spots, specks, flashing lights, glaucoma, cataracts.

Ears. Hearing, tinnitus, vertigo, earaches, infection, discharge. If hearing is decreased, use of hearing aids.

Nose and Sinuses. Frequent colds; nasal stuffiness, discharge, or itching; hay fever, nosebleeds, sinus trouble.

(continued)

CHART 5-1
Comprehensive History: Adult Patient (continued)

Mouth and Throat. Condition of teeth and gums, bleeding gums, dentures, if any, and how they fit, last dental examination, sore tongue, dry mouth, frequent sore throats, hoarseness.

Neck. Lumps, "swollen glands," goiter, pain or stiffness in the neck.

Breasts. Lumps, pain or discomfort, nipple discharge, self-examination.

Respiratory. Cough, sputum (color, quantity), hemoptysis, wheezing, asthma, bronchitis, emphysema, pneumonia, tuberculosis, pleurisy; last chest x-ray film.

Cardiac. Heart trouble, high blood pressure, rheumatic fever, heart murmurs; chest pain or discomfort, palpitations; dyspnea, orthopnea, paroxysmal nocturnal dyspnea, edema; past electrocardiogram or other heart test results.

Gastrointestinal. Trouble swallowing, heartburn, appetite, nausea, vomiting, regurgitation, vomiting of blood, indigestion. Frequency of bowel movements, color and size of stools, change in bowel habits, rectal bleeding or black tarry stools, hemorrhoids, constipation, diarrhea. Abdominal pain, food intolerance, excessive belching or passing of gas. Jaundice, liver or gallbladder trouble, hepatitis.

Urinary. Frequency of urination, polyuria, nocturia, burning or pain on urination, hematuria, urgency, reduced caliber or force of the urinary stream, hesitancy, dribbling, incontinence; urinary infections, stones.

Genital

Male. Hernias, discharge from or sores on the penis, testicular pain or masses, history of sexually transmitted diseases and their treatments. Sexual preference, interest, function, satisfaction, and problems.

Female. Age at menarche; regularity, frequency, and duration of periods; amount of bleeding, bleeding between periods or after intercourse, last menstrual period; dysmenorrhea, premenstrual tension; age at menopause, menopausal symptoms, postmenopausal bleeding. If the patient was born before 1971, exposure to DES (diethylstilbestrol) from maternal use during pregnancy. Discharge, itching, sores, lumps, sexually transmitted diseases and their treatments. Number of pregnancies, number of deliveries, number of abortions (spontaneous and induced); complications of pregnancy; birth control methods. Sexual preference, interest, function, satisfaction; any problems, including dyspareunia.

Peripheral Vascular. Intermittent claudication, leg cramps, varicose veins, past clots in the veins.

Musculoskeletal. Muscle or joint pains, stiffness, arthritis, gout, backache. If present, describe location and symptoms (e.g., swelling, redness, pain, tenderness, stiffness, weakness, limitation of motion or activity).

CHART 5 – 1

Comprehensive History: Adult Patient (continued)

Neurologic. Fainting, blackouts, seizures, weakness, paralysis, numbness or loss of sensation, tingling or "pins and needles," tremors or other involuntary movements.

Hematologic. Anemia, easy bruising or bleeding, past transfusions and any reactions to them.

Endocrine. Thyroid trouble, heat or cold intolerance, excessive sweating; diabetes, excessive thirst or hunger, polyuria.

Psychiatric. Nervousness, tension, mood including depression; memory.

(Source: Bates B: A Guide to Physical Examination and History Taking, 6th ed. 1996.)

be quiet, afford privacy, and be comfortable for both the RNFA and the patient. Note-taking should be done in brief, short phrases or words; it should not distract attention from the patient or from following the patient's leads. Asking general questions at the beginning of the interview (e.g., "What brings you here today?" "How can we help you?") allows the patient freedom of response. The patient's interpretations of his or her own symptoms is critical in understanding individual response and subsequent planning of interventions.[5] A symptom is the physical or psychological feeling that the patient describes to the RNFA. The RNFA follows the patient's lead by actively listening and watching for important cues. Patients are often reluctant to verbalize their emotions and feelings about their health problem directly; the empathic skill of recognizing when an emotion may be present but not directly expressed is critical to exploring and acknowledging these feelings.[6] The RNFA may guide the patient by using facilitation (encouragement without specifying the topic), reflection (a repetition of the patient's words to encourage further information), clarification (a request for the meaning of a statement), and empathic confirmation (a response that indicates understanding and acceptance).

Interviewing and communicating with a patient, and the family or significant other if present, is further guided by an understanding of theories of stress and coping, human growth and development, and patient confidentiality. Patients have the right to expect that their confidentiality and privacy will be maintained. Treating patients with dignity and preserving their privacy is one of the ethical standards of a professional. Adherence to these concepts is upheld in the Code for Nurses, with underlying values of fidelity (keeping promises), respect for persons, and nonmaleficence (avoiding harms or burdens).[7] The AORN's Standards of Perioperative Professional Performance further clarify this responsibility by noting that the nurse acts as patient advocate, maintaining patient confidentiality and delivering care that is nonjudgmental, nondiscriminatory, and sensitive to cultural, racial, and ethnic diversity while preserving patient autonomy, dignity, and rights.[8]

Theories of Stress and Coping

Various nursing models can serve as frameworks for understanding stress, coping, and adaptation. Whichever model is chosen to guide nursing practice, the RN first assistant may consider stress to be a state produced by some change in the internal or external environment that the patient perceives as threatening, challenging, or damaging to his or her sense of well-being. Each patient is unique in his or her perception of a stressor and in the adaptive mechanisms used to cope with it. Coping has both cognitive and behavioral aspects; the ability to cope effectively is influenced by the patient's resources. Important coping resources include health, energy, problem-solving skills, social skills, support, and the ability to access and afford external resources. Figure 5–1 provides a simplified diagram of the stress and coping process.

Ineffective coping results when the patient is unable to manage internal or external stressors adequately.[9] The patient may verbalize an inability to cope or may use defense mechanisms inappropriately, as in defensive coping (repeated projection of falsely positive self-evaluation in response to an underlying perceived threat to positive self-regard) or ineffective denial (minimization or disavowal of symptoms or situations detrimental to health). The following outcome criteria and sample nursing interventions by the RNFA may be selected with patients exhibiting ineffective coping:

Desired outcomes: The patient will verbalize feelings, identify coping patterns and their consequences, identify personal strengths, accept support through the nursing relationship, make decisions, and follow through with appropriate actions.

RN first assistant interventions:

1. Determine causative and contributing factors
2. Assess for risk factors for poor coping
3. Validate the patient's present coping status
4. Assist the patient with constructive problem-solving techniques
5. Encourage the patient to develop appropriate strategies based on personal strengths, abilities, resources, and previous experiences
6. Appraise the patient's understanding of diagnosis, treatment, and prognosis; provide factual information as appropriate
7. Initiate referrals as indicated[10]

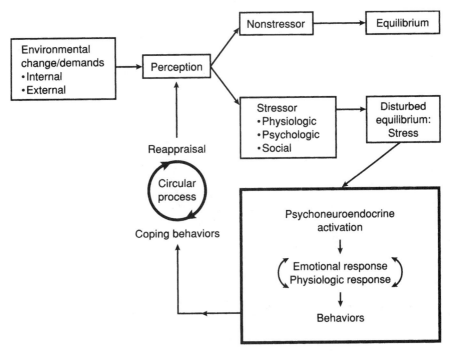

FIGURE 5–1

The stress–coping model. When an environmental change is perceived by the brain as stressful, psychoneuroendocrine activation occurs, eliciting emotional and physiological responses that are manifested in objective and subjective behaviors. As the individual copes, reappraisal will occur again and again, providing feedback to the perception of the situation. RNFAs should use coping enhancement strategies by assisting the patient to adapt to perceived stressors, changes, or other threats by identifying and encouraging the use of self-strengths, resources, and support systems.

Human Growth and Development

Maturational factors are also relevant when obtaining the patient history. A holistic nursing framework acknowledges the patient's developmental stage, appraises the patient's requisite life tasks and values, reinforces the patient's strengths and assets, and assists the patient in determining problems or dominant issues. Various nurse experts have built on Erikson's stages of development; Chart 5–2 summarizes these stages for the adult patient. Part of coping enhancement is the RNFA's contribution to the patient's ability to analyze and explore stressors and changes, build on adaptive strengths, and improve coping ability.

Skills in obtaining a history must be flexible and sensitive. It is not only the symptoms themselves that must be understood; the personal and cultural meanings attached to them are also important in fully understanding the patient. Symptoms are multidimensional, representing a combination of physio-

CHART 5-2

Erikson's Stages of Development for Adults

STAGE	AGE	TASKS	LACK OF ACHIEVEMENT
Early Adult	20-45	*Intimacy vs Isolation*	
		Increases independence	Avoids intimacy
		Establishes career	Is isolated
		Forms intimate bonds	Is promiscuous
		Chooses mate, significant other	Exhibits "character problems"
			Repudiates relationships
		Sets up, manages household	
		Establishes friendships, social networks	
		Assumes civic/community responsibility	
		Initiates parenting	
		Develops meaningful life values and philosophy	
Middle Adult	40–65	*Generativity vs Stagnation*	
		Adjusts to physical changes of aging	Is egocentric
			Is nonproductive
		Reviews/redirects career	Becomes an early invalid
		Develops hobby/leisure activity/organizational affiliations	Exhibits self-love
			Becomes impoverished
			Is self-indulgent
		Helps children/aging parents	
Late Adult	60+	*Integrity vs Despair*	
		Adjusts to physical and health changes	Feels that time is too short
		Forms new roles	Feels that life has no meaning
		Adjusts to retirement, loss of income, friends, significant others	Has lost faith in self/others
			Wants second chance
		Develops activities that enhance self-worth, usefulness	Lacks spirituality
			Fears death
		Prepares for death	

logical, psychological, and situational factors. Thus, the RNFA should assess symptoms across several dimensions, including intensity (strength or severity), timing (duration and frequency of occurrence), level of perceived distress (degree of discomfort and bothersomeness), and quality (what it feels like and its location).[11] Most health care facilities have forms that specify the content of the history. Although such forms can be useful, the RNFA should be guided just as much by what the patient says and the interview skills necessary to elicit this information.

■ PERFORMING THE PHYSICAL EXAMINATION

The RN first assistant uses four routine techniques during physical examination: inspection, palpation, percussion, and auscultation. These techniques are discussed in general in this section; the RNFA will need to modify and adapt them to specific body systems. Chart 5–3 provides an overview of a comprehensive physical examination.

Inspection

Inspection involves detailed observation; it begins with the initial patient contact. Throughout the history and physical examination, the RN first assistant should observe for and note the patient's body posture and stature, gait and stance, body movements, speech patterns, body temperature, skin color and moisture, any unusual odor, and general state of nutrition. Preliminary observations provide basic information that can influence the remainder of the examination. Unlike other physical examination techniques, inspection continues throughout the examination. With this kind of continuity, the RNFA constantly subjects to confirmation or dispute what is "seen" about the patient. The right and left side of the body should be compared; they should be nearly symmetrical.

As the RNFA gains clinical practice in inspection, visual acuity and sense of sight become trained to focus in on detail. Specific inspection will be directed to the focused part of the physical examination. During focused inspection, good lighting, either daylight or artificial light, is required. At times, such as during inspection of abdominal or precordial movement, directing light from an adjustable lamp at a right angle (tangential lighting) produces shadows that are useful in assessing movements.

Palpation

Palpation involves feeling through the use of touch. The RN first assistant confirms points noted during inspection, assessing temperature, texture (roughness, smoothness), size, swelling, rigidity, lumps or masses (motility and configuration), and the presence of tenderness or pain. Different parts of the hand are better suited to certain assessment parameters. The fingertips are tactile discriminators, good for noting skin texture, swelling, pulsatility, consistency, moisture, and shape of lumps or masses. To further detect the position, form, shape, or consistency of a structure or mass, a gentle grasping by the fingertips is used. The dorsum (back) of the hand or fingers, where the skin is thinner than on the palms, is best for assessing temperature. The ulnar

(text continues on page 118)

CHART 5–3

Overview of a Comprehensive Examination

GENERAL SURVEY. Observe the patient's general state of health, height, build, and sexual development. Weigh the patient, if possible. Note posture, motor activity, and gait; dress, grooming, and personal hygiene; and any odors of body or breath. Watch the patient's facial expressions and note manner, affect, and reactions to the persons and things in the environment. Listen to the patient's manner of speaking and note state of awareness or level of consciousness.

The survey continues throughout the history and examination.

VITAL SIGNS. Count the pulse and respiratory rate. Measure the blood pressure and, if indicated, the body temperature.

SKIN. Observe the skin of the face and its characteristics. Identify any lesions, noting their location, distribution, arrangement, type, and color. Inspect and palpate the hair and nails. Study the patient's hands. Continue your assessment of the skin as you examine other body regions.

The patient is sitting on the edge of the bed or examining table, unless this position is contraindicated. You should be standing in front of the patient, moving to either side as you need to.

HEAD. Examine the hair, scalp, skull, and face.

EYES. Check visual acuity and screen the visual fields. Note the position and alignment of the eyes. Observe the eyelids and inspect the sclera and conjunctiva of each eye. With oblique lighting, inspect each cornea, iris, and lens. Compare the pupils and test their reactions to light. Assess the extraocular movements. With an ophthalmoscope, inspect the ocular fundi.

The room should be darkened for the ophthalmoscopic examination.

EARS. Inspect the auricles, canals, and drums. Check auditory acuity. If acuity is diminished, check lateralization (Weber test) and compare air and bone conduction (Rinne test).

NOSE AND SINUSES. Examine the external nose, and with aid of a light and speculum inspect the nasal mucosa, septum, and turbinates. Palpate for tenderness of the frontal and maxillary sinuses.

MOUTH AND PHARYNX. Inspect the lips, oral mucosa, gums, teeth, tongue, palate, tonsils, and pharynx.

NECK. Inspect and palpate the cervical lymph nodes. Note any masses or unusual pulsations in the neck. Feel for any deviation of the trachea. Observe the sound and effort of the patient's breathing. Inspect and palpate the thyroid gland.

BACK. Inspect and palpate the spine and muscles of the back. Check for costovertebral angle tenderness.

POSTERIOR THORAX AND LUNGS. Inspect, palpate, and percuss the chest. Identify the level of diaphragmatic dullness on each side. Listen to the breath sounds, identify any adventitious sounds, and, if indicated, listen to the transmitted voice sounds.

Move behind the sitting patient to feel the thyroid gland and to examine the back, posterior thorax, and lungs.

BREASTS, AXILLAE, *AND* EPITROCHLEAR NODES. In a woman, inspect the breasts with her arms relaxed, then elevated, and then with her hands pressed on her hips. In either sex, inspect the axillae and feel for the axillary nodes. Feel for the epitrochlear nodes.

Move to the front again.

CHART 5-3

Overview of a Comprehensive Examination (continued)

By this time you have made some preliminary observations of the musculoskeletal system. You have inspected the hands, surveyed the upper back, and, at least in women, made a fair estimate of the shoulders' range of motion. Use these and subsequent observations to decide whether a full musculoskeletal examination is warranted.

MUSCULOSKELETAL SYSTEM. If indicated, examine the hands, arms, shoulders, neck, and temperomandibular joint while the patient is still sitting. Inspect and palpate the joints and check their range of motion.

BREASTS. Palpate the breasts, while at the same time continuing your inspection.

Ask the patient to lie down. You should stand at the right side of the patient's bed.

ANTERIOR THORAX *AND* LUNGS. Inspect, palpate, and percuss the chest. Listen to the breath sounds, any adventitious sounds, and, if indicated, transmitted voice sounds.

CARDIOVASCULAR SYSTEM. Inspect and palpate the carotid pulsations. Listen for carotid bruits. Observe the jugular venous pulsations, and measure the jugular venous pressure in relation to the sternal angle.

Inspect and palpate the precordium. Note the location, diameter, amplitude, and duration of the apical impulse. Listen at the apex and the lower sternal border with the bell of a stethoscope. Listen at each auscultatory area with the diaphragm. Listen for physiologic splitting of the second heart sound and for any abnormal heart sounds or murmurs.

Elevate the head of the bed to about 30° for the cardiovascular examination, adjusting it as necessary to see the jugular venous pulsations. Ask the patient to roll partly onto the left side while you listen at the apex. Then have the patient lie back while you listen to the rest of the heart. The patient should sit, leaning forward, and exhale while you listen for the murmur of aortic regurgitation.

ABDOMEN. Inspect, auscultate, and percuss the abdomen. Palpate lightly, then deeply. Assess the liver and spleen by percussion and then palpation. Try to feel the kidneys, and palpate the aorta and its pulsations.

Lower the head of the bed to the flat position. The patient should be supine.

RECTAL EXAMINATION IN MEN. Inspect the sacrococcygeal and perianal areas. Palpate the anal canal, rectum, and prostate. If the patient cannot stand, examine the genitalia before doing the rectal examination.

The patient is lying on his left side for the rectal examination.

GENITALIA AND RECTAL EXAMINATION IN WOMEN. Examine the external genitalia, vagina, and cervix. Obtain Pap smears. Palpate the uterus and the adnexa. Do a rectovaginal and rectal examination.

The patient is supine in the lithotomy position. You should be seated at first, then standing at the foot of the examining table.

LEGS. Examine the legs, assessing three systems while the patient is still supine. Each of these systems will be examined further when the patient stands.

The patient is supine.

Peripheral Vascular System. Note any swelling, discoloration, or ulcers. Palpate for pitting edema. Feel the dorsalis pedis, posterior tibial, and femoral pulses, and, if indicated, the popliteal pulses. Palpate the inguinal lymph nodes.

(continued)

CHART 5-3

Overview of a Comprehensive Examination (continued)

Musculoskeletal System. Note any deformities or enlarged joints. If indicated, palpate the joints and check their range of motion.

Neurologic System. Observe the muscle bulk, the position of the limbs, and any abnormal movements.

EXAMINATION WITH PATIENT STANDING. Assess the following:

Peripheral Vascular System. Inspect for varicose veins.

Musculoskeletal System. Examine the alignment of the spine and its range of motion, the alignment of the legs, and the feet.

Genitalia and Hernias in Men. Examine the penis and scrotal contents and check for hernias.

Neurologic System. Observe the patient's gait and ability to walk heel-to-toe, walk on the toes, walk on the heels, hop in place, and do shallow knee bends. Do a Romberg test and check for a pronator drift.

The patient is standing. You should sit on a chair or stool.

ADDITIONAL NEUROLOGIC EXAMINATION, as indicated:

Cranial Nerves not already examined: sense of smell, strength of the temporal and masseter muscles, corneal reflexes, facial movements, gag reflex, and strength of the trapezii and sternomastoid muscles.

Motor. Muscle tone, muscle strength, rapid alternating movements, and point-to-point movements.

Sensory. Pain, temperature, light touch, position, vibration, and discrimination. Compare right with left sides and distal with proximal areas on the limbs.

REFLEXES

MENTAL STATUS. If indicated and not done during the interview, assess the patient's mood, thought processes, thought content, abnormal perceptions, insight and judgment, memory and attention, information and vocabulary, calculating abilities, abstract thinking, and constructional ability.

The patient is sitting or supine.

(Source: Bates B: A Guide to Physical Examination and History Taking, 6th ed. 1996, pp 118-121.)

surface of the hand or palmar aspects of the metacarpophalangeal joints (ball of the hand) is best for detecting any vibrations.

Palpation should be slow and systematic. The hands should have well-trimmed nails and be warmed before touching the patient. Gloves should be worn for any contact with mucous membranes or where contact with body fluids or drainage is likely. Light palpation, gently pressing in to a depth up to 1 centimeter, is used for most of the physical examination. Heavy, continuous pressure will blunt the sense of touch. Any tender areas should be palpated last. Bimanual palpation, the use of both hands to capture or envelop a body part or structure, is used in breast or pelvic examination. Deep palpation, pressing in to a depth up to 4 centimeters, is used to assess the size and contour of specific structures, such as the liver, kidney, and other abdominal organs. During deep palpation, intermittent pressure is often better than one continuous palpation.

Percussion

The hands are also used for percussion, wherein the application of a physical force translates into sound. The feel and sound assist in depicting location and size by a change in the percussion note between two borders and in determining the density of a structure by a characteristic note. Figure 5–2 shows the procedure for a right-handed RN first assistant; a left-handed RNFA should reverse the hand positions.

The distal phalanx of the middle finger (sometimes referred to as the pleximeter) of the nondominant hand is placed firmly on the body surface being percussed. The remaining fingers and palm are raised off the surface to prevent dampening of sound vibrations. A sharp, crisp, rapid, light tap with the middle finger (sometimes referred to as the plexor) of the dominant hand, or the index and middle fingers together, is made using wrist action. Thus, in this technique one finger acts as the hammer and the other acts as the strik-

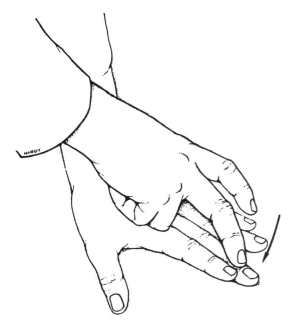

FIGURE 5–2

Percussion technique. A right-handed RNFA places the distal phalanx of the left middle finger firmly against the area to be percussed. The other fingers should be held away so as to not dampen or mute any sound produced. The middle finger of the right hand is then used to strike the terminal phalanx of the left hand middle finger, just behind the nail bed. When striking, the forearm is held steady; the motion of the hand should be predominantly a wrist motion.

ing surface. The shoulders and elbow should remain stationary; the downward snap of the striking finger (or fingers) should originate from the wrist. The tap of the hammering finger should be quick. The finger strikes, the wrist snaps back, and the finger is lifted off by this wrist action to prevent dampening the sound. The striking finger should hit at a right angle to the stationary finger with just enough force to achieve a clear note. The thickness of the body part being percussed is a factor in determining this force. Percussion tones usually arise from vibration 3 to 5 centimeters deep in body tissue. A stronger percussion stroke may be required for patients who are obese or who have a very muscular body wall.

The sound produced by percussion reflects the density of the underlying structure. From the least to the most dense, these sounds are called tympany (over air-filled viscus), hyperresonance (over lungs with an abnormal amount of air, as with emphysema), resonance (over normal lung tissue), dullness (over dense organs, such as the liver), and flatness (no air present, as over thigh muscle). Changes in sound assist in mapping the location and size of an organ and in detecting superficial masses. The RNFA should evaluate the intensity (loudness, characterized as very loud, loud, moderate, or soft), pitch (frequency of the sound, characterized as high, moderate, low, or very low), quality (timbre or tone of the sound, such as hollow, flat, or drumlike), and duration of the sounds heard.[12] Percussion may elicit pain if an underlying structure is inflamed. A percussion instrument, such as a percussion hammer is used to elicit deep tendon reflexes.

Auscultation

The final technique in physical assessment, auscultation usually is accomplished through the use of a stethoscope. The RNFA should select a good quality stethoscope with the correct size earpiece (one which fits snugly in the external meatus, occluding it and thus blocking extraneous sound). The direction of the angle of the metal tubing can usually be adjusted by the tension on the spring; it should angle slightly toward the nose to project sound correctly on the tympanic membrane. The diaphragm of the stethoscope has a flat edge used to auscultate high-pitched sounds, such as heart, breath, and bowel sounds and friction rubs and crepitus. The diaphragm should be warmed and then placed firmly against the patient's skin, creating a seal between the patient's skin and the diaphragm of the stethoscope. Application of a water-soluble lubricant to the diaphragm can improve the transmission of sound. Firm placement will leave a slight ring on the skin when the diaphragm is removed. The stethoscope's bell endpiece detects soft, low-pitched sounds such as heart murmurs, stenotic arteries, venous hums, and bruits. The bell is held lightly against the skin with only enough pressure to form a seal; if the bell is applied with too much pressure, it stretches the skin, inhibiting vibrations. The RNFA uses the stethoscope to listen for intensity (loudness), frequency (pitch), and quality (overtone). Special applications of auscultation depend on specific organ systems.

PREOPERATIVE TESTING

Demands for quality, effectiveness, appropriateness, and cost containment have altered past practices of prescribing a battery of routine screening tests for surgical patients. In the 1990s, preoperative testing should be based on clinical relevance, with a goal of ensuring that the operative or other invasive procedure is performed with minimal risk (and maximum benefit) to the patient. Laboratory studies should be based on the patient's age, sex, the presence or absence of coexisting diseases or conditions, and the type of surgery planned. The RN first assistant should understand each test's predictive value in detecting a disease or condition and its specificity in confirming whether the patient has the disease or condition. Appendix III provides a review of common diagnostic tests and their significance.

INFORMED CONSENT AND PATIENT SELF-DETERMINATION

Informed consent is an agreement reached between a physician and a patient as a result of a discussion between them. It is a physician's legal requirement to disclose information to the patient that enables that patient to understand the procedure, its risks, and its potential outcomes before consenting to it.[13] Implicit in such discussion is that information is presented in consideration of the patient's ability to understand it; thus, consideration must be given to the patient's age, education, and competence.[14] A consent form provides evidence of such an agreement. The RNFA is held to a nursing standard of care requiring that the nurse advise a superior or the physician if the nurse has reason to believe that consent was not obtained or was not adequately "informed."[15] RNFAs who are participants on quality improvement committees might wish to undertake an assessment of the readability of the surgical consent forms used in their practice setting. While the average patient reads at less than an eighth grade level, surgical consent forms are usually written at a far higher level and in a type size small enough to affect legibility.[16] A patient's right to self-determination is protected through the informed consent process. This process requires that the patient be capable of giving consent, understand the advantages and disadvantages of consenting, and not be coerced.

The Patient Self-Determination Act (PSDA) further enunciates patients' rights to make decisions concerning their medical care. It represents the first federal legislation to address advance directives and the rights of individuals to make health care decisions. The PSDA requires that all health care institutions participating in Medicare and Medicaid maintain written policies and procedures to inform adult patients of their rights to formulate advance directives, to document on the medical record whether or not they have executed advance directives, to ensure compliance with state laws regarding advance directives, and to provide education for staff members and the public concerning advance directives.[17] The Joint Commission on Accreditation of Healthcare Organizations defines an advance directive as written or verbal statements made by the patient indicating treatment wishes in the event the patient becomes incapacitated; these may include living wills, durable powers of attorney, or similar documents or documentation conveying the patient's preferences.[18] The RN first assistant should review these institutional policies and procedures, as well as the written information that must be provided to patients on admission. Part of the RNFA's patient assessment should include assessment of the patient's emotional status, values orientation, and willingness and capability to execute an advance directive. Patients may need assistance in reading and understanding an advance directive document; many of these documents are above reading levels recommended for patient materials.[19] Diplomacy, compassion, sensitivity, and empathy are required when assisting the patient, family, and health care staff in implementing PSDA protocols. Issues related to end-of-life decisions and withholding or withdrawing treatment represent an opportunity for RNFAs to assume a role in an area that has great potential for advancing patient autonomy and patient care.[20]

▨ SUMMARY

Trust, respect, and empathy underpin the creation of a therapeutic relationship between the RN first assistant and the patient. Productive communication that is free of imposed values or judgments facilitates the health assessment process. People communicate in a variety of ways, and the RNFA must listen actively to understand what the patient is really saying. As the RNFA collects subjective and objective data about the patient, the health state is assessed to uncover and diagnose health problems. At the same time, the patient's strengths and health assets are acknowledged and nurtured. Relevant data should be fit into the patient's developmental stage. The rapport built during the history and physical examination establishes and facilitates the continuing RN first assistant–patient relationship. As expert nurses, RNFAs learn to combine their practical experience and textbook knowledge in quantifying and responding to patient care needs. Central to their practice is their concern for responding to patients as persons, respecting their dignity and caring for them in a way that protects their personhood during the vulnerable time of diagnosing and intervening in a health problem that requires an operative or other invasive procedure.[21]

■ Review Questions

1. Subjective data are obtained
   a. As the RN first assistant develops from novice to expert.
   b. From what the patient says.
   c. As part of the RN first assistant's intuition.
   d. As the RN first assistant observes the patient.

2. One of the most important points to keep in mind while taking a history is
   a. That each patient is an individual.
   b. To make use of some of the time to teach correct health behaviors.
   c. That using a preprinted form expedites the process.
   d. That it should result in an index of operative risk.

3. It is common and desirable to describe which component of the health history in the patient's own words?
   a. Source of referral
   b. Chief complaint
   c. History of present illness
   d. Current health status

4. Relevant data from the patient's chart, such as laboratory reports, belong in which section of the history?
   a. Chief complaint
   b. History of present illness
   c. Current health status
   d. Past history

5. As part of a holistic framework, during the psychosocial history the RN first assistant will query the patient regarding:
   a. The use of alcohol, drugs, and related substances.
   b. Age and health/cause of death of immediate family members.
   c. Cultural and religious beliefs.
   d. Exercise and leisure activities.

6. To allow the patient some freedom of response, it is helpful to begin the history interview by
   a. Providing information about the RN first assistant's role on the health care team.
   b. Having the patient complete a health questionnaire.
   c. Reassuring the patient that all information will be kept confidential.
   d. Asking general, open-ended questions.

7. A useful interviewing technique that repeats the patient's words to encourage further information is termed

   a. Facilitation.
   b. Reflection.
   c. Clarification.
   d. Empathic confirmation.

8. The AORN Standards of Perioperative Professional Performance set the expectation that the RN first assistant will

   a. Assist the patient in adapting to stressors.
   b. Preserve the patient's autonomy, dignity, and rights.
   c. Make referrals when the patient requires access to external resources.
   d. Interpret relevant findings in the context of the patient's growth and development.

9. A utilitarian definition of stress views it as a patient state produced by

   a. Some change in the internal or external environment.
   b. Inability to cope.
   c. Psychoneuroendocrine activation.
   d. Cognitive perception and behavioral change.

10. A desired patient outcome for a nursing diagnosis of ineffective coping might be

   a. Assess for risk factors.
   b. Teach constructive problem-solving.
   c. Minimize symptoms; focus on positive results of treatment.
   d. Verbalize feelings and personal strengths.

11. The usual sequence in physical examination is

   a. Inspection, percussion, palpation, auscultation.
   b. Inspection, palpation, percussion, auscultation.
   c. Palpation, inspection, auscultation, percussion.
   d. Auscultation, palpation, percussion, inspection.

12. Focused visual attention best describes the technique of

   a. Auscultation.
   b. Palpation.
   c. Percussion.
   d. Inspection.

13. Information from resonance sounds is obtained through

   a. Auscultation.
   b. Palpation.
   c. Percussion.
   d. Inspection.

Column A lists findings from palpation. Column B lists the areas of the hand that are most sensitive to a specific finding. Match the finding (Column A) with the appropriate area of the hand (Column B).

Column A—Finding   Column B—Area of the hand

14. _____ skin texture   A. Fingertips

15. _____ pulsatility   B. Dorsum

16. _____ temperature   C. Ulnar surface

17. _____ consistency

18. _____ vibrations

19. _____ swelling

20. _____ shape of mass/lump

21. Light palpation presses in to a depth up to

    a. 1 centimeter.
    b. 3 centimeters.
    c. 4 centimeters.
    d. 6 centimeters.

22. During percussion, the middle finger of which hand is used to perform a light, rapid tap?

    a. Dominant
    b. Nondominant

23. The percussion tone expected over normal lung tissue is

    a. Dullness.
    b. Flatness.
    c. Resonance.
    d. Tympany.

24. The _____ of the stethoscope should be placed _____ against the patient's skin

    a. Diaphragm; lightly
    b. Diaphragm; firmly
    c. Bell; firmly
    d. Bell; flatly

25. The Patient Self-Determination Act enunciates the patient's right to

    a. Read and obtain a copy of his or her medical record.
    b. Be informed of the inherent risks and benefits of treatment.
    c. A private and confidential physician relationship.
    d. Make decisions regarding his or her health care.

Answer Key

1. b	6. d	11. b	16. b	21. a
2. a	7. b	12. d	17. a	22. a
3. b	8. b	13. c	18. c	23. c
4. b	9. a	14. a	19. a	24. b
5. c	10. d	15. a	20. a	25. d

REFERENCES

1. Curtin LL: Whatsoever you do. . . . Nurs Management 28(6):7–8, 1997
2. Schuster J: Wholistic care: Healing a sick system. Nurs Management, 28(6):56–59, 1997
3. Christou NV, Reiling RB: Nonemergency surgery: Initial evaluation and preoperative planning. In: American College of Surgeons: Care of the Surgical Patient. New York, Scientific American, 1997
4. O'Connell B: Diagnostic reliability: A study of the process. Nurs Diagn 6(3): 99–107, 1995
5. Teel CS, Meek P, McNamara AM, Watson L: Perspectives unifying symptom interpretation. Image 29(2):175–181, 1997
6. Suchman AL, Markakis K, Beckman HB, Frankel R: A model of empathic communication in the medical interview. JAMA 277(8):678–682, 1997
7. Rushton CH, Infante M: Keeping secrets: The ethical and legal challenges of confidentiality and privacy. Communique 5(1):7–9, 1996
8. Association of Operating Room Nurses: AORN Standards and Recommended Practices. Denver, Colo, Association of Operating Room Nurses, 1997
9. Carpenito LJ: Nursing Diagnosis: Application to Clinical Practice. Philadelphia, Lippincott-Raven, 1997
10. McCloskey JC, Bulechek GM: Nursing Intervention Classification (NIC). St Louis, Mosby–Year Book, 1992
11. Lenz ER, Pugh LC, Milligan RA, Suppe F: The middle-range theory of unpleasant symptoms: An update. Adv Nurs Sci 19(3):14–27, 1997
12. Barkauskas VH, Stoltenberg-Allen K, Baumann LC, Darling-Fisher C: Health and Physical Assessment. St Louis, Mosby–Year Book, 1994
13. Pape T: Legal and ethical considerations of informed consent. AORN J 65(6): 1122–1127, 1997
14. Brazell NE: The significance and application of informed consent. AORN J 65(2):377–386, 1997
15. Pryor F: Key concepts in informed consent for perioperative nurses. AORN J 65(6):1105–1110, 1997
16. Curtis D: The readability of surgical consent forms in US hospitals. AORN Congress Resource. Denver, Colo, Association of Operating Room Nurses, 1995, pp 294–295
17. Medicare and Medicaid Programs: Advance Directives; Final Rule. Fed Reg, June 27, 1995
18. Joint Commission on Accreditation of Healthcare Organizations: Comprehensive Accreditation Manual for Hospitals. Chicago, Joint Commission, 1996
19. Ott BB, Hardy TL: Readability of advance directive documents. Image: 29(1): 53–56, 1997
20. Johns JL: Advance directives and opportunities for nurses. Image: 28(2):149–153, 1996
21. Benner P, Tanner CA, Chesla CA: Becoming an expert nurse. Am J Nurs 97(6): 16–17, 1997

PERIOPERATIVE PATIENT PREPARATION

JANE C. ROTHROCK

■

As part of perioperative nursing, the RN first assistant is involved with the patient preoperatively, intraoperatively, and postoperatively. In a practice setting providing optimum continuity of care, the RNFA and patient would establish a relationship that originated at the time the decision for surgical intervention was made. The RNFA would begin patient assessment, identify and assist the patient and family/significant others to meet learning needs, initiate dialogue and plans for home care, and work in partnership with the patient to see that he or she was prepared emotionally, physically, spiritually, and in whatever other way the patient needed preparational assistance. In the operating area, be it an acute care or ambulatory surgery setting, the RNFA would assist in admitting the patient to the operating room and then assist during the patient's surgery. The RNFA would accompany the patient to the perianesthia care unit (PACU), give a nursing report, and follow the patient through the hospital stay, making home visits if necessary, seeing the patient postoperatively in the physician's office, and collecting data to determine the effectiveness of patient education and discharge planning. This chapter reviews preoperative education, pain management, admission to the operating room, skin preparation, and creation of a sterile field with surgical barriers.

■ PREOPERATIVE PATIENT EDUCATION

Quality surgical care encompasses more than the safe performance of a surgical intervention with the achievement of its physiological intent. Patient preparation, for the surgical intervention itself and for the ability to participate in rehabilitation and self-care at home, are important responsibilities of the RN first assistant. To underscore the importance of patient education, in 1994 the Joint Commission on Accreditation of Healthcare Organizations created a separate chapter and set of standards (Table 6–1) for patient and family education. To meet the intent of these standards, RNFAs and the institutions in which they work need to become proficient in the assessment of learning needs, teaching patients in short periods of time, organizing patient education materials, accessing community resources, and designing creative and innovative ways to incorporate the results of research into ongoing improvement efforts.[1] The general objectives of perioperative patient education include interactive communication, participation in decision making, enhancement of self-care skills, increasing coping abilities, and the provision of specific, concrete information regarding pre-admission events, the sequence of perioperative activities, and discharge instruction.[2] Patient education is a multidisciplinary effort; the RNFA participates in contributing to such an effort by selecting nursing interventions from a nursing framework.

A prevalent mechanism for designating the role and domain of nursing, and nursing knowledge, is the use of nursing diagnoses. This classification system provides nurses with a common frame of reference for providing and directing patient care, identifying nurses' accountability. As defined by the North American Nursing Diagnosis Association (NANDA), a nursing diagnosis is a clinical judgment about individual, family, or community responses to actual or potential health problems/life processes. Nursing diagnosis provides the basis for selecting nursing interventions to achieve outcomes for which the nurse is accountable; by linking nursing diagnosis, nursing interventions, and nursing-sensitive outcomes, RNFAs can contribute to the ongoing effort to develop nursing information systems.[3]

There are five types of nursing diagnosis: actual, high risk, possible, wellness, and syndrome. Actual nursing diagnoses must be clinically validated by identifiable characteristics. In 1992, NANDA changed the former terminology of "potential" nursing diagnosis to high risk; this diagnostic category is used when the RNFA makes a clinical judgment that a particular patient is more vulnerable to develop a problem than are others in a similar situation. Possible nursing diagnoses describe suspected problems for which additional data are required. Wellness diagnoses describe a transition from one level of wellness to a higher level. The use of wellness diagnoses assists both the RNFA and the patient in focusing on progress and not only problems.[4] Syndrome diagnoses are clusters of actual or high-risk nursing diagnoses that are predicted to be present because of a certain event or situation.

TABLE 6–1. JCAHO STANDARDS FOR PATIENT/FAMILY EDUCATION

Standard	Targets	Evidence*
Standard PF.1 Patient and family provided with appropriate education and training to increase knowledge of illness and treatment needs, and skills/behaviors to promote recovery and improve functions.	▪ Patient and family understanding of current health problem and reason for admission ▪ Patient informed consent re: treatment ▪ Patient and family understanding of treatment plan and the role they will play ▪ Overview of the survival skills needed for safe discharge	▪ All patients receive instruction. ▪ Priorities for education are identified by the organization.
Standard PF.2 Patient and family receive education specific to patient's assessed needs, abilities, readiness, and appropriate to length of stay.	▪ Safe and effective use of medications ▪ Medical equipment ▪ Potential drug-food interactions, modified diets ▪ Rehab techniques ▪ Community resources ▪ How to obtain further treatment ▪ Ongoing health care needs	▪ Patient assessment ▪ Information understandable to patient ▪ Teaching is culturally appropriate.
Standard PF.3 Any discharge instructions given to the patient and family are provided to the organization responsible for patient's continuing care.	▪ Written discharge instructions, understandable to patient, include targets for PF.2. ▪ Continuing care provider identified ▪ Instructions provided to continuing care providers	▪ Discharge planning involves patient and family. ▪ Discharge instructions clear: who is to do what?
Standard PF.4 The organization plans and supports the provision and coordination of patient and family education activities and resources.	▪ Classes ▪ Community resources access ▪ Closed circuit TV ▪ Multimedia library ▪ Patient education materials data base ▪ One-on-one presentations ▪ Interdisciplinary educational process	▪ Provision and coordination of patient education activities and resources ▪ Resources selected based on patient needs ▪ Health care team involvement ▪ Educational formats based on specific needs

*Policies and procedures, progress notes, flowsheets, referral and consultation notes, interviews with staff, written information given to patients and families.
(Source: Rankin SH, Stallings KD: Patient Education: Issues, Principles, Practices, 3rd ed. Philadelphia, Lippincott-Raven Publishers, 1996. Adapted from Joint Commission on the Accreditation of Healthcare Organizations: 1995 Comprehensive Accreditation Manual for Hospitals. Chicago, Joint Commission, 1995.)

Knowledge Deficit and Anxiety

Most RN first assistants would begin their approach to patient education with consideration of the nursing diagnosis of Knowledge Deficit. This state exists when a patient exhibits a deficiency in cognitive knowledge or psychomotor skills regarding his or her condition or treatment plan. The RNFA must not assume that a knowledge deficit is present; the patient should verbalize a lack of knowledge or skills, request information, express an inaccurate perception regarding surgery or required care, or incorrectly perform a care requisite. The patient and family/significant others should be involved in identifying vital areas of learning need and skill mastery (Box 6–1), and patient/family teaching should correspond to these needs.[5] Too often, nurses have assumed and directed what the patient should know without determining what the patient needs or wants to know. Such assumptions are not part of a nursing plan that respects the patient as an individual who is capable of self-determination and participation in the plan of care.

The term care is used in different ways in nursing. In some instances nurses "take care of"; this is an act of tending for another or doing something for the other. "Caring for" is often expressed in terms of physical needs. Care can also be "caring about"; in this sense, it is an attitude or emotional investment in another person. "Taking care" indicates a caution or concern, a guarding against harm, as in prevention of injury. The care processes engaged in by the RNFA may involve comforting, supporting, providing direct helping behaviors, assisting with coping and stress reduction, or offering empathy or compassion.[6] As part of his or her patient interaction, the RNFA should understand that caring is an interpersonal experience involving moment-to-moment human encounters between two people. Patient education may involve *taking care of* dressings until the patient can perform self-dressing changes; it may involve *caring about* the patient's anxiety and fears; and it may involve *taking care* that the patient does not suffer an injury or harm due to lack of instruction.

BOX 6–1

Questions to Keep in Mind While Assessing Learning Needs

- What information does the patient need?
- What attitudes should be explored?
- What skills does the patient need to perform health care behaviors?
- What factors in the patient's environment may pose barriers to the performance of desired behaviors?

(Source: Rankin SH, Stallings KD: Patient Education: Issues, Principles, Practices, 3rd ed. Philadelphia, Lippincott-Raven Publishers, 1996.)

Rather than knowledge deficit, another appropriate nursing diagnosis for surgical patients is Anxiety Related to Insufficient Knowledge of Perioperative Events (preoperative routines, postoperative exercises/activities, or postoperative alterations/sensations). In a study of select nursing diagnoses in an acute care setting, the three most frequent related factors for the nursing diagnostic label Anxiety were unfamiliar surroundings/procedures/test, undergoing a surgical procedure, and uncertain discharge plans.[7] Nearly 50% of the nursing interventions for anxiety are related to patient education. RNFAs can contribute enormously to intervening in the identified related factors with their perioperative patients. In other research, an analysis of studies indicated that knowing what to expect before, during, and after surgery allayed patient apprehension and improved overall recovery from surgery.[8] Anxiety should be confirmed by patient verbalization or the RNFA's observation of anxious behaviors such as restlessness, inability to concentrate and retain information, increased verbalization, poor eye contact, facial tension, extraneous movements, quivering voice, and tremulousness. This vague uneasiness that characterizes anxiety is usually due to the situational event of surgery and its perceived threats. The RNFA seeks to intervene by providing information related to preparation for, need for, and expectations for diagnostic studies, the surgical procedure, postoperative treatment regimens, pain management, discharge planning, and follow-up care.

RN First Assistant Interventions

Patient education can occur in various settings by various methods. It may be through discussion, printed materials, video, computer disk, or demonstration; it may be planned or spontaneous; it may be formal or informal. Whichever method is selected, certain general premises of adult education should guide the RN first assistant in planning and delivering patient education (Table 6–2).

At the outset, the RNFA should determine what the patient needs to know and wants to know. Because the patient may not know exactly what information he or she needs, it is helpful to ask about past experiences with surgery and positive or negative perceptions. Directed questions such as "Can you tell me what you are most concerned about?" may help the patient focus on worries and fears. This focused assessment will assist the RNFA and patient in determining sources of anxiety and direct some of the teaching plan; the plan should take into consideration the patient's level of understanding of the planned surgical procedure and its associated events, as well as the patient's level of education and preferred learning style. It is desirable to involve the patient and family/significant others in developing content area; there may be an area not identified by the patient that is of concern to a family caregiver. RNFAs should also consider specific concerns of family members and caregivers. During interactions with the patient, the RNFA may note stress on the part of a spouse, family member, or significant other; support in

**TABLE 6-2. APPLICATION OF ADULT LEARNING THEORY TO PATIENT
AND FAMILY EDUCATION**

Assumption About Learner	Applications
Self-concept moves from dependency toward self-direction; sees self as capable of making own decisions, taking responsibility for consequences, managing own life	Acknowledge learner's desire to articulate own needs, make choices, and gain respect for own ability to manage life; create psychological climate that communicates acceptance and support; help learner to feel comfortable expressing thoughts and ideas without fear of shame or embarassment; remember that adults are motivated to learn when they realize that they have a need to learn.
Growing reservoir of life experience is a resource for learning	Use past experiences as a resource for learning; remember that adults experience positive feelings of support and recognition when their experience is acknowledged; relate new learning to old; have adults teach other adults in a group setting; be aware that negative past experiences may pose barriers for learner and teacher.
Readiness to learn is strongly influenced by social roles and developmental tasks	Recognize social role of patient (e.g., father, mother, husband, wife, worker) and developmental tasks; relate learning to ability to become, to succeed in these roles.
Time perspective changes; orientation to learning shifts; needs immediate application of new knowledge and problem-centered learning	Give adults practical answers to their problems; help them to apply new knowledge immediately through role play or hands-on practice (i.e., return demonstration); remember that adults are particularly motivated to learn at times of crisis or when problems arise; prioritize learning activities by immediacy of need and patient-family perception of need; reinforce learning and promote problem-solving skills.

(Source: Rankin SH, Stallings KD: Patient Education: Issues, Principles, Practices, 3rd. ed. Philadelphia, Lippincott-Raven Publishers, 1996. Adapted from Knowles MS: The Modern Practice of Adult Education. New York, Association Press, 1970.)

coping should be provided.[9] Plans should be undertaken to communicate with these important persons during the surgical waiting period; research supports the contribution of progress reports to reducing anxiety in family members during this period of waiting.[10]

Teaching should begin with the most relevant and important information, with simple but clear explanations.[11] At appropriate intervals, the RN first assistant should have the patient restate information or demonstrate what has been taught. Positive reinforcement and affirmation are important; the RNFA should not assume that a patient knows that he or she is doing something correctly or well. Pacing during education is important; too much information in too little time is liable to stimulate anxiety, not reduce it. Providing written material can reinforce verbal teaching. Caution should be used in developing or selecting patient education materials; studies indicate that many of these materials require reading ability at the 10th-grade level and some require completion of the first year of college for reading comprehension.[12] The patient and family/significant others can refer to such written material and identify areas that are still unclear, but the RNFA should not rely on these materials as a substitute for nurse-facilitated patient education. It is critical to listen actively to a patient and redesign material to incorporate any concerns or anxieties. As necessary, and with the patient's agreement, the RNFA should initiate appropriate referrals to other assistive resources when preparation for discharge indicates unmet critical learning needs (Box 6–2).

Outcome Criteria: Knowledge Deficit and Anxiety

Establishing and evaluating outcomes is part of the accountability associated with nursing diagnoses. By knowing what is expected to result from a nursing intervention and determining whether this expectation was achieved, the RNFA validates that the problem is either resolved or that further intervention is required. Because access to patients for follow-up in assessing and measuring outcomes has become increasingly difficult with short-stay and ambulatory surgery, RNFAs need to participate in the development and effectiveness evaluation of creative methods for reaching patients after discharge.[13] Appropriate outcome criteria for the nursing diagnosis Anxiety Related to Insufficient Knowledge of Perioperative Events might include the following:

The patient will verbalize what to expect during the perioperative period.
The patient will demonstrate postoperative regimens and home care requirements.
The patient will relate/report less anxiety following teaching.

The first and third of these outcome criteria might be measured during the perioperative period. The second requires more than a simple demonstration of the care requirements during a teaching/learning episode. The RNFA should have a mechanism for determining that the patient is successfully handling postoperative regimens and home care requirements after discharge.

BOX 6–2

Critical Learning Needs:
Preparing for Discharge

1. What potential problems are likely to prevent a safe discharge?
2. What potential problems are likely to cause complications or readmission?
3. What prior knowledge or experience does the patient and family have with this problem?
4. What skills and equipment are needed to manage the problem at home?

(Source: Rankin SH, Stallings KD: Patient Education: Issues, Principles, Practices, 3rd ed. Philadelphia, Lippincott-Raven Publishers, 1996.)

Patient Education for Pain Management

It has been estimated that approximately 29 million people experience postoperative pain each year.[14] Surgery initiates the biological and physiological stimulus for pain. When tissue is injured, special nerves, the A-delta fibers and c-fibers, send electrical signals to the dorsal horn of the spinal cord; various chemical mediators exist, such as histamine, acetylcholine, and substance P. Prostaglandins can further stimulate nerves near the area of injury.[15] An incoming pain message is processed in the spinal cord's control center, then relayed to the brain. If pain persists, mediators build up and sensitize spinal nerves; eventually even harmless signals from the injured area become painful. Pain is felt once the nerve signal reaches both the thalamus and cortex of the brain. In 1992, the Agency for Health Care Policy and Research (AHCPR) issued a clarion call to practitioners involved with surgical patients, suggesting that more than half of postoperative patients experience unrelieved pain due to inadequate medication.[16] Since that time, RNFAs and their perioperative colleagues have focused part of preoperative patient education efforts on discussions of postoperative pain and its control.

Pain rating scales have been recommended as an important tool in helping patients identify the intensity of their pain, with the goal being achievement of enough pain relief for the patient to perform activities related to a satisfactory recovery or improved function. McCaffery and Pasero recommend the following steps in educating patients about managing their pain.[17] The purpose of a pain rating scale should be explained; the patient should understand that it is his or her right and responsibility to communicate when pain levels are personally unacceptable. The specific pain rating scale that will be used should then be reviewed; there are many scales available, and if one scale cannot be used by the patient, alternative scales should be considered (Figure 6–1). When introducing the pain rating scale, the concept of pain should be discussed, so that the patient understands that pain is not only an experience that is severe or intolerable but can range from mild to moderate to severe. It is helpful to have the patient give examples of kinds of pain experienced in the past, then use one of those examples as practice in using the pain rating scale. The final step involves having the patient set goals for comfort and his or her personal optimal recovery. The RNFA should focus with the patient on comfort levels that allow for important postoperative activities such as deep breathing, coughing, and early ambulation, and that are personally and culturally satisfactory.

Both pharmacological and nonpharmacological pain control measures should be reviewed. There are a number of easy-to-teach and easy-to-learn therapies that patients can use to assist in controlling their pain and anxiety about it. Relaxation techniques such as slow, rhythmic breathing, listening to music of the patient's choice, distraction, guided imagery, aromatherapy, and massage can all help with mild to moderate pain.[18–20] These rarely, however, can substitute for pharmacological control of severe pain.

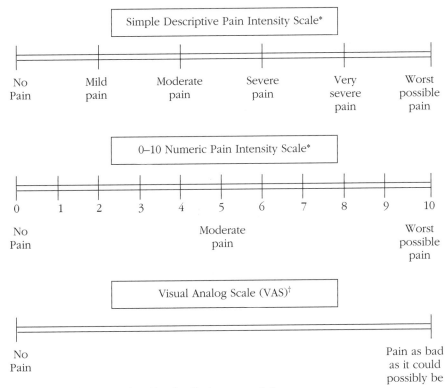

*If used as a graphic rating scale, a 10-cm baseline is recommended.
†A 10-cm baseline is recommended for VAS scales.

FIGURE 6–1

Examples of pain intensity scales. (Source: Agency for Health Care Policy and Research: Acute Pain Management: Operative or Medical Procedures and Trauma. Clinical Practice Guidelines. Rockville, Md, Agency for Health Care Policy and Research, US Department of Health and Human Services, 1992.)

The focus of pharmacological relief should be on prevention of pain. Whether this is via nurse-administered analgesics or patient-controlled analgesia (PCA) therapy, the goal of pain management is to alleviate the peaks and valleys in blood level concentrations. Thus, the suggestion that pain relief be administered "prn" is an outdated concept; by the time it is "needed," the pain has already become higher on the intensity scale and the analgesic is at a subtherapeutic level. Thus, around-the-clock or set-interval pain relief schedules are more likely to provide effective pain control. Balanced analgesia is a multimodal approach to postoperative pain relief, combining opioids, nonsteroidal anti-inflammatory drugs (NSAIDs), and local anesthetics.[21] Each of these agents acts by a different mode to interfere with the physiological pain sequence: NSAIDs act by inhibiting pain mediators at the injury site, opioids attach to receptor sites in the spinal cord and brain, and local anesthetics block sensory inflow. When used by the anesthesia provider preoperatively, this concept is referred to as preemptive analgesia.

RNFAs should choose to be part of pain management task forces, keep informed of recent research on postsurgical pain, and consider pain-reducing strategies such as using lidocaine when they are preparing for insertion of an intravenous catheter, talking with the pharmacist about providing buffered lidocaine solution to reduce the burning and stinging, and utilizing correct techniques when injecting the local anesthetic. The challenge of educating patients for enhanced pain management is a priority for RNFAs seeking to improve the quality of patient care.

Admission to the Operating Room

Whether the patient is an ambulatory surgery patient or an inpatient, the RN first assistant should make every attempt to greet the patient on his or her arrival in the surgical suite. In the holding area, the RNFA may assist the admitting nurse in the routine admission procedures of patient identification, operative site/side verification, allergy verification, and so forth. The RNFA should take the time to briefly review the patient's medical record for any recent reports that have not previously been reviewed and to assess the patient's emotional status. The rapport begun during the history, physical examination, and patient education facilitates the ongoing interpersonal relationship between the RNFA and the patient.

The RN first assistant should attempt to remain with the patient for preanesthesia preparation. As an experienced perioperative nurse, the RNFA is invaluable to the patient, anesthesia staff, and perioperative nursing colleagues during insertion of lines, transfer to the operating bed, and anesthesia induction. This versatility and multidimensionality in the nursing role are critical and essential contributions of an RNFA. Because the RNFA is well acquainted with patient care routines, productivity is enhanced, patient care quality improved, and risk managed.

▓ SKIN PREPARATION

All surgical patients have a high risk for infection related to impaired skin and tissue integrity. The RN first assistant's skill and knowledge of the origin of and containment methods for exogenous microorganisms by antiseptic skin preparation aid in protecting the patient from serious complications of wound infection.

Vitalized tissue has enormous resistance to infection. It takes a significant microbial deposit in the tissue to cause an infection; when bioburdens of 10^5 microorganisms per cubic millimeter are left in wounds, wound infection rates increase dramatically. Bacteria are commonly found on skin surfaces, especially in the moist areas of the axillae, the mouth, and the perineum. These areas are ideal incubators for microbes. Other body areas such as the trunk and extremities have negligible numbers of microbes. On the other hand, exposed body parts such as the face, hands, and feet can harbor up to 10^3 microorganisms per cubic millimeter. These bacteria are commonly found on the top, horny layer of the skin and around the entrance to hair follicles. For these reasons, the effectiveness of an antimicrobial chemical agent is critical to microbial destruction on the skin. Through proper skin antisepsis, the RN first assistant can rid the skin of these superficial microbes.

Anatomy and Physiology of the Skin

Intact skin and mucous membranes are the body's first line of defense against infection. The skin has two specific layers: the outer epidermis and the deeper dermis. Stratified squamous tissue that varies in thickness from 0.06 to 0.10 millimeters, the epidermis functions as a barrier to protect inner tissues, as a receptor for a range of sensations, and as a regulator of temperature. Essentially avascular, the multiple levels of epidermal cells progressively die as they reach the surface; this tissue layer constantly sheds cells, which are replaced from the dermal layer. The hair follicles and sweat glands pass through the epidermis. The dermis is a layer of fibroelastic connective tissue that contains lymphatic vessels, blood vessels, nerves, hair follicles, and sebaceous and sweat glands (Figure 6–2).

Bacteria are prevalent on all skin layers and are categorized as either transient or resident flora. The transient flora are those in loose contact with the skin, such as grease, sweat, and oil particles. Because they are in loose contact, these organisms are easily removed by gentle mechanical friction. The resident flora, on the other hand, are found in and around the glands and hair follicles. They are carried to the surface and shed with perspiration and skin cells. Examples of resident flora include *Staphylococcus epidermidis*, aerobic and anaerobic diphtheroid bacilli, aerobic spore-forming bacilli, aerobic and anaerobic streptococci, and gram-negative rods. Because the surgical incision breaks the continuity of the skin, skin preparation must be directed at removing transient flora and suppressing the activity of resident flora.

Objectives of Skin Preparation

General considerations in the preparation of skin include the surgical site, condition of the site, the numbers and kinds of contaminants, skin characteristics, the patient's overall condition, the use of aseptic technique, and the selection of effective antimicrobial agents and application techniques. The primary purpose of perioperative skin preparation is to remove the transient dirt, oil, and microorganisms from the epidermis and to prevent the growth

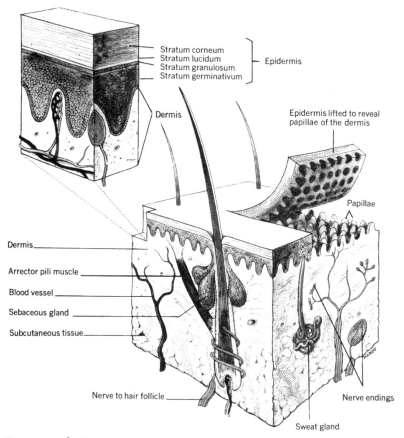

FIGURE 6-2

Anatomy of the skin. (Source: Chaffee EE, Lytle IM: Basic Physiology and Anatomy, 4th ed. Philadelphia, JB Lippincott, 1980.)

and multiplication of the dermal microbes. According to the Association of Operating Room Nurses (AORN) Recommended Practices for Skin Preparation of Patients, three objectives should be met:

1. to remove soil and transient microbes from the skin
2. to reduce the resident microbial count to subpathogenic amounts in a short time with the least amount of tissue irritation
3. to inhibit the rapid rebound growth of microbes.[22]

Nursing Diagnoses

Basic nursing diagnoses that guide nursing intervention during skin preparation activities include:

1. High Risk for Infection related to impaired skin integrity: a state in which the patient is at risk for invasion by an opportunistic or pathogenic agent from external sources
2. High Risk for Injury related to use of chemical agents for skin preparation: a state in which the patient is at risk for harm because of a lack of awareness of environmental hazards
3. Possible Anxiety related to loss of privacy during skin preparation procedures: a state in which the patient experiences a feeling of uneasiness

Outcome Criteria

Identification of potential patient problems assists the RNFA in planning prevention strategies that offer the patient an injury-free outcome from the nursing activities involved in skin preparation. For the above-listed nursing diagnoses, appropriate outcome criteria might be stated as follows:

The patient will demonstrate progressive healing at the surgical site.
The patient will be free of injury associated with chemical antisepsis.
The patient will relate/report decreased anxiety following measures to promote privacy.

Management of Hair in the Operative Area

The purpose of perioperative skin preparation is to reduce the number of existing microorganisms on skin surfaces and to prevent their entry into the surgical wound. The recommendation that hair not be removed preoperatively is supported by a broad, heterogeneous body of research.[23] Shaving of hair causes skin damage and has been associated with a relatively high incidence of wound infection.[24] If hair removal is absolutely necessary for accurate approximation of wound edges, using sterile clippers (or clippers with a disinfected head) in the operating room is suggested. Meticulous care should be taken with the clippers to avoid skin injury and irritation.

Before beginning to clip the hair, the RN first assistant should assess the patient's general skin condition, ensuring that the skin is dry and healthy. Good hand-washing technique and wearing gloves prevent cross-contamination. Hair removal should be documented in the patient's record.

Antimicrobial Agents for Skin Preparation

The numbers and kinds of microorganisms cultured from surgical sites vary according to wound classification, wound location, host susceptibility and resistance, and other endogenous and exogenous factors. *Staphylococcus au-*

reus and *Staphylococcus epidermidis* are highly implicated in surgical site infection. Gram-negative aerobes are frequently seen. Studies indicating the kinds and numbers of microorganisms found in wound sepsis form the basis for the selection criteria for antimicrobial agents. Groah lists seven criteria that should characterize agent effectiveness:

1. act rapidly
2. have a residual effect
3. reduce resident microbes
4. contain a nonirritating antimicrobial preparation
5. inhibit rebound growth of microbes
6. affect a broad spectrum of microbes
7. be nontoxic[25]

Antimicrobial agents from which the RNFA might select are described in the following sections.

Iodine and Iodine-Containing Compounds.

Masterson recommends painting the skin with povidone-iodine solution (10% available povidone iodine and 1% available iodine) and letting it dry. If the surgical area contains intertriginous folds or the umbilicus, the same solution should be used to mechanically cleanse these areas.[26] Iodine-containing agents are bactericidal against gram-negative and gram-positive organisms, providing microbicidal activity for up to eight hours. The combination of an iodine complex plus a detergent, such as found in the iodophors, produces an excellent cleansing agent. The slow release of iodine following application of an iodine-containing solution, often referred to as "paint," provides sustained antisepsis at the operative site. This brown stain outlines the prepared area in light-skinned patients, clearly demarking for the RN first assistant the anatomically aseptic landmarks. Pooling of iodine solutions at the bedlines can cause skin maceration and chemical contact dermatitis; absorbent towels should be placed at the bedlines of the prep area prior to preparation and carefully removed at the conclusion of skin preparation. Demling cautions that iodine should not be used on the perineum, genitalia, irritated or delicate skin, or when the patient has a history of iodine sensitivity.[27]

For an awake patient, the RNFA is often concerned about the discomfort of cold antiseptic solutions. Labels on povidone-iodine solutions should be read to determine whether warming is advised. Heating in a closed container can decrease iodine concentration in the solution, decreasing its effectiveness. Heating in an open container can result in water evaporation, resulting in increased iodine concentration.

Chlorhexidine Gluconate.

Chlorhexidine gluconate offers a broad spectrum of bactericidal action. It is highly effective against a variety of organisms. It has a relatively low skin reaction history with patient use and maintains microbial inhibition for up to six hours after application. It is colorless and does not stain skin or clothing. These latter properties are considered highly desirable in certain surgeries, especially in aesthetic surgery, and in certain practice settings, such as the ambulatory surgical unit. Chlorhexidine should not be used in the ear or eye.

Ethyl Alcohol. Used in a 70% solution, alcohol may be applied as a degerming agent. It is bactericidal for many gram-negative and gram-positive organisms. However, alcohol coagulates tissue protein and cannot be applied on open wounds or mucous membranes. Its potential flammability needs to be considered; pooling must not occur, and surrounding table covers must not become saturated, especially when an electrosurgery unit is being used as a surgical adjunct. Consideration also must be given to the storage of potentially flammable solutions in the operating room. Because of the risks from the flammability and volatility of alcohol and alcohol-based solutions, many operating rooms no longer use them for patient skin preparation.

Triclosan. Triclosan is a broad-spectrum antimicrobial agent combined with oils and lanolin to provide a detergent effect. It is safe for use around the eyes but develops a cumulative suppressive action after prolonged use.

Technique for Preparing the Surgical Site

Policies and procedures for skin antisepsis vary according to institutional protocol and physician preference. Nonetheless, the broad general principles of reducing the microbial count in the shortest time, suppressing regrowth, using aseptic technique, and attending to patient safety and privacy are applicable to any practice setting.

Before initiating any skin preparation procedure, the RNFA should verify landmarks denoting skin preparation for the intended surgical procedure. The next step is to inspect the patient's skin, noting any irritation, rashes, abrasions, or localized infection. Skin preparation accessories vary but usually include gloves, forceps, sponges, absorbent towels, cotton applicators, and solution cups. Maintaining a separate table for skin preparation instruments is the best approach, confining and containing instruments and supplies used on the skin so that there is no transfer from the prep table to the sterile instrument table.

If a disposable prep tray is used, it may or may not contain prep solution. If prep solution needs to be added to disposable or in-house setups, an adequate but not wasteful amount of solution should be poured. After doing this, the RNFA dons sterile gloves and tucks absorbent towels at the bedline.

These towels absorb excess solution to prevent possible skin excoriation and chemical contact dermatitis from pooled solution.

Cleansing begins with the detergent solution applied in a circular fashion from clean to dirty areas. If an abdominal prep includes the umbilicus, the umbilicus is considered potentially contaminated. Some detergent is squeezed into the umbilicus, and the prep is begun immediately outside it. As the rest of the abdomen is prepped, the antiseptic softens the detritus. The umbilicus should be cleansed last, then the sponge discarded. Cleansing is done to rid the skin of transient microorganisms; a gentle mechanical action is all that is necessary to remove these loosely attached bacteria. As the sponge reaches the wound periphery, it is discarded; a sponge that reaches the bedline should not be brought back to the incision site.

In some instances, only antimicrobial paint is applied. This single application may be sprayed on, or a sponge forceps may be used. The sponge on the forceps is dipped in the solution, gently squeezed of excess, and applied to the skin in a circular fashion from incision line to periphery. A prepped area should not be retraced. The solution should be applied at least twice. After application, the bedline towels are removed and gloves and prep table contents are disposed of.

There are some exceptions to the standard skin prep principles. Infected or draining wounds, open trauma, body orifices, or ostomy sites are considered potentially contaminated areas. For surgical interventions that involve such a contaminated site, the prep technique is reversed. Skin antisepsis begins with the peripheral areas and moves circularly to the center. If a skin graft is being done, the recipient site is considered the contaminated site. If more than one incision is being made, it is safest to use separate prep trays to minimize any cross-contamination.

The goal for the patient during skin antisepsis can be stated as follows: The patient will be free from any adverse conditions resulting from skin preparation. The criteria by which this goal is judged include the selection of an agent that rapidly decreases bacterial counts, allows for quick application and prolonged activity, does not cause skin irritation or sensitivity, is not rendered ineffective by alcohol or the presence of organic matter, and is easily removed from skin and fabrics. Patient privacy is considered throughout the preparatory process. Documentation includes hair clipping, if done, the anatomically prepped area, the prep agent, and the skin condition before and at completion of the procedure.

■ DRAPING THE OPERATIVE SITE

Draping is the procedure of covering the patient and surrounding areas with a sterile barrier to create and maintain an adequate sterile field during surgery. The role of the barrier material used in operating room gowns and drapes has received a good deal of attention in the nursing literature, especially with the development of synthetic and new reusable materials. The physical and bacteriological barrier characteristics of draping materials, as well as environmental considerations in the disposal of biohazardous waste, need to be considered by the RN first assistant when participating in the selection of barrier materials.

As in many perioperative patient procedures, in draping the surgical patient common nursing diagnoses are used as the basis for nursing actions. Consideration must be given to providing a sterile, safe environment for surgical intervention, as well as one that is comfortable and private for the awake patient. The risk for infection, possible loss of dignity, and possible anxiety all characterize patient problems for which nursing interventions might be developed.

Qualities of Barrier Material

Barrier materials are a key factor in the effort to decrease airborne contamination of the surgical wound. With the disrupted integrity of the patient's skin, the risk for infection is greatly increased. The proper use of surgical drapes and the creation of a sterile field are essential protective measures against this threat of infection. The RNFA initiates patient care measures by using surgical drapes to create a wide margin of sterility between the operative site and the surrounding unsterile area. Principles of infection control guide the RNFA and surgical team in creating the sterile field. The goal is to interrupt the transmission of microorganisms by establishing an aseptic area through the use of surgical barriers that isolate the operative site.

The materials used to create the sterile field will vary according to physician preference, agency policy, and characteristics of the operative site. The selection of a barrier material must be guided by a thorough knowledge of the criteria that characterize an effective barrier. These materials must be resistant to blood, body fluids, and aqueous solutions; must remain intact for the duration of the surgical procedure; should be nonabrasive and lint-free; should not possess memory; and should be drapable, easily fitting the contours of the patient and equipment. Dyes, often used to reduce glare, should be nontoxic. Material must be antistatic, meeting the standards of the National Fire Protection Association. It must also be sufficiently porous to allow temperature regulatory mechanisms to function to keep body temperature normothermic. The safety and efficacy of the material should be documented by the manufacturer's performance standards.

Reusable Drapes. Reusable barrier materials are usually composed of chemically treated 100% cotton with a 288-thread count per square inch. These materials are porous, eliminating heat buildup. They should be used with nonpenetrating clamps. These materials are considered advantageous in terms of institutional cost. They have a number of disadvantages, however. Consideration must be given to the amount of time, personnel, and equipment needed to reprocess reusable drapes. They must be inspected for holes, washed after every use, refolded, sterilized, and stored. Heavily soiled drapes present contamination hazards to the personnel who must handle them. Additionally, hospital laundering systems must be effective in reducing the pathogenic organisms that colonize the surface and interstices of cotton drapes. A system must be devised for tracking the number of times these drapes are reprocessed, for their barrier effectiveness can diminish with repeated use. The manufacturer's standards in defining barrier quality and reprocessing limitations must be strictly adhered to.

Single-Use Drapes.   Since the wick phenomenon was first shown to be a potential mechanism in microbial transport and subsequent wound infection, efforts have been undertaken to improve the barrier qualities of draping materials. The evolution of synthetic, disposable draping systems has resulted in the production of soft, lint-free, nonirritating, static-free, flame-resistant, and moisture-resistant materials. Many of these disposable drapes have an inner layer of spun-bonded fibers that have been frozen and broken, resulting in a web of right-angled fibers that retard microbial migration. The outer layer of the disposable drape has properties similar to cloth. These drapes have the advantage of being lightweight, easily handled, and time-saving. Standardization of product line and consistency of packaging are additional benefits. Nonetheless, disposable drapes have disadvantages in terms of environmentally safe disposal, cost, inventory levels, and storage space.

Draping Techniques

Whether using reusable cotton drapes or disposable synthetic drapes, the RN first assistant will encounter various types of drapes. Draping is a procedure in which the RNFA must be an expert.

In draping the patient, one of the most familiar steps is applying the towel drape used to demarcate and limit the operative parameters. The conventional four-towel method uses four surgical towels placed around the operative site. These may be fully opened or folded in half lengthwise and placed next to the skin. If reusable, the towel should be secured with nonperforating towel clamps. The disposable draping towel has an adherent sticky strip for fixation.

Some surgeons prefer a plastic incise drape to the use of four towels. If a plastic incise towel drape is used, two sterile team members are required. The drape, made of impermeable polyvinyl with adhesive on one side, is carefully applied and pressed firmly into place; a sterile rolled towel or lap sponge may be used to minimize air pockets and wrinkles. These self-adhering draping materials may be used instead of the towel drape, in combination with the towel drape, as aperture drapes, or as plastic sheets. They are controversial in terms of claims for microbial inhibition. Advocates of this type of drape claim that its advantage is in preventing lateral migration of skin microorganisms. In opposition are those who claim that the heat and moisture buildup under the draped area promotes microbial growth. Some of the larger plastic drapes are available with antimicrobial agents impregnated into the drape. Plastic incise drapes are commonly used in orthopedics and implant surgery, where their usefulness is apparent in keeping the implant from any contact with skin surfaces. These drapes are also helpful in isolating surgical anatomy where a high occurrence of microorganisms is expected, such as with stomas.

Following application of towels or plastic incise drapes, a large fenestrated sheet may be applied. Fenestrated sheets are most commonly used in surgical interventions in the abdomen, chest, flank, and back. The fenestration is modified in terms of length and width to accommodate approaches to the abdomen, thyroid, breast, kidney, hip, and perineum. The fenestrated sheet is placed over the towels and incision site. The drape should be of adequate size to provide a wide margin of sterility between the operative site and surrounding unsterile areas.

Principles of Aseptic Technique in Draping

The procedure for draping the patient follows principles of basic aseptic technique. Drapes should be handled as little as possible. The sterile field should be kept in view throughout the draping procedure. The RN first assistant must protect the gown and gloves from coming in contact with unsterile, undraped areas. Maintaining an adequate distance from unsterile areas, cuffing hands with drapes, and walking around the patient rather than leaning over an unsterile area are all ways of protecting the sterile self. The drape must be controlled during the draping process by holding it in its compact shape, to prevent it from unfolding or flipping down. The drape must be carried above waist level. Once placed on the patient, the drape is unfolded from center to periphery. The edges of the drape that fall below bed level are considered unsterile. Once the drape is placed, it cannot be moved. If a sterile drape becomes unsterile, or if sterility is questionable, the drape should be replaced.

All members of the surgical team are responsible for maintaining the integrity of the sterile field during the operative procedure. The RNFA, along with circulating and scrub personnel, monitors this integrity. Movements of team members are carefully coordinated as the nursing team provides a method of confining and containing supplies and instruments used in patient care.

Basic principles of aseptic technique guide the RNFA during patient draping procedures. Knowledge of the existing body of literature regarding barrier materials is essential in product selection and application. Professional development should include both a current knowledge base and a willingness to participate in nursing research that continues to evaluate barrier materials, both reusable and disposable, and their effectiveness in reducing surgical wound infections.

▨ SUMMARY

A genuine bond of communication and caring underpins the relationship between the RNFA and the surgical patient. The patient's participation in this relationship should be active. The patient should understand, to the extent desired, the nature of perioperative events and participate with the RNFA in developing a teaching plan and meeting its objectives. Education for pain management with pharmacological and nonpharmocological therapies should routinely be included in preoperative patient education. Because infections that develop in clean surgical wounds are primarily caused by exogenous microbial sources, proper preparation of the patient's skin before the surgical incision is made is one of the most important ways to decrease infection in clean operations. The most commonly used antimicrobial agents for skin antisepsis are the iodophors. The RNFA must use a skin preparation technique that prevents chemical injury. Sterile drapes are then applied to define and maintain the sterile field during the operative procedure. Drapes should preserve their barrier characteristics, even when wet. The sterile field must be closely monitored for barrier integrity during the procedure. Prevention of surgical site infection is a multifaceted, ongoing process that requires the RNFA to pay particular attention to details of technique. The RNFA's commitment to preventing any potential adverse consequences for the patient, however, makes meticulous technique a naturalized component of skill proficiency.

▨ Review Questions

Answer questions 1 through 10 in relation to the following patient situation: Mrs. Thomas is scheduled for a modified left mastectomy. She is a morning admission. RN first assistant Hutt is meeting her for the first time to complete a perioperative assessment and begin patient education.

1. Following the assessment, RNFA Hutt begins to develop a teaching plan with Mrs. Thomas. Which of the following would be most appropriate for inclusion in the teaching plan?
    a. The possibility of a skin graft.
    b. Dimpling and nipple changes.
    c. Incisional approaches to breast lesions.
    d. Self-care measures for the incision and relief of discomfort postdischarge.

2. As RNFA Hutt is explaining the surgical skin preparation, she notices that Mrs. Thomas is clenching and unclenching a tissue and has tears in her eyes. What would RN first assistant Hutt's most appropriate response/action be at this point?
    a. Suggest that they stop the discussion for a while.

   b. Ask Mrs. Thomas to pay attention.
   c. Recognize Mrs. Thomas' apparent distress and ask if she wants to talk about what she is feeling.
   d. Simply continue with the discussion.

3. An actual nursing diagnosis represents a state that has been clinically validated by major defining characteristics. Mrs. Thomas exhibits symptoms from the emotional category. Which of the following symptoms would RNFA Hutt look for from the cognitive category?
   a. Trembling
   b. Inability to concentrate
   c. Inability to relax
   d. Self-depreciation

4. A focused assessment for the nursing diagnosis of Anxiety includes a determination of the patient's usual _____ behaviors. To do this, RNFA Hutt might ask, "How do you usually handle (the particular situation)?"
   a. Coping
   b. Lifestyle
   c. Communication
   d. Religious

5. If major defining characteristics of a nursing diagnosis are present, it is what type of nursing diagnosis?
   a. Actual
   b. Potential
   c. High risk
   d. Possible

6. An appropriate nursing intervention during patient education is to explain:
   a. The reason for, anticipated outcome, and risks involved in the surgical procedure.
   b. The type of anesthesia and the patient's ASA classification.
   c. Perioperative routines, reasons for them, and their importance.
   d. Postoperative complications and their expected incidence.

7. For Mrs. Thomas, which of the following would most likely best meet critical needs for discharge planning?
   a. Providing written materials for her to read.
   b. Continuing one-on-one encounters with RN first assistant Hutt.
   c. Receiving a referral to an assistive resource.
   d. Participating with RNFA Hutt in developing a pain management plan.

8. An expected outcome of a teaching plan for Mrs. Thomas's anxiety related to knowledge deficit of perioperative routines would be that she
   a. Has a good cry and gets it out of her system.
   b. Verbalizes her anxiety.

   c. Thanks RN first assistant Hutt for her assistance.

   d. Verbalizes anticipated routines and what to expect.

9. The use of outcome criteria and their evaluation is an indication of RNFA Hutt's

   a. Understanding of the nursing process.

   b. Accountability for patient care.

   c. Participation in medical effectiveness initiatives.

   d. Compliance with quality indicator development.

10. In collaborating with the surgeon in writing postop orders, RNFA Hutt would recommend that pain medication be administered

   a. PRN, as requested.

   b. Prior to activities such as coughing and ambulating.

   c. Via a PCA pump.

   d. Based on Mrs. Thomas's use of a pain rating scale.

11. Skin bacteria are most commonly distinguished as

   a. Resident or transient.

   b. Pathogenic or nonpathogenic.

   c. Parasitic or commensal.

   d. Endogenous or exogenous.

12. When a patient is at risk for invasion by an opportunistic or pathogenic agent from an external source, then

   a. Prophylactic antibiotics should be initiated.

   b. The nursing diagnosis of High Risk for Infection is present.

   c. Repeated preoperative showers with an antimicrobial agent are recommended.

   d. The surgery should be postponed until the patient's status improves.

13. According to AORN Recommended Practices for Patient Skin Preparation:

   a. Iodine-containing compounds are the most effective preparation agents.

   b. A paint, not a detergent, should be used if a plastic incise drape will be applied.

   c. One of the objectives is to inhibit rapid rebound growth of microbes.

   d. Soil and transient microbes should be eliminated from the dermis.

14. There is a broad body of research that indicates that hair at the operative site should

   a. Not be removed unless absolutely necessary.

   b. Be shaved as close to the time of surgery as possible.

   c. Be removed in a wide margin near the incision site with a depilatory.

   d. Be removed in the operating room after the patient is anesthetized.

15. If hair must be removed from the operative site, then
    a. A razor with a recessed blade should be used.
    b. The patient should do this in a private area.
    c. It should be done immediately before wound closure.
    d. Sterile or disinfected clippers should be used.

16. For the awake patient, the antimicrobial skin agent should be warmed
    a. In a closed container.
    b. In an open container.
    c. Only after consulting the manufacturer's recommendations.
    d. In a sterilizer.

17. To prevent chemical contact dermatitis, the RN first assistant should
    a. Place absorbent towels at the bedlines.
    b. Test for skin reaction before application.
    c. Use antimicrobial agents only on intact skin.
    d. Blot the area dry following application.

18. Which of the following agents carries a disadvantage because it develops a cumulative suppressive action after prolonged use?
    a. Alcohol
    b. Hibiclens
    c. Triclosan
    d. Betadine

19. If both a detergent and a paint are being used to prepare the skin, which is applied first?
    a. Detergent
    b. Paint
    c. The order is inconsequential.
    d. These agents should not be used in combination.

20. A general maxim for patient skin preparation is:
    a. Start at the bedline, squaring off the area to be prepped.
    b. Progress from clean to dirty.
    c. Start in the center; progress to the periphery.
    d. The 5-minute scrub should suffice.

21. Documentation of skin preparation should include:
    a. The patient's consent for hair removal.
    b. The area prepped and agent used.
    c. The skin condition before and after preparation.
    d. Both b and c.

22. When participating in the institution's selection of barrier materials, the RN first assistant should consider
    a. Recommending antiseptic-impregnated incise drapes.
    b. Delegating this purchasing decision.
    c. Environmental disposal of biohazardous waste.
    d. Conducting a survey of local community standards.

23. A prime consideration in selecting any barrier material for perioperative use is that it meet what standards?
     a. NFPA
     b. OSHA
     c. ACS
     d. CDC

24. If towel drapes do not have an adhesive backing, what should be used to secure them?
     a. Allis clamp
     b. Skin staple
     c. Nonperforating towel clamp
     d. Simple silk suture

25. Drapes should be
     a. Unfolded from periphery to center.
     b. Unfolded toward a sterile person, then away.
     c. Handled as little as possible.
     d. Replaced at frequent intervals.

Answer Key

1. d	6. c	11. a	16. c	21. d
2. c	7. b	12. b	17. a	22. c
3. b	8. d	13. c	18. c	23. a
4. a	9. b	14. a	19. a	24. c
5. a	10. d	15. d	20. b	25. c

REFERENCES

1. Miller B, Capps E: Meeting JCAHO patient-education standards. Nurs Management 28(5):55–58, 1997
2. Cassidy J, Marley RA: Preoperative assessment of the ambulatory patient. J Perianesth Nurs 11(5):334–343, 1996
3. Coenen A, Ryan P, Sutton J, Devine EC, Werley HH, Kelber S: Use of the nursing minimum data set to describe nursing interventions for select nursing diagnoses and related factors in an acute care setting. Nurs Diagn 6(3):108–114, 1995
4. Stolte KB: Wellness nursing diagnosis: Accentuating the positive. Am J Nurs 97(7):16B–16N, 1997
5. O'Halloran VE: Defining educational settings to improve client health teaching. Medsurg Nurs 6(3):130–136, 1997
6. Morse JM: The science of comforting. Reflections 22(4):6–8, 1996
7. Coenen et al, 1995, p 111
8. How to prepare your body and mind for surgery. Consumer Rep Health 9(8):85–89, 1997
9. Trimm D: Spousal coping during the surgical wait. J Perianeseth Nurs 12(3):141–145, 1997

10. Leske JS: Effects of intraoperative progress reports on anxiety levels of surgical patients' family members. Appl Nurs Res 8(4):169–173, 1995

11. Katz JR: Providing effective patient education. Am J Nurs 97(5):33–36, 1997

12. Albright J, deGuzman C, Acebo P, Paiva D, Faulkner M, Swanson J: Readability of patient education materials. Appl Nurs Res 9(2):139–143, 1996

13. Reilly P, Iezzoni LI, Phillips R, Davis RB, Tuchin LI, Calkins D: Discharge planning: Comparison of patients' and nurses' perceptions of patients following hospital discharge. Image 28(2):143–147, 1996

14. Ferrell BR: Pain management: A moral imperative. Communique 5(2):4–5, 1996–97

15. Barber D: The physiology and pharmacology of pain: A review of the opioids. J Perianesth Nurs 12(2):95–99, 1997

16. Acute Pain Management: Operative or Medical Procedures and Trauma. AHCPR publication no. 92-0032. Rockville, Md, Agency for Health Care Policy and Research, 1992

17. McCaffery M, Pasero CL: Pain ratings: The fifth vital sign. Am J Nurs 97(2):15–16, 1997

18. Smith N: Using breathing to supplement pain control. Am J Nurs 97(2):16, 1997

19. Good M: A comparison of the effects of jaw relaxation and music on postoperative pain. Nurs Res 44(1):52–57, 1995

20. Smith NK, Pasero CL, McCaffery M: Nondrug measures for painful procedures. Am J Nurs 97(8):18–19, 1997

21. Pasero CL, McCaffery M: Using balanced analgesia for postoperative pain. Am J Nurs 96(12):17, 1996

22. Association of Operating Room Nurses: Recommended Practices for Skin Preparation of Patients. In: AORN Standards, Recommended Practices, and Guidelines. Denver, Colo, Association of Operating Room Nurses, 1997, pp 253–256

23. Meyer GM: Recommendation for surgical skin preparation: An integrative review of the literature. Online Journal of Knowledge Synthesis for Nursing, 2, Document 10, Online no. 22, 1995

24. Quebbeman EJ: Preparing the operating room. In: American College of Surgeons: Care of the Surgical Patient. New York, Scientific American Medicine, 1993, Chap 5, pp 1–13

25. Groah LK: Perioperative Nursing. Stamford, Conn, Appleton & Lange, 1996, p 202

26. Masterson BJ: Skin preparation. In: Care of the Surgical Patient, New York, Scientific American Medicine, 1996, Chap 2, pp 1–9

27. Demling RH: Preoperative care. In: Way LW, ed: Current Surgical Diagnosis and Treatment. Norwalk, Conn, Appleton & Lange, 1994, pp 6–14

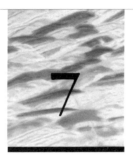

ANESTHESIA AND
PATIENT POSITIONING

JAMES E. RASINSKY D.O., M.S.W.

■

Anesthesiology is a fascinating specialty that closely coordinates pharmacology, physiology, and internal medicine. It aims, in a general sense, to provide anesthesia, analgesia, amnesia, and muscle relaxation (when appropriate) to patients undergoing surgical procedures. The anesthesia provider, whether anesthesiologist or certified registered nurse anesthetist (CRNA), also has the responsibility of monitoring the surgical patient according to guidelines established by the American Society of Anesthesiologists (ASA), which focus on circulation, oxygenation, ventilation, and temperature. This is done with the use of various monitors that have been developed over the years to ensure patient safety. Monitors also allow the anesthesia provider to observe and manipulate the surgical patient's physiological status to make it appropriate for the procedure being performed (Table 7–1).

■ EARLY HISTORY

Prior to the mid-1800s, surgery performed without anesthesia was a painful and rather barbaric affair. The risks of surgery were significant and included pain, hemorrhage, shock, and postoperative infection.[1] The administration of whiskey was one of the more common methods of providing sedation and analgesia prior to the introduction of inhalational ether by William Morton in Boston on October 16, 1846. It was within this same period of time that the anesthetic properties of chloroform and nitrous oxide were also recognized.

**T A B L E 7 – 1 . MONITORS USED IN ANESTHETIZED
SURGICAL PATIENTS**

Circulation
   Electrocardiogram
   Blood pressure (Dinemap or invasive arterial line)
   Central venous pressure
   Swan Ganz catheter (pulmonary artery occlusion pressure)
   Esophageal stethoscope
   Precordial Doppler imaging
Oxygenation
   Pulse oximetry
   Oxygen sensor (in circuit of anesthesia machine)
   Direct observation of patient color
Ventilation
   Capnometry/capnography
   Tidal volume monitor
   Esophageal stethoscope
   Precordial stethoscope
Temperature
   Esophageal stethoscope
   Skin temperature probes
Miscellaneous
   Foley catheter (measures urine output)
   Suction apparatus (measures blood loss)
   Surgical sponges (measures blood loss)

The goal of monitoring the anesthetized patient is to recognize and evaluate potential physiological problems. Standards adopted by the American Society of Anesthesiologists for intraoperative monitoring focus on the continual evaluation of the patient's oxygenation, ventilation, circulation, and temperature.

Toward the end of the 19th century, the local anesthetic properties of cocaine were discovered, followed by the description of epidural and subsequently spinal anesthesia. As time went on, the practice of anesthesia included the development and use of newer local anesthetics, opioids, volatile inhalational anesthetics, muscle relaxants, and improved methods to deliver them. The tracheal tube was introduced by Magill in 1920 for the delivery of inhalational anesthesia.[2] In 1945, tubocurarine was approved for human use, allowing the anesthesia provider to use less inhalation anesthesia, yet maintain a motionless surgical field.[3] The 1950s saw the introduction of fluroxene, halothane, halopropane, and methoxyflurane; enflurane was introduced in 1972, isoflorane in 1981, desflurane in 1992, and sevoflurane in 1995. The inhalational agents used most frequently today include nitrous oxide, halothane, isoflurane, desflurane, and sevoflurane.[4] Although the exact mechanism of action of the inhaled anesthetics is not conclusively known, they all produce unconsciousness in a dose-dependent fashion and have dose-dependent and drug-specific effects on the cardiovascular and respiratory systems. In the early 1990s, the concept of preemptive analgesia began to emerge as an area of clinical research; studies have provided good evidence that administering local anesthetics, opioids, and nonsteroidal anti-inflammatory agents before various operations can reduce pain in the postoperative period.[5] RNFAs should anticipate continued investigations of preemptive analgesia and incorporate the results of those clinical investigations into their understanding and management of pain in the surgical patient.

As a result of these rapid advancements in anesthesia, surgery has become safer and more tolerable to the patient. General, regional, and topical/local anesthesia are all employed for a range of surgical procedures, enabling the surgeon to operate while the patient remains free from pain. Standards of safety are constantly being improved, and the improvements are incorporated into the anesthesia delivery systems presently in use. Anesthesia providers are educated through residency and fellowship training for anesthesiologists and master's degree programs for CRNAs.

PRE-ANESTHESIA ASSESSMENT AND TYPES OF ANESTHESIA

Prior to the provision of any anesthetic, it is imperative to perform a preanesthesia assessment. The Joint Commission on the Accreditation of Healthcare Organizations standards require an evaluation of the patient and all pertinent data to determine the risk for and type of anesthesia while allowing time to discuss information with the patient to meet requirements for consent.[6] The history and physical examination are a good place to begin, although that may not be possible in emergency situations. In emergency situations or when the patient suffers from altered or obtunded mental status, the history is obtained from immediately available resources, such as emergency room physicians, fire rescue personnel, paramedics, family, and friends.

Past medical history, previous surgery, and previous experience with anesthesia and sedation/analgesia are an important guide in the safe delivery of anesthesia. Present medications, allergies to medications, foods, and latex, and social history (i.e., use of tobacco, alcohol, or recreational drugs) must also be obtained. If the patient has soy or egg allergies, propofol (Diprivan) should not be selected as an induction agent.[7] A focused physical assessment includes a review of the cardiac and respiratory systems, with attention paid to factors that may be associated with difficult airway management. These include previous problems with anesthesia or sedation, stridor, sleep apnea, snoring, advanced rheumatoid arthritis, significant obesity (especially involving the head and neck), a short neck, cervical spine disease or trauma, limitations in neck mobility, and neck masses, as well as an assessment of the mouth and jaw.[8]

One of the most important issues for the anesthesia provider is to determine when the patient last ate. Patients should have had no solid food intake for at least eight hours prior to elective surgery. If they have consumed any food substance within eight hours of pending surgery, including full liquids, they are considered to have "full stomachs." This will affect not only the timing of surgery but, in emergencies, how the anesthesia is conducted and possibly the type of anesthesia.

Conditions that predispose patients to the status of "full stomach" are those in which there is a decrease in gastric motililty and emptying or an increase in gastric acid secretion and volume. Pregnancy, obesity, bowel obstruction, diabetes mellitus, renal failure, head trauma, and patients admitted through the emergency room are categorically included. If a patient has been identified as a "full stomach" precaution, most anesthesia providers opt for a rapid sequence induction of general anesthesia; manual pressure is exerted against the cricoid cartilage to prevent aspiration. Atelectasis and chemical pneumonitis are the two serious complications of aspiration that affect morbidity and mortality. The rationale behind manual cricoid pressure is that the cricoid cartilage is the only tracheal cartilage that forms a complete ring around the trachea. When manual pressure is applied, it compresses the esophagus posteriorly at the level of the sixth cervical vertebral body. This prevents regurgited gastric contents from coming up to the oropharynx and rerouting back down past the epiglottis into the trachea and subsequently the lungs.

Pharmacological manipulation of gastric acidity (pH) can be performed with the use of H_2 receptor antagonists (cimetidine, ranitidine, famotidine, nizatidine) or proton pump inhibitors (omeprazole, lansoprazole). The use of oral, nonparticulate sodium citrate also decreases stomach acid content by neutralization and increasing pH. Metoclopramide and cisapride are drugs used to increase gastric motility and decrease emptying time within the gut. They also increase lower esophageal sphincter pressure, therefore minimizing regurgitation.

The ultimate object of rapid sequence induction is to preoxygenate the patient and induce general anesthesia quickly to place a cuffed endotracheal tube distal to the vocal cords. The cuff is then inflated, preventing any material in the mouth from entering the lungs.

If the patient has none of the "full stomach" considerations, induction of general anesthesia can be done without cricoid pressure in a more leisurely manner. Maintenance of general anesthesia can be performed with either inhalational or intravenous anesthetics in combination with narcotics to manage pain (Table 7–2). Pain during general anesthesia is manifested by an increased sympathetic response (i.e., increased blood pressure and heart rate).

At the end of the operation all anesthetics should be discontinued and muscle relaxation pharmacologically reversed. When the anesthesia provider determines that the patient is able to protect the airway by following commands and shows the ability to hold the head up against gravity for five sec-

T A B L E 7 – 2. ANESTHETIC DRUGS

Induction agents
  Sodium pentathol
  Thiamylal
  Propofol
  Etomidate
  Ketamine
Opioids
  Morphine
  Fentanyl
  Sufentanyl
  Alfentanyl
  Remifentanyl
Amnestics/anxiolytics
  Midazolam (Versed)
  Diazepam (Valium)
  Lorazepam (Ativan)
  Oxazepam (Serax)
  Alprazolam (Xanax)
Muscle relaxants
  Short acting
    Succinylcholine
    Mivacurium
  Intermediate acting
    Vecuronium
    Rocuronium
    Cisatracurium
    Atracurium
  Long acting
    d-Tubocurarine
    Pancuronium
    Pipercuronium
    Doxacurium
Inhalational anesthetics
  Enflurane
  Halothane
  Isoflurane
  Nitrous oxide
  Sevoflurane
  Desflurane

The dictionary definition of anesthesia (a loss of sensation) is expanded on by anesthesia providers to include blockade of sensory (minimal response to pain), reflex (cardiovascular, respiratory, and gastrointestinal reflexes), mental (sedation, amnesia, and deep sleep), and motor (muscle relaxation) functions. To achieve this desired effect, anesthesia providers use a combination of agents and techniques during general anesthesia.

onds, the patient may be safely extubated and be taken to the perianesthesia care unit (PACU). Obviously, other factors must be considered as well, such as hemodynamic stability, the absence of major acid–base disturbances, and a relative return to preoperative physiological parameters.

Regional anesthesia is just that—providing anesthesia to the specific region of the body where the operative procedure is being performed. This is done with the use of local anesthetics that are injected to provide analgesia and muscle relaxation. The injection can be made anywhere from head to toe. Retrobulbar blocks are performed for surgery to the eye just as ankle blocks can be performed for surgery to the foot. Interscalene blocks are used for shoulder surgery just as axillary blocks are used for surgery to the hand.

Epidural and spinal anesthesia are probably the best-known examples of regional anesthesia, also known as conduction anesthesia. Local anesthetic agent injected into the epidural space can provide analgesia or surgical anesthesia for labor and delivery as well as thoracic surgery and orthopedic surgery on the lower extremities. Spinal anesthesia or a subarachnoid block provides dense motor blockade as well as surgical anesthesia for urological procedures or any procedure from the perineum to the lower extremities. Epidural and spinal anesthesia are commonly used for cesarean births in obstetrics (Figures 7–1 and 7–2). Regional anesthesia is usually complemented by sedation to produce anxiolysis and amnesia. The patient's vital signs are also monitored, as in general anesthesia, and recorded on the anesthetic record.

Monitored anesthesia care or straight local anesthetic procedures involve the injection of local anesthetic agent with or without sedation, respectively. The decision is based on the extent and nature of the surgical procedure and the preference of the patient and surgeon. Local anesthetics (Table 7–3) are

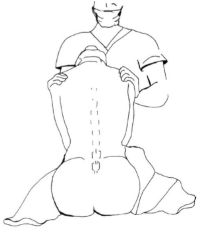

FIGURE 7–1

The patient is placed in the sitting position for induction of a subarachnoid block (spinal) or epidural catheter. The iliac crest, usually located at the level of L4, is an important landmark. The L3–4 and L4–5 interspaces are commonly used for placement of regional anesthesia. (Illustration by Ronnie Sklar.)

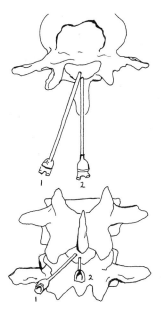

F I G U R E   7 – 2

(1) Paramedian approach for placement of subarachnoid (spinal) block. It is commonly used for patients with spondylitic changes in the vertebrae, making a midline approach difficult. (2) Midline approach for placement of spinal or epidural needle. (Illustration by Ronnie Sklar.)

T A B L E   7 – 3 . LOCAL ANESTHETICS

Amides
    Lidocaine
    Prilocaine
    Bupivicaine
    Etidocaine
    Mepivicaine
    Ropivicaine
Esters
    Cocaine
    Chloroprocaine
    Tetracaine
    Procaine
    Benzocaine

Local anesthetics block the generation and propagation of nerve impulses. The choice of a local anesthetic depends on the duration of the surgery (influences choice of short-acting, long-acting), the regional anesthetic technique used (such as subcutaneous infiltration, peripheral nerve block, central neural blockade), and the potential for local or systemic toxicity (the ester-type local anesthetics are hydrolyzed by cholinesterase enzyme and have a more rapid clearance than most amides).

often classified into three groups according to their potency and duration of action: (1) low potency and short duration (e.g., procaine, chloroprocaine), (2) moderate potency and intermediate duration (e.g., lidocaine, mepivacaine, prilocaine), and (3) high potency and long duration (e.g., tetracaine, bupivacaine, etidocaine).[9] The use of epinephrine with a local anesthetic agent prolongs the duration of effect. However, RNFAs should not use epinephrine with anesthetic agents at sites where the vascular supply distal to the site of infusion is marginal, such as the nose, toes, fingers, or external ears. RNFAs should also recognize that whenever local anesthetic agents are used, the possibility of systemic toxicity and allergic reaction exists.

■ POSTIONING THE ANESTHETIZED PATIENT

The desired outcome of patient positioning during surgery is to provide optimum exposure of the operative site to the surgical team while simultaneously preventing any potential patient complications related to the selected surgical position. The RNFA should be aware that positioning can profoundly affect the patient in many ways. Care must be taken to protect the patient and ensure that the physiological status remains as close to preoperative values as possible. Positioning is a collaborative effort by all surgical team members (i.e., the anesthesia provider, surgeon, RNFA, and circulating RN). Prevention of injury to the patient is paramount. While positioning a patient, the relationship between certain positions and risks for injuries specific to those positions must be understood. It is also important to understand the physiological changes that occur with a position change.

Injuries that can occur range from temporary to permanent. Superficial injuries to skin as well as injuries caused by stretching a nerve plexus or hyperflexion or extension of joints may not be noticed until an awake patient is evaluated in the PACU. The RNFA should remember that a patient under general anesthesia is unable to communicate that something is wrong, uncomfortable, or painful. Patients receiving a regional anesthetic with significant sedation are also unable to describe painful or uncomfortable stimuli that may accompany inappropriate or unprotected positioning.

The RNFA must take a proactive stance to ensure a patient's safety and protection. One of the first precautions is to determine that the patient is adequately secured on the operating table to prevent the patient from falling at any time during the procedure. A review of the positioned patient should include adequate padding to areas of pressure. Pressure from gravity, friction from the patient's skin rubbing against stationary surfaces, and shear forces that occur when the patient's skin remains stationary while underlying tissue shifts can combine to produce pressure ulcers.[10] Pressure necrosis can be caused by inadequate blood flow to the skin or peripheral nerves; the principal cause of peripheral nerve injuries in anesthetized patients is ischemia of the intraneural vasa nervosum.[11] Both pressure and stretching the nerve and its blood supply lead to ischemia and possibly permanent injury.

The brachial plexus is one of the most susceptible and common sites for nerve injuries in surgical patients. Its course along the axilla is superficial, and it is easily stretched if the arms are abducted greater than 90 degrees; this is exaggerated if the head is turned to the opposite side (Figure 7–3). The individual nerves of the brachial plexus may be injured when the pressure points at the elbows and wrists are inadequately padded and secured. A poorly cushioned arm can be the cause of compression injury from the sharp edges on the sides of the operating table.

Nerves to lower extremities can also be injured by inadequate padding and incorrect positioning. Stretching of the sciatic nerve or direct compression of the common peroneal nerve (at the head of the fibula) against leg supports used in the lithotomy position can easily occur. Scissoring injuries to fingers at the leg section of the table can be avoided by wrapping the digits in towels or having the arms abducted on arm boards at an angle less than 90 degrees.[12]

Position also alters pulmonary function. Adult patients can experience a decrease in functional residual capacity (FRC) by 0.5 to 1.0 liters when assuming the supine position.[13] In patients with compromised pulmonary function caused by obstructive or restrictive disease, this can cause a decrease in pulmonary reserve. If the patient is placed in a Trendelenburg position, the abdominal contents move cephalad against the diaphragm, further altering the ventilation/perfusion (V/Q) relationship.

Alteration of hemodynamic status occurs to varying degrees, depending on position. Trendelenburg or head-down positions usually increase venous return to the heart and may help to elevate blood pressure when necessary. Head-up positions produce an uphill gradient for the arterial blood supply

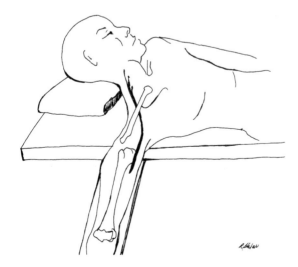

FIGURE 7–3
Stretching of the brachial plexus occurs with the arm abducted to 90 degrees or greater while the head is turned to the opposite side. These nerves (C5–T1) provide sensory and motor innervation to the upper extremity. (Illustration by Ronnie Sklar.)

and therefore may decrease blood pressure. This may be helpful in the prevention of postoperative cerebral edema following brain surgery.

The reverse Trendelenburg position enhances venous blood pooling in the lower extremities. This reduces circulating blood volume to the heart and head. Head-up positions may be helpful in determining a patient's volume status. If the head is elevated to 75 degrees for several minutes and the patient experiences an increase in heart rate with a concomitant decrease in blood pressure when compared to the supine position, the patient's circulating volume is significantly decreased. This would be considered a positive tilt test.

Supine Position

In the supine position, also known as the dorsal decubitus or dorsal recumbent position, the patient is positioned lying on the back. The arms should be abducted less than 90 degrees to prevent injury to the brachial plexus and placed on padded arm boards. If the position of the arms interferes with the comfort and position of the surgeon during the procedure, the arms can be tucked at the patient's sides. Care must be taken to ensure that the pressure points from head to toe are well padded (Figure 7–4).

Proper padding at the head improves patient comfort by preventing either hyperextension or hyperflexion of the neck. Pressure on the occiput is also prevented. The elbows must be evaluated to determine whether padding is necessary to prevent ulnar nerve compression between the ulnar groove and the side of the operating table or arm boards. If the arms are tucked at the sides or sleds are used to maintain the arms at the sides, the RNFA should also check the patient's fingers to prevent any damage that can be caused by catching them in any part of the operating table. The fingers should remain in a neutral position if possible (not hyperflexed or extended). Care should be taken to see that the wrists are also in a neutral position.

Some patients may need a pillow just above the knees, slightly flexing the hips and knees to improve the level of comfort. This position is more physio-

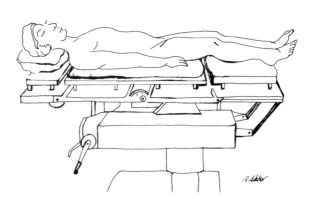

F I G U R E   7 – 4

Supine position. The patient's arms are at the sides with padding under the dorsal surface of the patient. (Illustration by Ronnie Sklar.)

logically neutral and takes extension stress off the knees. The heels are a source of pressure discomfort due to their bony prominence pressing against the operating table. Damage to the skin and pain at the heel postoperatively can be prevented by the use of foam rubber (egg crate) or other padding. The longer the procedure, the greater is the propensity for problems to arise.

In the supine position, gravity has minimal effects on circulation. Little arterial perfusion gradient is present for the upper or lower part of the body. Venous return to the heart is enhanced by chest excursion during respiration, altering intrathoracic pressures. Trendelenburg and reverse Trendelenburg positions alter these relationships and change circulatory patterns, as previously described.

Functional residual capacity is the combination of residual volume and expiratory reserve volume. This is responsible for pulmonary reserve in the anesthetized patient and acts like a spare tank to be filled with 100% oxygen by mask prior to inducing general anesthesia. In the supine position, FRC can be reduced by 500 to 1,000 cc. In patients with severe preexisting pulmonary disease (e.g., emphysema, asthma, congestive heart failure), the supine position can compromise oxygenation and ventilation.

Administration of general anesthesia with muscle relaxants inhibits excursion of the diaphragm. In the supine position, the abdominal contents then move cephalad, pressing against the diaphragm and further decreasing FRC. Relaxed chest wall muscles are overcome by the elastic recoil of the lungs, further reducing lung volumes. Positive-pressure ventilation partially reverses and improves this picture to decrease the V/Q mismatch.

Trendelenburg Position

The Trendelenburg position is a modification of the supine position, with the head down. This position is used during abdominal surgery to improve surgical access to lower abdominal viscera.[14] Improved access to the surgical field is accomplished with the help of gravity pulling the abdominal contents cephalad (Figure 7–5). The Trendelenburg position has also been used to increase blood pressure in cases of volume depletion by increasing central blood volume. Patients receiving spinal or epidural anesthesia are prone to sympathectomy and vasodilation, causing an abrupt decrease in blood pressure. This can be minimized with volume repletion, vasoconstriction, and placement in the Trendelenburg position. Trendelenburg positioning can also help facilitate the placement of a central line by increasing central venous pressure (CVP). Increased CVP helps to distend the veins to provide an easier target for the initial venipuncture.

The Trendelenburg position helps to decrease bleeding at the site of surgery. Arterial and venous pressures are decreased by gravity's effect on blood. The steeper the angle of the Trendelenburg position, the greater is the gravitational effect, increasing the gradient imposed on blood flow.

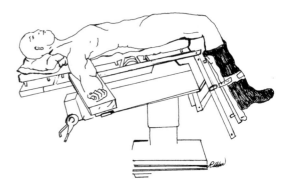

FIGURE 7-5

The OR bed is tilted head down, with a 10–15 degree tilt.
Angling the OR bed at the knees, and adding well-padded
ankle or chest restraints, maintains the position without the
use of shoulder braces. Antiembolism stockings or
sequential compression hose are often added to prevent
deep vein thrombosis. (Illustration by Ronnie Sklar.)

All pressure points must be protected as described in the section on the supine position. The operating table is tilted head down, with a 10- to 15-degree head-down tilt, rather than the former steep tilt. Angling the table downward at the knees and placing a well-padded ankle or chest restraint will maintain the patient in the tilt position without the use of shoulder braces as long as the flexed knee joint is sufficiently caudad of the leg–thigh hinge on the operating bed. This prevents the adjacent firm edge of the depressed leg section of the bed from indenting the patient's calf.

Pulmonary mechanics and the V/Q relationship are altered greatly in this position. Abdominal contents pressing against the diaphragm at the bases of the lungs decreases FRC and increases the work of breathing in a spontaneously ventilating patient. Under general anesthesia, greater positive inspiratory pressures are required during mechanical ventilation to maintain adequate tidal volume.

Blood flow to the head is also increased, raising intracranial pressure. In patients with preexisting intracranial pathology, limited surgical time is best to prevent positional sequelae. The aim is to minimize the cerebral edema that can be caused by extended placement in the head-down position.

Reverse Trendelenburg Position

The reverse Trendelenburg position is the opposite of the Trendelenburg position. The patient lies supine with the head up. All pressure point considerations are the same, and the patient must be secured on the operating table by a lightly placed, well-padded restraint across the chest. Blood flow to the head is decreased, as are central venous pressure and venous return to the heart. External pneumatic compression (EPC) sleeves or graduated compression stockings (GCS) may be used to minimize pooling of blood in the lower extremities and the potential for deep vein thrombosis (DVT). Risk factors for developing DVT and subsequent pulmonary embolism are fairly well established for surgical patients. In addtion to assessing for risk factors in the clotting cascade, the RNFA should consider recommending the use of EPC or GCS in patients who are elderly, have cancer or sepsis, are taking estrogen therapy, are immobilized, are obese, have varicose veins, have a history of cardiovascular disease, have inflammatory bowel disease, have previously had thromboembolism, or are undergoing surgery that is expected to last more than two hours.[15]

In the reverse Trendelenburg position, gravity pulls the abdominal contents away from the diaphragm and helps to improve FRC. Under general anesthesia, positive inspiratory pressures generated by the ventilator are decreased. Ventilation/perfusion relationships are closer to normal, preferentially increasing blood flow and ventilation to the base of the lungs. This position is common for laparoscopic procedures of the upper abdomen, where abdominal contents impede visualization of the surgical site.

Lithotomy Position

In the lithotomy position, the patient is supine with the legs elevated and flexed at both the hips and the knees. The legs are separated to provide surgical access to the perineum. This position is used for portions of colorectal surgery, urological procedures, gynecological procedures, and obstetrics (Figure 7–6). One of the complications that may occur perioperatively due to placement in this position is peripheral nerve damage. The sciatic nerve can be overly stretched when flexion at the hip is exaggerated and combined with extension at the knees and external rotation. This is manifested by sensory and motor deficits in the distal lower extremities below the knees.

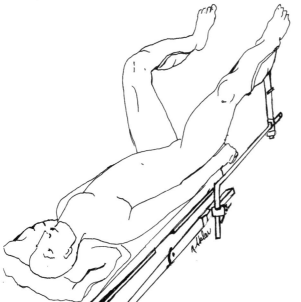

FIGURE 7–6

Lithotomy position. The patient's legs are flexed at the hips and knees. The arms can be placed across the abdomen with the elbows placed on a padded surface. The lower extremities are supported by leg supports. (Illustration by Ronnie Sklar.)

The sciatic nerve bifurcates laterally at the head of the fibula, giving rise to the common peroneal and the tibial nerves. The common peroneal nerve can be damaged by compression against leg supports that are placed lateral to the knee. Proper padding and distal placement of padded leg supports by the RNFA can help prevent such an occurrence. Common peroneal nerve damage is manifested by foot drop.

The femoral nerve, which supplies motor innervation to the anterior femoral muscles, can be damaged by hyperflexion at the hip. This can be observed when the patient loses the ability to extend at the knee or flex at the hip. Damage to its articular branches may cause sensory loss to the anteromedial portion of the distal lower extremity (calf).

Obturator nerve damage due to hyperflexion at the hip can cause deficits in abduction of the flexed thigh and lateral rotation of the extended thigh.[16]

The saphenous nerves need to be protected by adequate padding placed between the distal lower extremity and the leg braces. Sensory deficits will be obvious at points of contact on the leg where nerve compression has occurred against medially placed leg supports (Figure 7–7).

As in the supine position, FRC is reduced in the lithotomy positon. When the lithotomy position requires the thighs to be flexed onto the trunk for surgical access to the retropubic space, the abdominal contents are compressed. Diaphragmatic excursion is inhibited and pulmonary compliance is decreased, contributing to any V/Q mismatch that may already exist. Under these circumstances, the patient is usually under general anesthesia and receiving positive-pressure ventilation through a cuffed endotracheal tube.

Raising and lowering the legs alters hemodynamic status by shifting the blood volume through the effects of gravity. As the legs are raised, venous blood is preferentially shifted to the central core, increasing venous return to

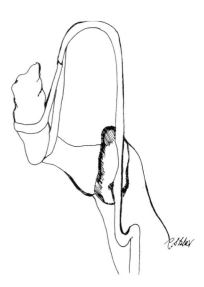

FIGURE 7–7

In the lithotomy positon the saphenous nerve is protected with padding against candy cane leg supports that have been placed medial to the lower extremity. (Illustration by Ronnie Sklar.)

the heart. Conversely, as the legs are lowered at the end of the procedure, blood shifts from the central core back to the legs. In patients who are volume depleted, hypotension can result. Volume repletion, vasoconstrictors, and a slow change in position back to supine can minimize this effect.

Leg support devices vary from ankle-strap stirrups and calf supports to total leg supports, which are preferred in longer procedures with a more exaggerated lithotomy position, such as abdominal perineal resections. During positioning it is best to raise the legs simultaneously. Care must be taken by the RNFA to secure the patient to the operating table and to protect all pressure points in both upper and lower extremities. Finger-wrapping with towels to prevent scissoring at breaks in the table, arm tucking with egg crate foam rubber padding at the elbows, or arms abducted less than 90 degrees all help to alleviate pressure and stress at vulnerable areas of the upper body.

Prone Position

The prone position, in which the patient lies face and chest down on the operating table, poses many challenges for the RNFA and the rest of the surgical team. Pressure point padding and improvement in physiological parameters must be attended to before proceeding with the surgical procedure.

With general anesthesia, the patient is intubated and the airway is secured with the patient in the supine position (usually on the transport vehicle). The anesthesia provider remains at the head of the patient, always controlling the airway. Other members of the team are positioned at the thorax, hips, and legs. The transport vehicle is locked in place. The patient is then slowly turned to the prone position in a coordinated, controlled manner, with the anesthesia provider directing the maneuver. As the patient is rolled over, he or she is simultaneously received on the far side of the table. Once the patient is prone, many things occur simultaneously.

The first, most important issue is protecting the airway. To determine that the endotracheal tube is still in place and secure, bilateral breath sounds must be auscultated and a positive end-tidal CO_2 must appear on the capnometer. The patient must then be secured to the OR bed with a gluteal safety restraint. As this is being attended to, the other team members place chest rolls on both sides of the patient that extend from the shoulders to the hips. A pillow may also be placed under the pelvis. This allows improved motion of the abdomen and anterior chest wall, improving FRC and pulmonary mechanics. The viscera can push the diaphragm in an uphill direction. Abdominal contents that may otherwise compress mesenteric and paravertebral vessels are allowed to move more freely, decreasing pressure on the inferior vena cava. Increased intra-abdominal pressure can cause increased intraoperative bleeding.

Pressure on facial structures can be relieved by placing the face down in a molded foam rubber head rest and padding the eyes. The eyes must be secured by tape or Tegaderm in the closed position to prevent corneal abrasions.

Lacrilube may also be placed in the eyes for corneal protection. Conjunctival edema secondary to the effects of gravity may be anticipated in the dependent eye. The molded foam rubber head rest alleviates pressure on the nose against the operating table. If the head is turned to the side, the ear must be checked to prevent undue compression or bending in the wrong direction.

The arms may be abducted at the patient's sides and bent at the elbows or tucked at the sides. As in all other positions, the elbows should be protected with the fingers and wrists checked to prevent hyperflexion or extension. Knees should have padding placed between them and the table while pillows are placed under the feet (Figure 7–8).

Extreme care must be taken to check and prevent compression of female breasts and male genitalia. It is easy to distort anatomy while placing the patient in the prone position. Before positioning the patient, all lines (i.e., intravenous, arterial, other monitors) must be freed to prevent tangling. As the patient is turned, the lines should be free and accessible for use by the anesthesia provider.

At the end of the procedure but before extubation, the sequence of events may occur in reverse. All lines and monitors are freed and accessible. The endotracheal tube is checked and the airway controlled by the anesthesia provider, who directs the placement of the patient into the supine position from the operating table to the locked transport vehicle. The surgical team members are on both sides of the thorax and hips with another at the feet. The patient is then carefully rolled in a coordinated fashion to the person on the far side of the locked transport vehicle, who accepts the patient. The airway is reconnected to the ventilator and bilateral breath sounds are auscultated. All pressure points are simultaneously checked. The patient may be extubated at this point if extubation criteria are met and taken to the PACU.

It should be noted that one must pay close attention to the patient's airway in the prone position. Should the endotracheal tube be dislodged and come out, it is virtually impossible to reintubate. The patient would have to be placed in either the lateral or supine position emergently to resecure the airway.

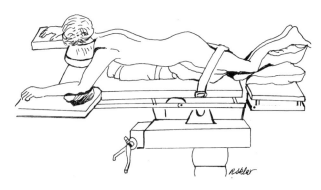

FIGURE 7–8

Prone position. The face is placed in molded foam padding to protect facial structures. The elbows are padded. Chest rolls and pelvic support improve functional residual capacity. Knees are padded and the legs are slightly flexed. (Illustration by Ronnie Sklar.)

Lateral Decubitus Position

In the lateral decubitus position the patient's left or right side is down. The position is designated by which side is down and flush against the operating table (i.e., left or right lateral decubitus position). Precautions must be taken, as in all other positions, to minimize pressure point compression and physiological changes that could compromise the patient's hemodynamic status and postoperative outcomes.

After safe anesthesia induction, the first challenge to the RNFA and the surgical team is to safely and properly reposition the supine patient. All team members work together and under the direction of the anesthesia provider, who maintains the airway and controls the patient's head. Team members assume positions on both sides of the patient while another person controls the legs.

The RNFA should place an arm under the patient's thorax while the circulating nurse simultaneously places an arm under the hips and thighs. With the legs also being controlled at the ankle, the patient is first positioned on command to the supine position, with the prospective dependent side brought to the midline of the operating table. The next step is to gently roll the patient into the lateral decubitus position, with the side at the bed's midline becoming the dependent side. This is also done on command as a coordinated effort. At this time the patient's airway is immediately checked for patency and resecured if necessary. The head is supported with padding to prevent undue flexion, extension, or side bending in either direction. The cervical spine should be aligned with the thoracic spine. The arms are placed at an angle less than 90 degrees anterior to the patient and flexed at the elbow to prevent stretching and subsequent damage to the brachial plexus. The nondependent arm may be supported by an arm support that attaches to the table or a padded Mayo stand. Either device must be sufficiently padded to prevent injury to the skin or ulnar nerve at the elbow. The dependent arm must also be protected with padding at the elbow to prevent compression of the lateral epicondyle against the operating table.

An axillary roll is placed at the dependent axilla while the RNFA and circulating nurse are positioned on both sides of the patient, gently lifting the thorax. As the airway is being securely held by the anesthesia provider, the axillary roll is placed by the fourth team member. The axillary roll slightly elevates the thorax and enhances excursion of the chest wall as well as minimizing compression on the axillary artery. It also decreases pressure and compression at the shoulder and the proximal humerus. A check of the radial pulse in the dependent arm by the RNFA will help determine if compression of the axillary artery has been alleviated (Figure 7–9).

The legs should be slightly flexed at the hips and knees with a pillow placed between the knees and ankles. The greater trochanter in the dependent femur as well as the head of the fibula in the dependent lower extremity must be padded adequately to prevent pressure necrosis of the skin and

FIGURE 7-9

Lateral decubitus position. A beanbag is placed under
the patient's dependent side to help support the patient.
An axillary roll is placed near or at the dependent axilla
to relieve pressure on the axillary artery and improve
pulmonary mechanics. Padding is also placed between
the knees. (Illustration by Ronnie Sklar.)

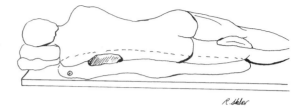

nerve damage. Damage to the common peroneal nerve, which bifurcates at
the head of the fibula, causes foot drop (inability to dorsiflex the foot at the
ankle). Egg crate foam rubber is commonly used for padding of dependent
portions of the body.

The patient must be secured to the operating table with restraints placed
across the hips or thighs. Positioning is also maintained with the use of a
"beanbag" device, which is placed on the table prior to the patient's transfer.
After the patient is positioned, the beanbag is formed around the patient and
suctioned through a special port to retain its molded position around the patient. Because the addition of a beanbag adds height to the table, care must
be taken to determine that the height of the locked transport vehicle is the
same, to facilitate safe patient transfer.

The lateral decubitus position may or may not alter hemodynamic status.
If the patient placed in the lateral position is on a level table parallel to the
floor, there will be few hemodynamic changes due to positioning. Very few
(if any) hemodynamic pressure gradients exist along the length of the body
in the long axis. It is important, though, to place pneumatic or compression
stockings on the lower extremities to minimize venous pooling. When the
kidney rest is raised for urological procedures (e.g., radical nephrectomy), the
body is also flexed laterally, which may cause increased pooling of blood in
the legs. This causes decreased venous return to the heart and may reduce
cardiac output. Therefore, these patients must have elastic or pneumatic
stockings placed on the lower extremities to decrease venous stasis and pooling and to improve venous return to the heart. Lateral flexion can decrease
venous return through the inferior vena cava.

Pulmonary relationships and mechanics are altered with the patient in the
lateral decubitus positon. The dependent hemithorax compresses the lung on
that side, decreasing FRC and chest wall compliance. At the same time, medi-
astinal structures under the influence of gravity further decrease dependent
lung volumes. Abdominal viscera press against the diaphragm in a cephalad
direction, adding to compression of the lungs. This is more of a concern in
mechanically ventilated patients than in spontaneously ventilating patients,
whose diaphragmatic movement improves the V/Q relationship.

Gravity effects on pulmonary blood flow preferentially favor the dependent (down side) lung. Less blood flows to the nondependent lung, which is
enclosed in the less restricted upper hemithorax. Chest wall compliance of

the nondependent (upper) hemithorax therefore is better, allowing more unrestricted mechanical ventilation. Ventilation/perfusion mismatch is magnified by a well-perfused dependent lung that is underventilated and an upper, nondependent lung that is better ventilated with decreased pulmonary blood flow.[17] This is most apparent in patients with pulmonary pathology, particularly those presenting for thoracotomy and subsequent lobe resections or pneumonectomies. Restraining straps should not be placed across the chest wall during nonpulmonary surgery, as this can hinder thoracic expansion, contributing to hypoventilation and hypoxemia.

Sitting Position

In the sitting position, the patient sits upright on an operating table that has been configured to resemble a chair. This position is rare in modern-day surgery but was used in the past for operations on the posterior fossa as well as for dental procedures and pneumoencephalography. The RNFA may never see this position in practice but should be aware that it may cause significant physiological changes that can have a negative impact on the patient.

Physiologically, gravity's effect on blood flow to the brain occurs by increasing the gradient against which blood must flow. As the sitting angle is increased, the gradient increases. Blood tends to pool in the lower extremities as it shifts away from the head. Baroreceptors in the carotid sinus and aortic arch sense the gravity-mediated shift of intravascular volume from the upper body and act to mediate a sympathetic increase in vascular tone while simultaneously inhibiting parasympathetic response.

Venous return to the heart decreases, as does cardiac output, despite an increase in heart rate.[18] Cardiac dysrhythmias (e.g., tachycardia, bradycardia, premature ventricular contractions) are possible during surgery, secondary to retraction on the cranial nerves. If dysrhythmia occurs, the surgeon must be notified and the dysrhythmia must be treated. Cerebral blood flow may decrease by approximately 20%, which may exacerbate preexisting cerebral pathology due to ischemia.

Pulmonary mechanics are more normal than in other positions. In the sitting position, gravity pulls the abdominal viscera downward, allowing improved excursion of the diaphragm. FRC increases, improving the V/Q relationship at the base of the lungs.

For patients undergoing neurosurgery on the posterior fossa, air embolism is potentially fatal. If the venous sinuses are opened during the procedure, air can be entrained, leading to eventual circulatory collapse. This is due to the difference between atmospheric pressure and venous pressure at the level of the head in the upright patient. Atmospheric pressure being greater than venous pressure enables air to enter the venous sinuses, which are tented open by their attachment to the cranium. The venous sinuses are not collapsible and pose a constant threat when the head is elevated above the heart. Air embolism is best monitored with the use of transeophageal echocardiography (TEE) or more commonly by a precordial Doppler monitor that is placed over the right side of the heart to listen for a "millwheel murmur."

If an air embolus is suspected during observation of monitors, unstable hemodynamic status, and a drop in end-tidal carbon dioxide levels, the surgeon must be notified immediately. At that time the surgery stops as the surgeon floods the operative site with sterile normal saline solution. The patient is simultaneously lowered to a position in which the head is at least at the level of the heart. Air should be aspirated via a central venus pressure monitor line which is placed at the junction of the superior vena cava and the right atrium prior to the beginning of surgery.

Induction of general anesthesia is conducted in the supine position and the airway is secured once the position of the endotracheal tube is confirmed. The position of the patient is then slowly changed to the head-up, sitting position in a controlled, coordinated manner with the anesthesia staff directing the action. All pressure points must be identified and adequately padded.

The head is usually placed in head pins whose frame is secured to the sides of the operating table with clamps. Padding is placed between the lower thoracic and lumbar spine, adding support to the patient at the lordotic curve. Padding is also placed under the buttocks and the plantar surfaces of the feet, which are placed against a well-padded foot rest to prevent the patient from sliding down during the surgery. The knees are slightly flexed and the legs are placed roughly at the level of the heart (Figure 7–10).

Arms should be placed across the abdomen with pads under the elbows, which rest against the back of the table. The torso should be secured with a

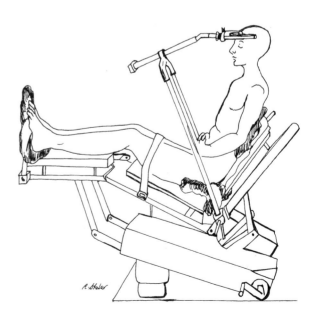

FIGURE 7–10

Sitting position. The head is secured with head pins. Padding is placed to support the lordotic curve in the spine and under the buttocks. Foot rests prevent the patient from sliding down on the operating table. (Illustration by Ronnie Sklar.)

restraining strap. Extremities at the joints should be in as neutral a position as possible to prevent injury from hyperflexion or hyperextension. Pneumatic or compression stockings should be applied to minimize venous pooling and stasis. Use of these stockings also improves venous return to the heart and therefore cardiac output.

When all these maneuvers have been completed, a final reexamination of the patient's airway, position, padding, monitors, and intravenous lines should be conducted to ensure patient safety and accessibility for the anesthesia and surgical teams.

■ SUMMARY

The practice of anesthesia developed into a distinct medical specialty beginning around the mid-1800s. Its aim is to relieve pain and awareness of the surgical procedure being performed while at the same time ensuring patient safety. In the 1990s, anesthesia providers continue to be interested in clinical investigations, innovations, and cost-effective patient management. Applications of music therapy, the nonpharmacological treatment of postoperative nausea (such as with elastic wrist bands that exert acupressure), and unexpected awareness and memory in perianesthesia patients are but a few of the topics of interest to these practitioners.[19-21]

Anesthesia training involves mastering the airway to protect the patient from aspiration and to provide controlled ventilation for procedures requiring general anesthesia. This can be accomplished by endotracheal intubation when aspiration is an issue, and with a laryngeal mask airway or face mask when aspiration is of little concern. After induction, general anesthesia can be maintained with inhalational or intravenous agents. Narcotics are given to manage intraoperative and perioperative pain and muscle relaxants are given to prevent inadvertent patient movement.

Knowledge of the patient should include medical and surgical/anesthetic history, allergies to any medications, foods, or latex, the present use of medications, and social history (i.e., the use of tobacco, alcohol, or recreational drugs). A physical examination is conducted and a determination is made that the patient's medical condition has been maximized for the planned surgical procedure. Before elective surgery, it is imperative to know when the patient last consumed solid food or full liquids; these should be restricted for at least eight hours prior to induction of anesthesia for elective surgery. If the patient is considered to have a "full stomach," a rapid sequence induction of general anesthesia is the preferred method. A regional or local anesthetic agent may be considered on its own merit or may be used to keep the patient awake and able to protect his or her own airway in urgent or emergency cases.

The RNFA should remember the following points, regardless of the procedure performed or surgical position:

1. All patient maneuvers in the operating room are a collaborative and coordinated effort.
2. Before the patient is transferred from the transport vehicle to the operating table, both vehicle and table should be locked into place to prevent the patient from falling.
3. Someone should always be on both sides of the patient during the transfer, with the transport vehicle side person bracing his or her body against the vehicle to prevent inadvertent movement. One person always receives the patient with hands on until the patient is safely positioned. The anesthesia staff control the head at all times, with a fourth person controlling the feet if necessary.
4. If an anesthetized patient is being transferred to the operating table, a secured airway is the first thing to be checked for adequacy and patency.
5. All patients must be appropriately secured to the locked operating table.
6. All monitors should be properly connected and intravenous lines clearly available to the anesthesia team.
7. Review the patient systematically from head to toe, identifying points of undue pressure or stress. Padding or repositioning may be needed to prevent skin or nerve injuries or joint stress. This may also improve physiological parameters that may have been negatively altered by position changes.

    a. Head: The occiput, eyes, ears, and nose should be checked.
    b. Neck: Neither hyperflexed nor hyperextended. No excessive side bending unless otherwise required. The cervical spine should align with the thoracic spine.
    c. Shoulders: Place an axillary roll if the patient is in a lateral position. Check the radial pulse in the dependent arm to determine patency of the axillary artery.
    d. Arms: Abducted less than 90 degrees on padded arm boards or tucked at the sides. Consider padding the elbows and wrapping the fingers. Observe wrists for hyperextension or hyperflexion.
    e. Chest: Observe chest excursion when the patient is in a lateral or prone position. Apply axillary or chest rolls where appropriate.
    f. Abdomen: Chest rolls for a prone patient help excursion of abdomen and minimize visceral compression against the diaphragm.
    g. Hips: Pad the dependent greater trochanter and coccyx as necessary. The hips should be slightly flexed when the patient is in a sitting, lateral, or supine position.
    h. Knees: Place a pillow at or between the knees. The fibular head must be padded in some lithotomy positions. The knees may be slightly flexed in some positions.
    i. Legs: Pneumatic or compression stockings may be applied, based on risk factors for DVT or anticipated physiological consequences of the surgical position.
    j. Feet: Place padding at the heels. The ankles should not be hyperflexed or hyperextended.

8. Transfer of the patient back to the transport vehicle from the operating table is a coordinated team effort. Patient care remains the same as in items 2 through 4.

This list is by no means all-inclusive but is meant to provide a framework for the RNFA. It is also important to recognize that, despite the best of efforts and diligence, a patient may suffer a nerve injury due to compression or stretching, as well as a pressure injury of the skin. Lengthy surgery with the patient remaining in one position increases the risk of damage to the skin, joints, and nerves. Preoperative patient condition and coexisting disease states may offset the best-laid plans for excellent patient care. Undernourished and cachectic patients whose dietary intake is deficient in protein are at increased risk for the development of pressure ulcers. Patients with diabetes mellitus are much more prone to the development of neuropathies than the normally healthy patient population. Not all perioperative complications are due to human error.[22] However, RNFAs who value teamwork and collaboration and who have a thorough knowledge of the principles of positioning and the equipment involved, patient assessment and identification of risk factors, and an understanding of the effects of anesthetic agents on the patient's physiological response to the surgical position will provide the patient with the greatest opportunity for a positive postoperative outcome.

▣ Review Questions

1. The injury mechanisms most likely to combine and produce a pressure ulcer are
    a. Poor nutrition, maceration, and pressure.
    b. Ischemia, stretching, and friction.
    c. External rotation, shearing, and ischemia.
    d. Friction, shearing, and pressure.

2. To recognize and evaluate potential physiologic problems, the ASA standards for intraoperative monitoring focus on
    a. Amnesia, analgesia, relaxation, and loss of sensation.
    b. Hypoxemia, fluid balance, acid–base disturbance, and dysrhythmias.
    c. Oxygenation, ventilation, circulation, and temperature.
    d. Capnography, end-tidal CO_2, FRC, and ECG.

3. The RNFA can collaborate in preventing brachial plexus injury by
    a. Modifying the straight supine position to a lawn chair position.
    b. Ssing padded wrist restraints if the arm is extended on an arm board.
    c. Pronating the palm when the arm is extended on an arm board.
    d. Ensuring that the arms are not abducted more than 90 degrees.

4. Prior to the induction of anesthesia:
    a. The patient may consume full liquids up to three hours before surgery.
    b. The patient should have no solid food intake for eight hours prior to elective surgery.
    c. The RNFA should review the past medical history and obtain consent for the type of anesthesia determined during the pre-anesthesia assessment.
    d. Patients need not be monitored for vital signs.

5. "Full stomach" precautions are taken for the following patients:
    a. Obstetric.
    b. Trauma.
    c. Insulin-dependent diabetes mellitus.
    d. Bowel obstruction.
    e. All of the above.

6. Induction of general anesthesia for patients with full stomachs includes
    a. Rapid sequence induction.
    b. The use of a laryngeal mask airway.
    c. Pretreatment with H_2 antagonists and Mylanta.
    d. Preoxygenation.
    e. Both a and d.

7. Spinal anesthesia is appropriate for
    a. Craniotomy.
    b. Shoulder surgery.
    c. Transurethral resection of the prostate.
    d. Carotid endarerectomy.
    e. All of the above.

8. The purpose of patient positioning is
    a. To make patients more comfortable for their surgery.
    b. To enhance surgical exposure.
    c. To provide easier access to the patient for the anesthesia team.
    d. To improve the patient's respiratory pattern.

9. For the supine patient, the RNFA should provide padding for the
    a. Dependent side of the patient.
    b. Occiput, ear, brachial plexus, sacrum, and heels.
    c. Shoulders, sacrum, popliteal space, elbows, and heels.
    d. Occiput, shoulders, elbows, sacrum, coccyx, and heels.

10. Damage to nerves and joints may be contributed to by
    a. The patient's preoperative medical condition and nutritional status.
    b. Hyperflexion or hyperextension at the site of injury.
    c. Inadequate padding of the nondependent greater trochanter in the lateral decubitus position.

    d. Both a and c.

    e. Both a and b.

11. The Trendelenburg position
    a. Increases venous stasis and pooling of blood in the lower extremities.
    b. Decreases venous return to the heart.
    c. Improves functional residual capacity.
    d. Can cause cerebral edema in patients with preexisting cerebral pathology.

12. Functional residual capacity increases in which position?
    a. Reverse Trendelenburg
    b. Sitting
    c. Lithotomy
    d. Prone
    e. Both a and b

13. One of the most susceptible and frequently occurring nerve injuries is to the
    a. Brachial plexus.
    b. Median nerve.
    c. Genitofemoral nerve.
    d. Posterior tibial nerve.

14. Pneumatic or compression stockings are used to
    a. Enhance blood flow to the lower extremities.
    b. Minimize pressue injuries to nerves in the legs.
    c. Decrease venous stasis and pooling of blood in the lower extremities.
    d. Enhance reduction of central blood volume.

15. In the lithotomy position
    a. Blood pressure may go down as the legs are lowered.
    b. No significant volume shifts occur.
    c. Fingers need to be protected from scissoring injury.
    d. Both a and c.
    e. Both b and c.

16. Chest rolls used in
    a. The lithotomy position enhance venous return to the heart.
    b. The prone position improve pulmonary mechanics by enhancing abdominal movement and thoracic excursion.
    c. The lateral positon are placed on the nondependent side to relieve pressure on the shoulder.
    d. The prone position relieve pressure on facial structures and improve tissue perfusion.

17. Knowledge about the patient's past medical history and preoperative physical examination

    a. Has little relevence for nurses in the perianesthesia care unit.
    b. Is important to the physicians only.
    c. Is unecessary for the anesthesia team after induction of general anesthesia.
    d. Helps in the evaluation of postoperative changes in the condition of the patient.

18. One of the most serious complications of the sitting position is
    a. Aspiration while the endotracheal tube is in place.
    b. Venous pooling and stasis in the lower extremities.
    c. Venous air embolism.
    d. Decrease in cardiac output.

19. Patients presenting for back surgery
    a. Risk dislodgment of the endotracheal tube and difficult reintubation.
    b. Must be repositioned by at least four people working as a unit.
    c. Need protection of facial structures.
    d. Need all of the above.
    e. Need none of the above.

20. Injury to patient nerves, skin, or joints
    a. Is always due to inadequate positioning or padding.
    b. May still occur, regardless of the precautions taken.
    c. Will not occur when experienced professionals are assigned to the patient.
    d. Can only occur through negligence and oversight.

Answer Key

1. d	6. e	11. d	16. b
2. c	7. c	12. e	17. d
3. d	8. b	13. a	18. c
4. b	9. d	14. c	19. d
5. e	10. e	15. d	20. b

REFERENCES

1. Calverly RK: Anesthesia as a specialty: Past, present, and future. In: Barash PG, Cullen BF, Stoelting RK, eds: Clinical Anesthesia, 2nd ed. Philadelphia, JB Lippincott, 1992, p 3
2. Stoelting RK, Miller RD: Basics of Anesthesia, 2nd ed. New York, Churchill Livingstone, 1989, p 2
3. Walker JR: Neuromuscular relaxation and reversal: An update. J of Perianesth Nurs 12(4):264–274, 1997
4. Walker JR: What is new with inhaled anesthetics: Part 2. J of Perianesth Nurs 11(6):404–409, 1996

5. Goldstein FJ: Preemptive analgesia: A research review. Medsurg Nurs 4(4): 305–308, 1995
6. Joint Commision on Accreditation of Healthcare Organizations: Joint Commission Comprehensive Accreditation Manual for Hospitals. Chicago, Joint Commission, 1996
7. Mathias JM: New anesthetics have fewer side effects. OR Manager 11(1):16–19, 1995
8. Recommendations for Safe Administration of Sedation and Analgesia (Conscious Sedation). Pittsburgh, Anesthesia Patient Safety Foundation, 1996
9. Reiling RB, Christou NV: Nonemergency surgery: Perioperative issues and postoperative care. In: American College of Surgeons: Care of the Surgical Patient. New York, Scientific American Medicine, 1997, sect V, chap 3, pp 1–10
10. McEwen DR: Intraoperative positioning of surgical patients. AORN J 63(6): 1059–1079, 1996
11. Stoelting and Miller, p 201
12. Martin JT: Patient positioning. In: Barash PG, Cullen BF, Stoelting RK, eds: Clinical Anesthesia, 2nd ed. Philadelphia, JB Lippincott, 1992, p 713
13. Benumof JL: Respiratory physiology and respiratory function during anesthesia. In: Miller RD, ed: Anesthesia, 3rd ed. New York, Churchill Livingstone, 1990, p 535
14. Willenkin RL: Management of general anesthesia. In: Miller RD, ed: Anesthesia, 3rd ed. New York, Churchill Livingstone, 1990, p 1345
15. Blondin MM, Titler MG: Deep vein thrombosis and pulmonary embolism prevention. Medsurg Nurs 5(3):205–208, 1996
16. Moore KL: Clinical Oriented Anatomy, 2nd ed. Baltimore, Williams & Wilkins, 1985, p 444
17. Benumof JL: Physiology of the lateral decubitus position, the open chest, and one lung ventilation. In: Kaplan JA, ed: Thoracic Anesthesia, 2nd ed. New York, 1991, p 202
18. Young ML: Posterior fossa anesthetic considerations. In: Cottrell JE, Smith DS, eds: Anesthesia and Neurosurgery. St Louis, Mosby, 1994, p 343
19. Eisenman A, Cohen B: Music therapy for patients undergoing regional anesthesia. AORN J 62(6):947–944, 1995
20. Ferrara-Love R, Sekeres L, Bircher NG: Nonpharmacologic treatment of postoperative nausea. J Perianesth Nurs 11(6):378–383, 1996
21. Kiviniemi K: Unexpected awareness and memory in the perianesthesia setting. J Perianesth Nurs 12(1):17–24, 1997
22. Warner MA, Warner ME, Martin JT: Ulnar neuropathy: Incidence, outcome and risk factors in sedated or anesthetized patients. Anesthesiology 81:1332–1340, 1994

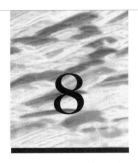

8

Principles of Tissue Handling

Rudolph C. Camishion
Arthur S. Brown

■

In the early part of the 19th century, the four most important problems confronting the surgeon were pain, hemorrhage, shock, and infection. In 1842 Crawford Long used ether as a general anesthetic to remove small skin tumors; thus began the solution to the control of pain during surgery. Treatment of hemorrhage by specific therapy had to await the development of blood typing and cross-matching in the early 20th century. Shock is still imperfectly understood. Before the time of Lister, most patients did not survive operative procedures or open traumatic wounds because of infection. With the use of carbolic acid and simple clean technique, the incidence of wound sepsis dropped precipitously. Eventually, carbolic spray was found to be unnecessary and perhaps even harmful, but better sterile technique evolved and proved to be one of the more important factors in avoiding infection. By the late 1980s, the incidence of wound infection following uncontaminated, clean operations had dropped to 1% or less.

Halsted was probably the first American physician to teach that both surgical antisepsis and gentle tissue handling during an operation helped decrease the incidence of wound infection. Adopting and amplifying Theodore Kocher's meticulous bloodless surgical techniques, Halsted developed an approach that mandates the following: tissues should be cut by scalpel or scissors whenever possible rather than bluntly dissected; with sharp dissection, less tissue is injured. Sutures are foreign bodies; the fewer left in the wound, the better. Small bleeding vessels will clot spontaneously if covered with a gauze sponge while the operation proceeds; direct pressure is an effective way to stop bleeding and to provide a clear operating field. The hemostat should clamp only the tissue to be ligated. Clamping and tying large amounts of tissue surrounding blood vessels causes excessive tissue necrosis and produces a fertile culture medium for bacterial growth. Unobliterated or undrained "dead space" in a wound quickly fills with blood or serum, inviting infection by providing bacteria with nutrient material in which to grow.

In the 1880s, when Halsted championed good surgical technique, little was known about the biology of wound healing. To practice surgery today, one must have a clear understanding of how wounds heal.

OVERVIEW OF WOUND HEALING

From the moment of injury, whether traumatically or surgically created, the body begins to repair itself. Events are taking place on a biochemical and microscopic level even though no gross changes are noted by the casual observer. Initially, capillaries dilate, with resultant increased blood flow to the injured area. Vasoactive substances (e.g., serotonin, histamine, kinins) are released to help promote this vascular response. In addition, platelets are mobilized, and the coagulation cascade is activated to promote hemostasis. Various types of white blood cells—polymorphonuclear leukocytes, monocytes, and macrophages—are also called forth to start the phagocytic process that helps clean the area of foreign matter and debris. A fibrin network is initiated, and coagulum is formed—all part of the body's means of self-preservation.

After the initial inflammatory phase, which can last up to three days or so, the second phase of wound healing begins. In this phase, the fibroblasts that have migrated into the wound start to produce collagen, the protein that gives the wound its strength. Also at this time, the squamous epithelium begins to migrate and replicate from the basal cell layer to restore the surface anatomy of the skin. Moisture, provided by damp dressings, promotes this epithelial migration and prevents dessication of these newly produced cells.

For optimal collagen synthesis, certain factors should be present in ideal concentrations. Among these are ascorbic acid (vitamin C), oxygen, zinc, amino acids, other vitamins and nutrients, and adequate blood flow. Other generalized conditions can interfere with wound healing. These conditions include malnutrition, anemia, the long-term use of anti-inflammatory medications (including corticosteroids), systemic illnesses such as malignancy, immunosuppression, and infection. Nevertheless, local factors at the wound site are considered to be more important in the overall healing process than are these other, less alterable conditions.

After the fibroblastic, scar-forming phase, which can last several weeks, the third phase of wound healing begins. Scar maturation and remodeling continue, albeit at a slow pace, for months to years. External forces, such as those provided by pressure garments, can be used to help in this remodeling phase. The maximum tensile strength of a skin and fascia wound is usually achieved at about six weeks, although this level of tissue strength never reaches that of unwounded tissue. During the remodeling phase, the wound begins to contract and reorganize along the direction of least resistance. It is necessary, therefore, to apply appropriate splints to counteract this contracting force when such forces could create scar contractures and their subsequent deformities, such as those seen over flexion creases (e.g., elbow, neck, axilla). A more detailed description of wound healing may be found in Chapter 11.

▨ PREPARATORY MANEUVERS

Despite the remarkable advances in surgical technology and scientific knowledge, there are no absolute methods at the surgeon's disposal to accelerate the orderly wound healing process. Although careful patient preparation and choice of the appropriate procedure are essential ingredients in a successful operation, a poorly prepared surgeon or assistant can nullify even the most meticulous planning and judgment. To be competent, the RN first assistant must master some basic techniques common to all operations. The RNFA's goals are to carefully consider the planned incision, to handle tissues properly, and to facilitate efficient surgery through manual and intellectual dexterity. With these competencies, iatrogenic tissue injury is reduced, fluid loss through evaporation, tissue drying, and dessication is decreased, and the amount of time the open wound is exposed to exogenous contamination is reduced. As a result, wound healing is facilitated.

Most surgeons are right-handed. Consequently, most operations have been designed to be done from the patient's right side, to facilitate use of the surgeon's right hand. The RNFA stands opposite the surgeon. Other assistants stand at the head or the foot with their bodies perpendicular to the surgeon's. Sometimes the surgeon can work better on the patient's left side—for example, during abdominal aortic surgery. Microsurgical procedures are best done with the surgeon and RNFA seated. By resting the arms on the operating table, gross motor movement can be minimized. Various magnifying devices, including flip-down loupes, lenses mounted on eyeglass frames, and operating microscopes, are available if needed.

The height of the operating table should reach the level of the surgeon's elbows; the RNFA should seek this same position in relation to the table height. This height allows the wrist to be in slight extension, the desired position of function. A table raised too high requires compensatory flexing of the wrists, elongating the long extensors and shortening the long flexors. In this position, these tendons are out of tonic balance, small muscle control in the hands is reduced, and fatigue is increased.

For an operation on a depressed body area or in the mouth or a deep cavity, the table is lowered. Lowering the field to below the surgeon's and RNFA's elbows allows the wrists to be kept relatively straight or in slight dorsal extension. This position improves dexterity and finger strength. Again, the goal is to seek a table height that does not require the wrists to be in a position of flexion.

Speed is not an essential element of good surgical technique, but it is generally true that the shorter the operating time, the better off the patient. A fast surgeon does not rush. All movements are economical and expertly made. Economy of time and motion is a principle that guides actions of both surgeon and RNFA during all phases of the surgical intervention.

Each operating room usually has two lights—one small, one large—mounted on tracks or swivels above the operating table. Because an operating room table can be moved, it is wise to check that it is centered under the lights before the patient is anesthetized. The best position for the lights is usually along the vertical axis of the patient's body—that is, one light at the head and one at the feet. Lights positioned behind the surgeon or the RNFA interfere with optimum illumination. In some instances, however, light from behind the surgeon and RNFA is preferred, as when operating within the mouth (e.g., cleft palate repair). The surgeon and the RNFA must learn to stand upright to avoid casting shadows. In cases where the incision is narrow (as in a thoracotomy) or where the structures are deep (as in an abdominal aortic aneurysm), it is wise to wear a headlight to illuminate the operating field.

■ SURGICAL APPROACHES TO THE ABDOMEN

The abdominal cavity is opened more frequently than any other area by the general surgeon. As with any incision, a primary goal for abdominal incisions is to provide safe access to underlying structures. Abdominal incisions are classified into four groups: rectus, midline, oblique, and transverse (Figure 8–1).

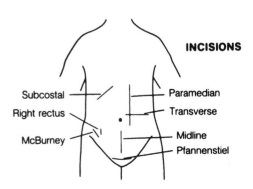

FIGURE 8–1

Incisions of the abdomen. (Source: The Lippincott Manual of Nursing Practice, 6th ed. Philadelphia, JB Lippincott, 1996.)

Rectus Incisions

Made lateral to the midline, rectus incisions can extend from above the umbilicus to the pubis. Paramedian incisions are placed at the medial rectus border; pararectus incisions, at the lateral border; and transrectus incisions, through the muscle belly. Of the three types, the paramedian approach is preferable, because it avoids nerves entering the rectus along its lateral border. Midway between the umbilicus and the pubis at the semicircular line of Douglas, the inferior epigastric artery emerges from the peritoneal cavity. Incisions through this point or excessive traction on the muscle may damage the artery, necessitating ligation. Transrectus incisions are bloodier and should be avoided when possible. Advocates of paramedian incisions believe that they produce strong incisions and scars because the wound is closed in three layers. Studies of bursting strength, not a totally reliable test, comparing paramedian to midline incisions, however, seem to indicate that the midline approach is stronger.

Standard Midline Incisions

The standard midline incision offers several advantages. It provides excellent access to all intraperitoneal structures. It is fast and requires less dissection. With one stroke of the scalpel blade above the midline, the surgeon can rapidly and safely open the abdominal cavity by incising skin, subcutaneous fat, linea alba, and peritoneum. By lifting the walls of the abdomen, the surgeon and the RNFA can extend the incision quickly under direct vision. If further exposure is needed, the midline incision can be extended as a median sternotomy in the chest. Because the linea alba contains no blood vessels or nerves above the umbilicus, the midline incision is almost bloodless and does not injure nerves. Below the umbilicus, the linea alba is a fine line and may be difficult to locate. Postoperative incisional hernias are more common above the umbilicus than below it, because the single-layer closure of the linea alba is weaker than the two-layer closure of the rectus sheath. In a review of wound dehiscence following midline laparotomy, variables significantly associated were hypoalbuminemia, anemia, malnutrition, chronic lung disease, and an emergency procedure.[1] As the frequency of the risk factors increased, so did the incidence of wound dehiscence. RNFAs may wish to consider using retention sutures for patients with three or more of these risk factors. The inexperienced surgeon has a tendency to bevel the edges of the incision around the umbilicus, which leads to ischemia of the skin. This, in turn, promotes wound infection and poor healing. By keeping the scalpel blade perpendicular to the skin at all times, this problem can be avoided.

Oblique Incisions

The most common oblique incisions are the McBurney, the Kocher, and the lower oblique incisions.

McBurney Incision. This standard appendectomy incision is made at the junction of the middle and outer thirds and at right angles to an imaginary line drawn between the anterior superior iliac crest and the umbilicus in the right lower quadrant. The incision is usually 4 to 5 inches long and is made in the direction of the fibers of the external oblique muscle. Muscle layers are split in the direction of their fibers down to the peritoneum. Splitting rather than incising muscles causes less damage and reduces postoperative incisional weakness. Use of the McBurney incision is limited to patients with appendicitis. The mobility of the skin and subcutaneous tissues in the lower quadrant allows the surgeon to place the skin incision below the bikini line. By retracting skin cephalad, the muscles overlying the appendix can be split easily. When the appendix has perforated, it is best to approach it through a McBurney incision, because the incidence of wound infection doubles if a paramedian or midline incision is used.

Kocher Incision. The Kocher, or right subcostal, incision is used to approach the gallbladder. A similar incision can be made on the left side for splenectomy. A chevron incision—right and left subcostal incisions joined across the midline—provides excellent exposure to the stomach, duodenum, pancreas, and portal structures. Oblique incisions take longer because the rectus muscle must be transected. However, they provide much better exposure to structures under the diaphragm than do midline or paramedian incisions.

Lower Oblique Incision. Long, lower abdominal oblique incisions are used in transplant, urological, and occasionally vascular surgery. These incisions require transection of the abdominal wall and flank musculature, which is best done with electrosurgery to minimize blood loss. Access to deep flank structures, including the aortic vessels, kidney, and retroperitoneal aorta, is facilitated using this approach. If needed, this incision can be extended into the chest to provide access to vessels at the hiatus of the diaphragm. The retroperitoneal approach to the abdominal aorta using this incision may result in fewer postoperative pulmonary problems.

Transverse Incisions

Like oblique incisions, transverse incisions follow Langer's lines of tension in the abdominal wall. Because they are made parallel to nerves and vessels, these structures are rarely injured. Vertical scars, such as those left by midline and paramedian incisions, stretch with time. Transverse scars usually heal with a more pleasing cosmetic result and are less conspicuous with time.

Pfannenstiel Incisions

Used most often in obstetric and gynecological surgery, the Pfannenstiel incision combines midline and transverse incisions, offering some advantages of both approaches. The skin and soft tissues are incised transversely below the bikini line, but the compartment is entered by incising the midline fascia. The end result is a strong, deep wound with a cosmetically acceptable superficial closure.

■ SHARP DISSECTION

Surgical dissection is a complex skill that cannot be learned simply by study. The wide range of tissue composition in the human body requires a variable response in selecting the most appropriate dissection technique. Dissection technique must be suited to the character of the tissue.

Dissection with the Scalpel

Of the various scalpel blades available, the general purpose no.10 and no.20 blades are used most often for skin incisions. They are designed with a wide blade and a straight cutting surface. Long skin incisions, such as an abdominal midline, are best made with the scalpel held between the thumb and the first two fingers like a violin bow (Figure 8–2). This allows the balance point to pivot on the middle finger while lateral movement is controlled by the index finger and thumb. In this position, the arm moves as a unit from the shoulder; downward pressure is controlled by using the weight of the arm. Sometimes the index finger can be placed directly on the back of the handle. By applying pressure on the top of the handle with the index finger, the depth of the incision can be varied. The scalpel handle is forced against the thenar muscles; lateral and vertical movement is controlled by the wrist.

Fine scalpel dissection depends on control by finger movement. The scalpel is held like a pencil, with the heel of the hand resting firmly on adjacent tissue for stability. One single controlled incision through the skin and subcutaneous tissues is preferred to multiple hesitation cuts. A single, smooth incision with the blade held perpendicular to the skin prevents beveled skin edges and sharply transects blood vessels, which allows them to retract effectively. When speed is mandatory, as in a ruptured abdominal aortic aneurysm or a thoracotomy for cardiac compression, this technique permits rapid, controlled entry into a body cavity.

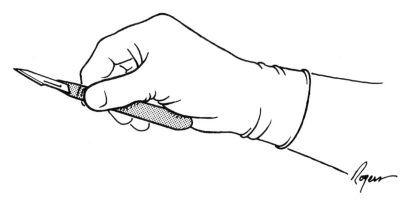

F I G U R E   8 – 2

Long skin incisions, such as the abdominal midline incision, are best made with the scalpel held between the thumb and the first two fingers like a violin bow. Holding the scalpel in this position allows the balance point to pivot on the middle finger while lateral movement is controlled by the index finger and thumb.

For small incisions in the skin or fine structures, the no.15 blade is more suitable. The smaller curve concentrates the short cutting surface at the tip of the scalpel blade. Holding the scalpel handle like a pencil, the surgeon has pinpoint control of the cutting surface.

The no.11 blade has a sharp, tapered point, making it useful for puncturing rather than incising. It is used most often for puncturing an abscess or a vessel wall. The sharp point of this blade also makes it useful for excising small skin lesions where full-thickness removal is required.

Many other blades are available for use in specialty work. Each is designed for a specific purpose.

Assisting During Scalpel Dissection. In preparation for skin incision, the RNFA should stretch and fix the skin. Sponges are useful in aiding this maneuver on a moist skin surface. Once skin tension is achieved, it should not be relaxed unless the surgeon pauses in the stroke or lifts the scalpel. As the incision is started, steadily increasing traction helps open the developing incision. Any inadvertent tightening or relaxing while the scalpel is cutting may result in a misdirected or beveled incision. A beveled skin edge results in uneven closure of skin margins and the risk of necrosis. Additionally, uneven pulling as the incision is deepened causes each sweep of the scalpel to fall in a different line, resulting in a terraced effect and subsequent poor wound healing. A long incision may require two or more resettings of the RNFA's hand to improve skin fixation. While resetting, the RNFA must be attentive to the surgeon's movements to avoid inadvertent injury from the scalpel when reaching across its path.

Scissors Dissection

Scissors come in all shapes and sizes, varying by tip (blunt or sharp), blade (straight or curved), and length. The Metzenbaum and Mayo scissors are the most commonly used types. The workhorse of the general surgeon, the Metzenbaum scissor is used for most sharp dissection. The heavier Mayo scissor is most useful in cutting through large or thick structures that would dull the Metzenbaum scissor. Both of these scissors have slightly curved tips and blades, allowing versatility in the angle of approach and the ability to lift and palpate tissue. This is not as possible with straight-tipped scissors. Although sharp dissection with a scalpel blade is an art that can be learned, many surgeons feel more comfortable using a good Metzenbaum scissor. Regardless of the instrument used, sharp dissection is preferable to blunt dissection in most situations.

Using Scissors for Dissection.   One of the first things the RNFA needs to learn about using scissors is the movement basic to all ringed instruments. By rotating the axis of the forearm, a full range of positions for the tips of the scissor is available. The RNFA's body should be turned to maintain the axial relationship between forearm and scissor. For good scissor control, the thumb and ring finger are placed through the rings, with the distal joints of the index and long fingers curling beneath the scissor's shank. This gives three points of fixation against the hand; the index and long fingers provide stability and control the direction of the tips. For extremely dense tissue, it may be necessary to extend the index finger along the shanks behind the scissor's fulcrum; the thumb comes through the ring to press down on one handle. With this grip, more downward pressure is exerted on the tips and blades while cutting.

The most natural and controlled cut is made away from oneself, from right to left. A left-to-right cut may necessitate cocking the wrist and rotating the body. Supination puts slightly more strain on fine hand control. Squeezing the blades of the scissor together will enable a clean cut to be made when the instrument is not sharp.

Accurate dissection requires exposure of the structure, good lighting, careful hemostasis, and two-point traction. One of these traction points is often a fixed feature of the anatomy, such as the adhesions between the gallbladder and liver bed. When the gallbladder is gently stretched, the liver bed becomes a fixed point. Stretching tissues allows a clean cut to be made. The anatomy should be clearly exposed to allow dissection under clear vision, which will help prevent injury to adjacent structures. The curve of the scissor follows the curve of the structure under dissection. If the structure is curved, as in a cyst, a small tunnel is created to follow the natural shape. Dissection continues one layer at a time.

Blunt dissection with the Metzenbaum scissor is used to define a natural tissue plane. Pressure is applied to the scissor's rings to keep the cutting edges firmly apposed. Only a gentle spread is needed to open space for a subsequent cut. Any forceful stretching tears adjacent vessels and structures. When the scissor is withdrawn, it is turned 90 degrees and the lower blade is inserted. With the structure held taut to ensure a clean cut, the tip is inserted only to the level of dissection; then the cut is completed in a single smooth motion.

ACCESSORIES USED IN TISSUE HANDLING

The RNFA must anticipate each step of the surgical procedure, responding to each of the surgeon's moves with the appropriate follow-up move. As the pattern of the surgeon's approach is observed, the RNFA anticipates the next move. A flowing synergy develops as move and countermove are synchronized appropriately. This occurs when the RNFA knows how to provide good exposure, how to handle tissues, and how to achieve hemostasis efficiently. A number of accessory surgical items are available to the skillful RNFA.

Retractors

Retraction should first and always be gentle to tissue. A retractor that exerts prolonged, excessive pressure destroys cells, injures small vessels, and damages nerves or other structures. A detailed discussion of retractors and retraction is presented in Chapter 9; the basic points are elucidated here. Retractors of all shapes and sizes are available for use in the operating room. Each has been designed for a specific purpose and obviously works best when used appropriately.

Deaver retractors are the most commonly used retractors in abdominal surgery. On this device, the handle is curved and constructed to be held with the hand under the handle, palm up. This keeps the tip of the retractor "toed-in" and lessens the need for strong pulling on the blade to provide retraction. The RNFA should be familiar with the various types of specialty retractors. Retractors used in a typical bowel resection include "army-navy" or small Kelly-Richardson retractors to hold back wound edges during the fascial incision. This can also be done with sponges. Once the peritoneal cavity is entered, intestines can be held down in the wound with either retractors or sponges. During closure, a flat, broad plastic wound retractor shaped like a flounder holds the intestines out of the way.

Several retraction devices that attach to the operating table are available. These have either separate, articulated metal arms or a large metal ring to hold retractors. The latter sometimes requires placement of opposing retractors to provide adequate exposure. The former, nicknamed the "iron intern," pulls against itself and can be positioned without the need for opposing forces. These devices can obviate difficult, inadequate exposure and eliminate the need for extra help. Once in place, the instruments generally do not move, unlike human assistants. The surgeon and RNFA can operate quickly without having to stop to readjust a retractor to regain exposure lost by a fatigued RNFA.

Sponges

Sponges are used (1) as padding to keep organs, usually intestine, out of the way, to protect solid organs, like the liver, from retractor injury; (2) to absorb blood, bile, and other sera that collect in the wound; and (3) as packs to provide hemostasis. Sponges should be placed, not shoved, into the wound to provide adequate retraction. The organs to be retracted are held back with the spread fingers of one hand. The opened sponge is placed over the hand with the operator's second hand or long forceps. The deep edge of the sponge is curled under the organs to be retracted at the level of the retroperitoneum. The upper edge of the sponge is tucked under the incision, between the organs and the anterior abdominal wall. Sponges placed in this way will maintain good exposure without the need for back-breaking retracting by the RNFA.

Bleeding from individual vessels or rapid, exsanguinating bleeding is best controlled by ligation. Oozing, especially in localized spaces in the retroperitoneum, can be stopped by packing moistened sponges into the area. Using dry sponges increases the risk that the adherent sponge surface will pull away freshly formed clots. The sponges should be left undisturbed for 5 to 10 minutes to allow blood in vessels to clot. Direct pressure over small areas, such as needle holes in vessels, is applied more effectively with the gloved finger without any intervening sponge. When the finger or sponge packing is withdrawn, the RNFA should be prepared to control any renewed bleeding.

During a skin incision, the assistant may place a moistened sponge against the opened ends of transected or bleeding vessels. Small clots will usually form in the ends of small vessels after 15 to 20 seconds of digital pressure. When the sponge is withdrawn, it must be done so as not to dislodge the fresh clot.

In a deep incision or recess, a sponge on a stick (a sponge grasped in a packing forceps or similar instrument) may be required to reach the vessel to apply pressure until the surgeon is ready to clamp and ligate it. The RNFA holds this stick sponge in position until the clamp is in the surgeon's hand. If necessary, the area should be cleared away by suction. When the field is clear and the surgeon ready, the stick sponge is slowly rolled off the vessel to expose it for clamping.

The RNFA may also need to remove clotted blood from a wound with a sponge. The sponge should be pressed firmly against the clot with a slight grasping or pinching movement of the fingers. The clot is then lifted away in one single motion. Heavy rubbing movements are avoided. If rebleeding occurs, or when blood is still liquid, the sponge should be used in a gentle blotting action.

A surgical procedure can be made technically easy or difficult on the basis of the incision made and retraction obtained. Occasionally, a surgeon tries to perform an operation through a poorly placed incision rather than extend it or close it and make another incision. Forceful retraction of an inadequate incision can be dangerous. The direction and force of retraction by the RNFA must be controlled by the surgeon. Care must be exercised to gain exposure without causing injury. During operations on extremities, a retractor may compress nerve against bone, causing serious injury. In the abdomen, improper retraction can tear the liver or spleen and avulse mesenteric vessels. Injury can be minimized by padding the retractor with a moistened, folded sponge. Sponges used to protect solid organs from retractor injury should be moistened and folded to double or triple thickness, then placed between the retractor blade and the organ. Improper retraction during abdominal operations can inadvertently compress the vena cava, diminishing venous return to the heart and decreasing cardiac output. In a fragile and marginally compensated patient, this could be harmful.

When the bowel must be displaced from the abdominal cavity during a procedure, the intestines must be protected. They may be wrapped with a sponge moistened in physiological saline solution, but a specially designed plastic intestinal bag is an easier and more desirable means of protection. The bag keeps the intestines together and out of the way while maintaining a humid atmosphere to prevent drying and injury to the serosal surfaces of the bowel. Bowel displaced in this way hangs over the end of the incision and is suspended by its mesentery. This impedes venous return and, if prolonged, may result in injury to the intestinal vascular supply. Frequent observation of the bowel and periodic temporary return of the bowel to the abdominal cavity will help prevent this problem.

Electrosurgery

Used properly, electrosurgery diminishes blood loss and decreases operating time. Dessication of large areas of tissue causes excessive damage and increases wound infection rates. Extensive tissue "frying" with the coagulation current set at maximum is unnecessary. Precise visualization, clamping, and electrosurgical coagulation of individual vessels is preferable. For pinpoint coagulation, short applications of high energy can be used. When blood loss must be kept at a minimum, subcutaneous tissue, fascia, muscle, and viscera can be incised with electrosurgery. Chapter 13 presents a detailed discussion of using electrosurgery to achieve hemostasis.

▓ WOUND CLOSURE

The goal of wound closure is to provide a secure, strong wound that will heal normally without infection or dehiscence and will form a cosmetically and functionally acceptable scar. Adequate preparation of the patient and surgeon to eliminate skin bacteria will reduce the incidence of wound infection. Good surgical technique is of paramount importance. A minor break, such as a torn glove, changes a clean case to a clean-contaminated case, doubling the risk of wound infection. Choice of the appropriate incision enhances wound healing. A midline incision can withstand three times the force capable of disrupting a paramedian incision. Mass closure of a midline incision has twice the bursting strength of a transverse incision or a linea alba closure.

The techniques used to close a wound depend in part on the type of wound. Most clean incisions and lacerations can be closed primarily; that is, all tissue layers are closed at the time of operation. The wound surface is quickly sealed with a coagulum that is resistant to bacterial penetration. If an abscess has been drained or if the wound is contaminated, the skin should be left open. By delaying closure for about four days, the wound is given enough time to develop resistance to infection.

The choice of materials for closing wounds is great and at times may be confusing. Should the RNFA staple, or sew, or tape, or glue? When the RNFA sews, which suture should be used? Nonabsorbable? 2-0? 4-0? Chapter 10 provides an in-depth discussion of sutures; here, we discuss only the two major classes: absorbable and nonabsorbable.

Absorbable Sutures

Absorbable sutures are natural or synthetic products that lose tensile strength in tissues within 60 days. The most traditional absorbable suture, catgut, is made from sheep submucosa. It may be treated with chromium salts to increase tensile strength and to diminish breakdown by collagenolysis. Catgut sutures are degraded by proteolytic enzymes and lose strength rapidly. Wet catgut may lose up to 30% of its strength after two hours. Compared to nonabsorbable sutures, it has less knot security, less tensile strength, and less strength retention.

Synthetic absorbable sutures are available; these include polyglycolic acid (Dexon), polydioxanone (PDS), polyglyconate (Maxon), and polyglactin 910 (Vicryl). Synthetic absorbable sutures are degraded by hydrolytic enzymes, producing only mild tissue reaction during absorption. Their tensile strength is retained for varying amounts of time.

Nonabsorbable Sutures

Nonabsorbable sutures are either natural (silk, cotton) or synthetic (nylon, Dacron, polypropylene [Prolene], wire). As a group, they are characterized by longer retention of tensile strength. Silk rapidly loses it strength after 60 days; the synthetics last longer and are not as irritating to tissue. Nylon loses only 16% of its tensile strength after 70 days, and polypropylene keeps its tensile strength for up to two years. Degradation products of both sutures may have some antibacterial properties. Nonabsorbable sutures may be monofilament or braided. Monofilament sutures are harder to handle and to tie. Braided sutures are more irritating to tissue and may trap bacteria, potentiating wound infection.

Clips, staples, tapes, and glue all can be used to close wounds. In the past, metal clips were commonly used to close head and neck incisions. They have the disadvantages of being less elastic and weaker than sutures. Instead of clips, most surgeons now use staples, which can be applied quickly, decreasing operating time. Most disposable appliers are designed to evert and appose skin edges automatically. A variety of stapling devices are available for gastrointestinal resection and anastomosis. Very adherent tapes can be used to close small wounds, particularly of the hands and face. Because they leave no needle tracks or staple puncture wounds, tape closures are the most resistant of all to infection, but most prone to wound disruption. Cyanoacrylate glues have a limited role in clinical general surgery because of their carcinogenic potential.

Selection of closure materials should be based on the state of the wound, the healing characteristics of the tissue being closed, the patient's condition, and properties of the closure material. The effects of both local and systemic factors on wound healing and the principle of delayed closure must be considered. In infected or contaminated wounds, the less suture the better. Absorbable sutures dissolve rapidly in infected wounds and should not be used. Monofilament nylon and polypropylene are the best sutures for closing contaminated wounds. Fascia and skin take longer to heal than visceral tissues; for this reason, the sutures of choice for fascial and skin closure are those that maintain their tensile strength. To avoid scarring from suture tracts, skin stitches and staples should be removed within three to five days. Because the skin wound strength is only 5% to 10% of normal at this time, the fascial and subcutaneous closures must be strong enough to support the wound. Alternatively, skin may be closed with a subcuticular absorbable suture or a pullout, nonabsorbable suture and reinforced with skin tapes.

The most common cause of wound dehiscence is faulty technique. Fascia should be closed with a nonabsorbable suture of appropriate gauge, such as a 0 or 1 nylon, placing each stitch 1.0 to 1.5 centimeters back from the wound edge and 1.0 centimeter apart. Knots tied too tightly do not allow for the normal 30% postoperative wound expansion, leading to tissue ischemia, suture pull-through, and dehiscence. Including muscle along with fascia in each stitch makes the wound stronger than does closing fascia only. A continuous or running suture closure is as good as interrupted closure and has the advantage of being faster. Too fine a suture (e.g., 4-0 instead of 0 nylon) may not be strong enough to support an abdominal wound. Damaged suture—either frayed nylon or polypropylene that has been fractured by grasping with needle holders—can break, leading to wound disruption. Monofilament sutures of nylon and polypropylene must be tied with multiple knots to prevent slippage.

Incisions in the biliary and genitourinary tracts should be closed with absorbable sutures. Nonabsorbable sutures in the common bile duct or the bladder can be a nidus for stone formation. Bowel anastomoses can be performed "by hand" with one- or two-layer closures using absorbable sutures such as catgut in the mucosal layer and nonabsorbable silk in the outer layer, or with staplers. The end-to-end stapler offers tremendous advantages over a hand anastomosis in the distal sigmoid colon and rectum, allowing the surgeon to save the anus when resecting low-lying tumors. Although the stapled anastomosis is probably no better or worse than a sewn anastomosis, it can be done faster.

The suture of choice in vascular surgery is polypropylene because of its lasting power, smoothness, strength, and especially its memory. Each stitch can be placed under direct vision in small, recessed vessels by leaving big loops of suture. On completion of the anastomosis, the entire suture can be pulled up and tied.

DRAINS

Drains are never a substitute for hemostasis or a replacement for meticulous technique. The drain material should be soft, nonirritating to tissue, firm enough to remain in the intended place, resistant to decomposing, and smooth for easy removal. Careful choice, placement, and care of drains are needed. Superficial wounds ordinarily do not need to be drained. In fact, the drain may provide a route for bacteria to gain access to the subcutaneous tissues. Subcutaneous tissues are particularly vulnerable to infection because fat is relatively avascular. If a drain is needed, one that can be attached to a source of suction in a closed system is preferred to one that drains passively.

Drains within the abdominal cavity are placed either for localized infection, such as an abscess cavity, or to drain raw surfaces that may slowly bleed or leak other types of fluid. Placing multiple drains throughout the abdominal cavity in an attempt to drain generalized peritonitis has been proved to be of little value. The drains quickly become isolated from the peritoneal cavity by the bowel and omentum and thus fail to achieve their goal.

When the RNFA is placing a drain, the shortest, most direct route to the skin is selected. The stab wound should be just large enough for unobstructed passage of the drain. Placing the stab wound separate from the main incision prevents its potential contamination. The drain is sutured to the skin at the egress site. When the drain is dressed, gauze is first applied, then the drain is taped in such a way that the tape can be removed without pulling the drain.

DRESSINGS

With so many products on the market for dressing the wound, choosing the best one for a specific wound can be difficult. The RNFA should base his or her decision on an assessment of the patient's general health status as well as the type of wound. Surgical wounds may be broadly classified as nondraining and draining. The nondraining wound includes most approximated surgical incision sites. For this type of wound, the RNFA should select a dressing that provides an optimal environment for epithelial migration at the wound edges and minimizes the likelihood of wound disruption. Draining wounds, where heavy serosanguineous or enzymatic drainage is present, require a dressing that minimizes tissue maceration.

The primary function of a surgical dressing is to protect the wound surface from exogenous contamination before reepithelialization occurs, thus providing an optimum environment for wound repair. In general, the RNFA evaluates and selects a product that supports moist wound healing; this environment enhances angiogenesis (the process of new capillary formation) and cellular tissue repair as well as epithelial cell migration. The product should not be traumatic to healthy granulation tissue or periwound tissue, should be comfortable and reduce or eliminate pain during dressing changes, and should be as easy as possible to apply during recovery at home.[2] Occlusive dressings, traditionally consisting of gauze dressings held in place with tape, are more commonly achieved today by application of a transparent, semipermeable film. More appropriately termed semiocclusive, this film is waterproof yet allows the skin to breathe because the film is permeable to water vapor and oxygen, while still provding a barrier to bacteria and contamination.[3] With this type of dressing, the RNFA can inspect the wound without dressing removal. The film prevents wound dehydration; a moist rather than dry environment is more conducive to reepithelialization. Before a semipermeable film dressing is applied, the wound and surrounding skin should be as clean as possible. This may be done by first swabbing the wound, then using a fresh swab with an iodophor for the surrounding area. A 70% alcohol swab can be used to remove excess iodophor solution. When the surface is dry, the dressing is applied. These dressings are intended for long-term application. However, excessive or prolonged accumulation of serum beneath the dressing surface must be avoided. This dressing is not recommended for infected wounds. The moist physiological environment, usually desirable for epidermal regeneration, would provide a growth medium for pathogens in an infected wound.

Highly absorbent, nonocclusive dressings are also used for nondraining wounds. After the wound is cleaned, a nonadhering dressing is applied. If light to medium drainage is anticipated, an impregnated gauze dressing is placed first, followed by general use dressing sponges.

Draining wounds require a dressing that will keep wound exudate from healthy skin. A nonadherent dressing is applied directly to the skin in a single layer, followed by a layer of general use dressing sponges to wick exudate. This may be covered with a secondary layer of dressings, added to absorb and contain drainage.

■ TRAUMATIC WOUNDS

The RNFA who works in collaboration with a physician or group practice may be called to assist with injured patients. Before closing any traumatic wound in an emergency department, several questions must be answered.

How long has it been since the time of injury? What was the nature of the wounding implement? Where is the wound located? What is the patient's overall condition? The longer the time between injury and wound closure, the greater the likelihood of bacterial infection. For most clean wounds, primary closure can be done safely six to eight hours after injury. This safe period can be extended several hours by using debridement and prophylactic antibiotics in some wounds. Unfortunately, there are no absolutes in dealing with the safety of wound closure, because the development of wound infection depends more on the total wound bacteria count than on time. Whenever there is any doubt about the safety of primary closure, the wound should be left open to heal by secondary intention.

Scalpel blades produce clean lacerations that can be closed primarily. Blunt trauma, such as that which occurs when the head strikes a dashboard, produces stellate laceration. This type of compression injury breaks the skin open and disrupts surrounding tissues, making them ischemic. Devitalized tissue provides an anaerobic culture medium that inhibits phagocytosis, thereby enhancing bacterial growth. Wounds contaminated with feces, saliva, soil, or clothing particles are more susceptible to infection. Before crush wounds or contaminated wounds are closed, all dead tissue must be debrided and all foreign matter removed.

Mechanical cleansing of contaminated wounds can decrease the incidence of infection. Simple flooding of the wound with saline or antibiotic-containing solutions is inadequate. Vigorous scrubbing of the wound with a surgical brush may lead to further damage. High-pressure irrigation that mechanically disrupts bacteria from the tissue surface can decrease bacterial wound counts to safe levels. The pressure exerted by saline squirted from a 35 milliliter syringe through an 18-gauge needle is sufficient to clean most small wounds. Extensive wound irrigation is more easily accomplished with a pulsating device, such as a Water-Pik. It is not necessary—and in fact may be harmful—to add an antibiotic agent to the cleansing solution. High concentrations of povidone iodine or hydrogen peroxide solutions kill human cells by damaging the fibroblasts that synthesize collagen for wound repair, as well as bacterial cells.[4] Neomycin, kanamycin, and similar antibiotics can be absorbed in large amounts from the wound, leading to renal and auditory impairment and respiratory depression. A nontoxic surfactant, such as Pluronic F–68, can help loosen bacteria from wound surfaces.

■ SUMMARY

The RNFA can have a major effect on the outcome of a surgical procedure. By understanding essential principles, the RNFA can be of immeasurable help in promoting a favorable result. Measures of wound care outcomes include wound healing, relief of discomfort, prevention of infection, and quality of life measures such as return to normal activity and functions.[5] Wound management, although the direct responsibility of the operating surgeon, is enhanced by the collaboration of a knowledgeable RNFA. The collegial relationship between surgeon and RNFA is initiated based on shared knowledge and complementary skills. As these are elucidated in patient care activities, mutuality and respect develop. Understanding the rationale for a particular surgical approach, implementing principles of tissue handling, and participating in the selection of a skin closure material are all characteristic activities of an RNFA whose contribution to patient care is marked by excellence.

Review Questions

1. Halsted developed an approach to tissue handling that suggests which of the following? (Circle all that are correct.)
   a. Sharp dissection is preferred over blunt dissection.
   b. The fewer sutures left in a wound, the more chance for wound disruption.
   c. Small vessels will clot with direct pressure.
   d. The hemostat should clamp the vessel and an adequate margin of surrounding tissue.
   e. Dead space invites infection.

2. In the inflammatory phase of wound healing, the vascular response is
   a. Vasoconstriction.
   b. Vessel retraction.
   c. Vasospasm.
   d. Vasodilation.

3. During a preoperative nutritional assessment, the RNFA will assess the patient's dietary intake of which important nutrient for wound healing?
   a. Vitamin K
   b. Vitamin E
   c. Vitamin C
   d. Fiber

Fill in the blanks in the following questions regarding surgical technique.

4. The height of the operating room table should reach the level of the RNFA's _____.

5. The desired position of the wrist of an assistant is slight _____.

6. If the operating room table is too high, the extensors are _____ and the flexors are _____, which reduces small muscle control and increases fatigue.

7. In general, lights positioned behind the surgeon or assistant _____ optimum illumination.

8. Lateral and vertical movement of the scalpel is controlled by the _____.

9. To prevent beveled edges, the scalpel blade should be held _____ to the skin.

10. In preparation for the skin incision, the RNFA should _____ and _____ the skin.

11. As the skin incision is started, the RNFA can _____ traction to assist in opening the developing incision.

12. During scissors dissection, the most natural and controlled cut is achieved when it is made _____ from oneself.

13. Holding a Deaver retractor with the hand under the handle, palm up, keeps the tip of the retractor _____, lessening the need for strong pulling.

14. To remove clotted blood from a wound with a sponge, the RNFA presses firmly against the clot with a slight grasping or pinching motion and _____ the clot away.

15. Placing a stab wound for drain insertion should be done _____ from the main incision.

16. _____ dressings are waterproof yet allow the skin to "breathe."

17. Mechanical cleansing of contaminated wounds can _____ the incidence of infection.

Answer the following questions about surgical incisions.

18. The _____ approach is preferable among the pararectus, paramedian, and transrectus, since it avoids nerves entering the rectus along its lateral border.

19. _____ rather than incising muscles causes less damage and reduces postoperative incisional weakness.

20. Following _____ in the abdominal wall assists in preventing injury to the vessels and nerves that run parallel to them.

Answer Key

1. a, c, e
2. d
3. c
4. elbows
5. extension
6. elongated, shortened
7. interfere with
8. wrist
9. perpendicular
10. stretch, fix

11. increase
12. away
13. toed-in
14. lifts
15. separate
16. Semipermeable or semiocclusive
17. decrease
18. paramedian
19. Splitting
20. Langer's lines

REFERENCES

1. Makela JT, Kiviniemi H, Juvonen T, Laitinen S: Factors influencing wound dehiscence after midline laparotomy. Am J Surg 170:387–389, 1995
2. Hahn JF, Olsen CL: Wounds: Nursing care and product selection. Nurs Spectrum 3(22):12–13, 1994
3. Tallon RW: Wound care dressings. Nurs Management 27(10):68–70, 1996
4. Schumann D: Reducing post critical care infection. Medsurg Nurs 5(3):169–176, 1996
5. Bolton LL, Rijswijk LV, Shaffer FA: Quality wound care equals cost-effective wound care. Nurs Management 27(7):30–37, 1996

PROVIDING EXPOSURE: RETRACTORS AND RETRACTION

NANCY B. DAVIS

■

The Association of Operating Room Nurses (AORN) Official Statement on RN First Assistant states that "the RN first assistant at surgery collaborates with the surgeon in performing a safe operation with optimal outcomes for the patient."[1] A major function of the RNFA is to provide exposure of the operative site.

Exposure is necessary for visualization of organs and tissues that are being inspected, dissected, repaired, or sutured. It is also necessary to prevent injury to tissues and other structures that are adjacent or close to the operative area by retracting them out of harm's way. Providing physical safety for the patient during the intraoperative period is essential and must involve all members of the surgical team.

■ NURSING DIAGNOSIS: PREVENTING INJURY

A judgment made by the RNFA related to the patient's problems, potential problems, needs, or health status is stated as a nursing diagnosis. When the RNFA determines that retraction will be necessary during the operative procedure, the nursing diagnosis could be stated as "High Risk for Injury (trauma) related to retraction of tissues during the operative procedure." A high risk for injury exists when the patient is at risk for harm; the risk factor in this nursing diagnosis is situational. The surgery and its required tissue manipulation pose hazards for which nursing intervention is required. In planning and implementing intraoperative care, the desired outcome is that the patient will be

201

free from injury. For outcome achievement, the RNFA must implement appropriate first assistant measures to protect the patient from known, possible injuries. This outcome would relate to AORN's Patient Outcomes: Standards for Perioperative Care, which state that the patient is free from signs and symptoms of physical injury and injury due to extraneous objects.[2] It is the RNFA's ethical responsibility to safeguard and promote the health, well-being, and safety of the patient.[3]

Standards of Care

For perioperative patients, there are a number of predicted care regimens indicated for specific situations. When such a nursing situation occurs, standards of care can be developed that contain detailed guidelines representing the predicted care required. The RNFA can participate in developing a set of problems, either actual or high risk, that typically occur during the intraoperative phase of first assisting. The associated standards represent the level of care the RNFA is responsible for providing. When the standards are designed to represent the predicted generic care for all intraoperative patients who receive care from an RNFA, they can become part of the perioperative nursing unit's standards of care. Because they apply to all patients receiving care from an RNFA during the intraoperative period, they do not need to be written on each patient's care plan. Instead, institutional policy can specify that the generic standard will be implemented for all perioperative patients. The prevention of injury during tissue retraction and the other potentially injurious perioperative patient care situations requiring nursing intervention by the RNFA should be part of the generic standards of care.

Providing exposure of the operative site is usually the first function that the RNFA performs. An experienced assistant makes this activity appear easy. The necessary skill and judgment needed for providing exposure are based on knowledge, which is why the AORN Recommended Education Standards for RN First Assistant Programs require formal education with structured didactic and clinical learning activities that prepare the RNFA with the necessary cognitive and psychomotor behaviors.[4] The assistant must be knowledgeable regarding the operative procedure and the potential injury to tissues and their underlying and surrounding structures. Proper selection and performance of exposure methods is essential. As the assistant becomes more skilled at providing exposure, the surgeon provides less direction to the assistant. Protecting the patient from injury becomes the standard of care and part of the quality improvement program.

Unfortunately, because the act of providing exposure may appear easy or be viewed as a simple task requiring "an extra pair of hands" that are positioned by the surgeon, some institutions may permit the use of unlicensed assistive personnel to act as "retractor holders." As teaching programs downsize their surgical residency slots so that fewer residents are available to assist in surgery, this "retractor holder" may appear even more utilitarian.[5] However, institutions cannot ignore their corporate liability, part of which is ensuring that there are adequate numbers of perioperative personnel with appropriate training to carry out the tasks they are assigned. In 1997, a verdict against a hospital clearly upheld this legal accountability on the part of an employer. In this case, a surgical technician was allowed to hold retractors during a pediatric hip arthroplasty. The technician was not trained for this procedure and was unaware of the risk of damaging the sciatic nerve resulting from a slight deviation from the surgeon's positioning of the retractor. The verdict against the hospital was in excess of $800,000; the court held that there was a necessity for surgical personnel to have specific training in the tasks and procedures they performed.[6] Thus, protecting the patient from injury is not only a standard of care, it is also part of the institution's legal accountability.

METHODS OF PROVIDING EXPOSURE

The most common method of providing exposure is by using retraction instruments. Other methods include using grasping instruments, sponges, sutures, tapes, Penrose drains, vessel loops, suctioning, the assistant's hands, or plastic bags.

When choosing the method of providing exposure, the RNFA must consider several factors. The major factors are the operative procedure and the stage of the operation. Physical characteristics of the patient that are considered include the patient's age, height, weight, body build, and any physical deformities or limitations. Also, the type of tissue and the location of vascular or nerve structures, as well as the presence of organs, must always be evaluated in relation to the exposure method used.

Traction on tissues is the mechanism that provides exposure. If traction is inadequate, then the operative site will be poorly exposed, which will impede the surgeon. Excessive traction could result in injury related to lacerations or pressure. The assistant must observe the operative site at all times to ensure effective exposure and prevent unnecessary tissue injury. Knowledge of how to provide the correct amount of traction is acquired through an understanding of surgical anatomy and an appreciation of the fragility of tissue structures.

Retractors

Retractors are instruments designed specifically for holding tissues or organs out of the surgeon's field of vision during the operative procedure. Many retractors are intended for use only in selected operative procedures; other retractors are more versatile and can be used for many different procedures.

Selection of a retractor is based on several factors, including:

- the operative procedure
- the stage of the operative procedure
- the tissues or organs being retracted
- the complexity of the operative procedure
- the length and depth of the wound
- the time necessary to perform the operation
- the amount of force (effort) needed to provide exposure.

Retractors are of two basic types: hand-held and self-retaining. Retractors come in several designs and may be sharp or blunt; large or small; flat, round, or curved; wide or narrow; short or long; malleable, hinged, or fixed; straight or angled; and composed of one solid piece or several parts. The assistant must know the types of retractors available, the name of each retractor, and how to use each retractor.

Hand-Held Retractors.   As the name implies, hand-held retractors are held continuously by the assistant during use. This is the major disadvantage of this type of retractor, because the assistant's hand or hands are not available to provide other assistance during the operation. In certain operations this may not be a problem, because the surgeon may need a minimal amount of assistance during the procedure. But in more complex operations, if the assistant is holding a retractor, more than one assistant may be needed for safe and efficient execution of the surgical intervention.

Nevertheless, the hand-held retractor has several advantages. It can be more quickly positioned, repositioned, and removed. It allows the alert RNFA to instinctively vary retractor position to provide more exposure or to let up on the pressure when the harder pull is no longer necessary. The amount of traction placed on the tissues can be altered as necessary, which allows the tissue beneath the retractor to get oxygen and nutrients to its capillary network. For very fragile tissue, the hand-held retractor may be essential to prevent injury. If access to the tissue needing retracting is difficult, a hand-held retractor may be the retractor of choice.

Hand-held retractors may be designed with or without handles. The handle is designed to provide the assistant with a firmer grip, but many are not designed for comfort. The handle may be round or flat and may have finger notches, rings, or curves (Figure 9–1). A flat handle is hard to hold for long periods. Retractors without handles usually have straight shafts that may have a different retracting surface at each end (Figure 9–2). Malleable retractors (ribbons) are flexible and may be bent into various angles. They are available in different lengths and widths (Figure 9–3). These are versatile retractors: in addition to retracting where a unique angle is needed, they can help hold in and protect the viscera during abdominal closure.

Retractors designed with prongs are usually used for retraction of shallow tissues, such as the skin or subcutaneous tissue. The prongs may be sharp or

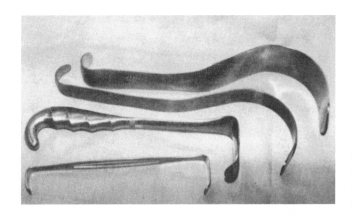

FIGURE 9–1

Examples of hand-held retractors. *Top to bottom:* two Deavers, Richardson, and army-navy.

dull, and there may be one prong or several (Figure 9–4). Sharp prongs cause more tissue trauma but hold better. The assistant must be careful when using the sharp-pronged retractor as it can easily puncture gloves or tissues, such as the bowel or blood vessels. For this reason, blunt prongs are preferred whenever possible.[7]

When placing the retractor, the RNFA must take care not to injure nerves, organs, or vascular structures. Circulation to the tissues should not be compromised. Pinching of tissues or organs can occur if the retractor is placed improperly. Underlying structures should be protected from excessive pressure or tension that could result in tissue damage.

The RNFA should hold the retractor in a position that causes the least amount of discomfort, strain, or fatigue. If the RNFA is retracting laterally or away from himself or herself, the retractor should rest comfortably in the hand with the palm supine and the arm flexed at the elbow (Figure 9–5). When retracting toward himself or herself, the RNFA is more comfortable holding the retractor with the palm in the prone position or toward himself or herself (Figure 9–6). The retractor should not be gripped any harder than necessary, because this only increases hand fatigue. It is important not to lean or rest the arm on the patient, as this could cause pressure injury to soft tis-

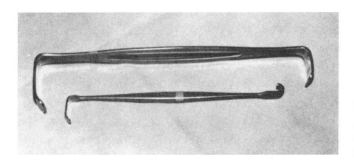

FIGURE 9–2

Hand-held retractors with different retracting surfaces at each end. *Top,* army-navy; *bottom,* Senn.

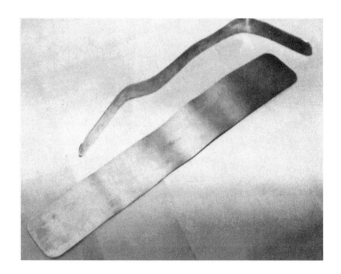

FIGURE 9–3
Malleable retractors. Note bend in narrow retractor.

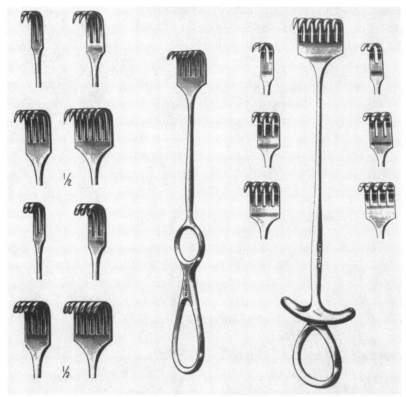

FIGURE 9–4
Rake retractors. *Left,* Volkman retractor; *right,* Murphy retractor. (Source: Smith EJ, Smith YR: Smiths' Reference and Illustrated Guide to Surgical Instruments. Philadelphia, JB Lippincott, 1983, pp 633, 646.)

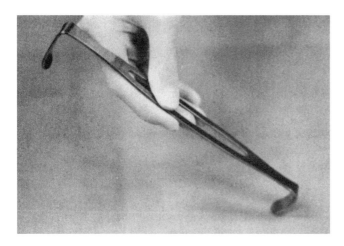

FIGURE 9–5
Position for holding retractor when retracting laterally or away from self.

sues or even interfere with respiration and circulation. The RNFA's hand should not obstruct the surgeon's view.

The pull on the retractor should provide adequate exposure of the operative field without distorting tissues that are being dissected or sutured by the surgeon. Excessive pulling on the retractor could result in tissue laceration or slipping of the retractor from the incision. Inadequate pulling results in poor

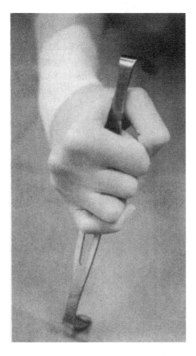

FIGURE 9–6
Position for holding retractor when retracting toward self.

exposure and may allow retracted tissues to slip into the field and obstruct the surgeon's visualization. The RNFA must observe the effect of the retraction and alert the surgeon if the retractor or tissues are slipping so that the retractor may be readjusted. The RNFA may tire with long or difficult retracting, and must advise the surgeon when this is occurring.

Self-Retaining Retractors.   The self-retaining retractor is designed to provide continuous and unchanging retraction of tissues. Once placed, this retractor does not need to be held, thereby freeing the RNFA's hands for other activities. Various self-retaining retractors are available, and the RNFA needs to be familiar with the commonly used ones. Some retractors are versatile; others are designed for a specific operative procedure. Self-retaining retractors are especially useful during long operations and are essential when much effort is needed to provide retraction (e.g., during thoracotomy).

Self-retaining retractors are more complex than hand-held retractors. Such a retractor may be designed as a frame with fixed blades or prongs (Figure 9–7), or the retracting surfaces may be detachable, with several variations available (Figure 9–8). The retracting blades or prongs may vary in width, depth, and angulation. The mechanical components of the retractor may include ratchets, springs, cranks, or nuts that open the retractor and hold it in the open position. Any removable parts must be accounted for and included in the formal instrument count.

Good visualization is necessary when placing the retractor. Care must be taken not to injure nerves, vascular structures, organs, or tissues by accidentally pinching them in or under the retracting surfaces or mechanisms. It is often necessary to protect the wound edges from the retractor blades by padding with a sponge. Moistening the sponge with warm saline solution can prevent drying of the tissues, tissue friction, and abrasion. The RNFA should keep in mind that the greater the exposure and the longer the procedure, the

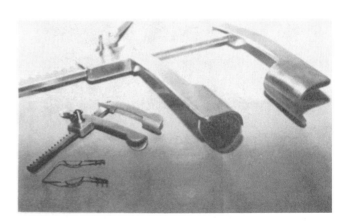

FIGURE 9–7

Examples of self-retaining retractors. *Left to right:* Parsonnet epicardial retractor, pediatric Cooley sternal retractor, and adult Cooley sternal retractor.

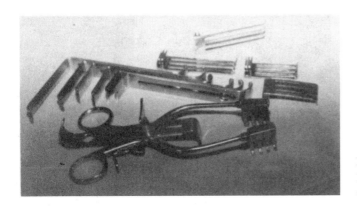

FIGURE 9 – 8

Henly retractor with various blades for altering depth of retraction.

more fluid loss and tissue dessication occur. The need to use and replace warm, moist pads is determined by these factors.

The retractor should be opened carefully and under direct visualization. It may be necessary to hold the wound edges in the retractor blades while opening the retractor to prevent slipping. With self-retaining abdominal wall retractors, the RNFA should keep a hand over each blade to avoid trapping viscera between the blade and the abdominal wall as the retractor is being opened. In operative procedures where retraction requires increased force, the retractor should be opened slowly and possibly in stages. The retractor should not be overexpanded, which will cause excessive pulling on tissues and, possibly, tearing lacerations. For extremely lengthy operations, the self-retaining retractor should be removed periodically to prevent ischemic injury to the wound edges.

Grasping Instruments

Several instruments may be used to provide a secure hold on tissues so that traction can be applied, thereby providing exposure. Grasping instruments cause varying degrees of tissue damage, depending on the type of tissue grasped, the instrument being used, how the instrument is applied to the tissue, and the amount of traction exerted on the tissue. Judgments made by the RNFA when using grasping instruments are based on knowledge and experience.

Tissue Forceps. Tissue forceps are instruments that provide an extension of the thumb and fingers for pinching-like action. Forceps are some of the most commonly used surgical instruments, and the RNFA must be skilled in using them with either hand. They are quick and easy to use once the skill has been acquired.

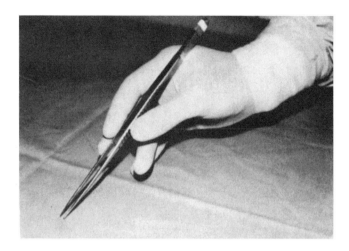

FIGURE 9–9
Position for holding tissue forceps (opened).

The forceps is held like a pencil (Figure 9–9), and the tips are forced together by applying pressure with the thumb and fingers (Figure 9–10). Grasping pressure must be sufficient to provide a secure hold with minimal damage to the tissues. With tissue forceps, pressure can be altered easily and with more precision than with a clamping type of instrument.

The tissue forceps is basically two blades joined at one end that spring apart at the other. The blades do not lock. The most commonly used forceps are straight, but they vary in length, width, and tip design. Some forceps are very delicate; others are bulky. Each forceps is designed for use on specific types of tissues, and the assistant must know which forceps is to be used where. Toothed forceps may have one tooth or several teeth at the tip. The teeth may be fine or heavy (Figure 9–11). Forceps without teeth, called "smooth forceps," are used to grasp tissues that might be easily perforated or torn, such as bowel.

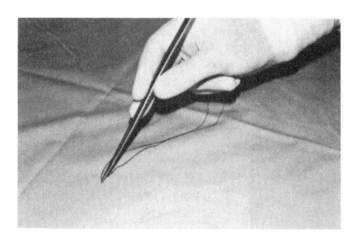

FIGURE 9–10
Tissue forceps closed, grasping suture ligature.

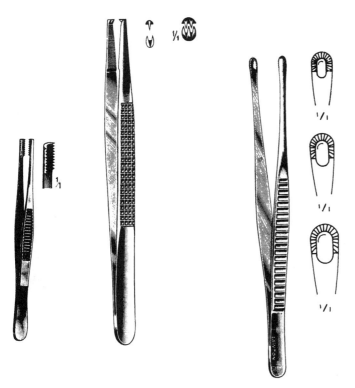

FIGURE 9–11

Examples of toothed tissue forceps. *Left,* Brown; *center,* Bonney; *right,* Russian. (Source Smith EJ, Smith YR: Smiths' Reference and Illustrated Guide to Surgical Instruments. Philadelphia, JB Lippincott, 1983, pp 183, 188, 350.)

Smooth forceps are also useful for holding gauze sponges, because the gauze material will not become caught in the tips (Figure 9–12).

When tissue forceps are used, tissue should not be held any longer or more firmly than necessary because this increases the damage to the tissues. The amount of traction used when holding tissue with the forceps must be appropriate for the type of tissue. If the traction is too great, the tissue may tear or the forceps may slip. The RNFA should carefully inspect the forceps to ensure that the tips meet correctly and that there are no barbs or hooks that could injure tissue.

Clamps. Several types of clamps are used to grasp tissue. These clamps are available in various lengths and may be straight, curved, or angled. They have ringed handles and ratcheted boxlocks to secure their grasp. Clamp structure varies from delicate to heavy, and the jaws may be smooth or serrated. The tip of the clamp may be fine, pointed, rounded, blunt, or triangular, or it may have interlocking teeth.

Delicate clamps cause less trauma to the tissues and are used for soft or fragile tissue, such as lung or bowel (Figure 9–13). Delicate clamps must not be used to grasp heavier tissues, because the clamp may slip when traction is

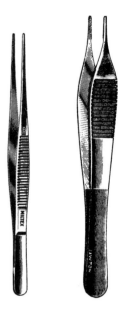

FIGURE 9–12

Examples of smooth forceps. *Left,* Semken; *right,* Adson. (Source: Smith EJ, Smith YR: Smiths' Reference and Illustrated Guide to Surgical Instruments. Philadelphia, JB Lippincott, 1983, pp 365, 417.)

applied. Also, the clamp will be damaged if forced to clamp heavy or bulky tissue.

Clamps with teeth are used only on tissues that will not be seriously injured by tooth perforation. The teeth increase the clamp's grasping power, so that greater amounts of traction can be applied (Figure 9–14). The tips may be very sharp; the RNFA must be careful not to perforate gloves or delicate structures like bowel or blood vessels.

Heavy clamps can cause crushing injury to tissues and must be used appropriately. Frequently, just the clamp's tip is used to grasp tissue and apply traction (Figure 9–15). Excessive traction will cause the clamp to slip or the

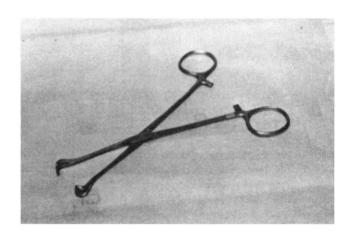

FIGURE 9–13

Babcock clamp. Note smooth grasping surfaces.

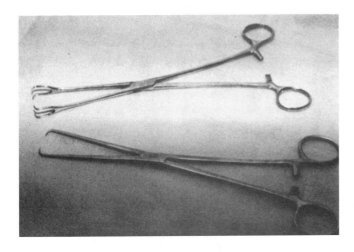

FIGURE 9–14
Tenaculum forceps (single- and double-toothed).

tissue to tear. The RNFA may need to simultaneously hold several clamps that are providing retraction at different points on a structure. When a clamp is attached to tissue, it should be held by the shaft rather than by the ring handles, because there is less chance of accidentally unlocking the clamp when it is held in this manner (Figure 9–16).

Sponges

Sponges are used in different ways to provide exposure. Several types and sizes of sponges are used in the operating room. Laparotomy sponges, gauze 4 × 4 × 8 inches, cottonoid pledgets, and "peanuts" (pills, kitners, pushers, dissectors) are the most frequently used types.

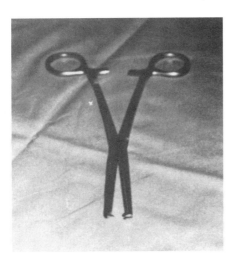

FIGURE 9–15
Ochsner forceps. Note grasping tooth at tip of clamp.

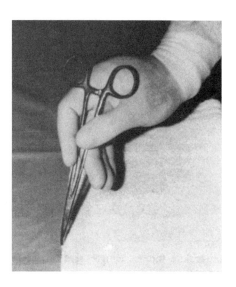

F I G U R E 9–1 6
Position for holding clamp by shaft.

The most common use of the sponge is to absorb fluid or blood that accumulates in the operative site and obstructs the surgeon's field of vision. Sponges are designed to soak up blood and should be used to blot tissues. Rubbing tissue with the sponges is abrasive and can remove clots, increase bleeding, and cause tissue damage.

Sponges may be used with an instrument to remove blood and fluids or as dissectors or retractors to gently push or pull tissues from the operative area. A 4 × 4-inch gauze pad can be folded and clamped into a sponge stick (stick sponge) (Figure 9–17), or a peanut may be clamped in the tip of a curved clamp, such as a peon (Figure 9–17). It is important that the sponges extend be-

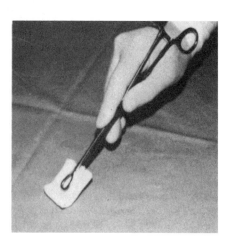

F I G U R E 9–1 7
Sponge stick holding folded gauze sponge.

yond the end of the clamp to protect tissue from injury by the clamp tips. The RNFA must be careful to not use excessive pressure with this type of sponge, or else tissue may be perforated or torn. Also, the blood supply can be compromised if pressure is applied too firmly or in the incorrect area.

Slippery structures (i.e., bowel or lung) can be held more securely by using a sponge under the fingers. The sponge's coarse fibers will increase the friction and improve traction. Dry sponges provide a better grip than wet ones but cause more tissue friction and abrasion. This tissue trauma can result in adhesion formation, which could cause postoperative complications, especially with abdominal surgeries. Using a sponge (4 × 4 × 8-inch or lap sponge) under the fingers may also reduce the likelihood of contaminating internal tissues with skin bacteria when retracting skin edges.

Sponges can also be used to stabilize tissues. Organs or tissues that would fall into the operative field and obstruct the surgeon's vision can be packed out of the way with sponges. Loose structures such as bowel can be better retracted if they are wrapped with moistened laparotomy sponges. Tissues can be protected from retractor blades by using sponges for padding.

Sutures

Sutures are frequently used to provide exposure. They are particularly helpful in everting or fixing small mobile structures, such as the inner surface of the eyelid. They also can be used to stabilize or hold tissues. Skin, pleural, pericardial, dural, peritoneal, and certain other tissue edges are commonly retracted with sutures (Figure 9–18). Suturing is frequently considered a retraction method when delicate structures require intermittent release and retraction over an extended period.

The amount of tension or pull that can be exerted on the suture depends on the tissue's fragility and the suture's tensile strength. Sutures must be placed securely in the tissue. Traction on the sutures is applied by the RNFA's hand or by clamping or suturing the stitch to the drapes, wound towels, or wound edges. When clamps are placed on the end of a retraction suture, the clamp should not be left unattended. Holding it or fixing it to a drape minimizes the risk that someone will mistakenly pick it up without realizing that its jaws are clamped to a suture. Once a suture is placed through a drape or wound towel, it cannot be removed and repositioned.

For very fragile tissues, the surgeon may use a pledget of Teflon felt (Figure 9–19). The felt keeps the suture from cutting into the tissue. When sutures are held with a clamp, the jaws might need to be shod to keep the suture from being cut. Various prepackaged, sterile shods are available. When the sutures are stitched to drapes or to other structures, tension must be appropriate for the tissue and the sutures, knots must be tied securely, and sutures must be cut close to the knot to prevent other sutures from catching on the knots.

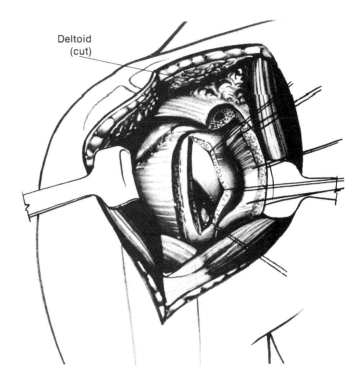

FIGURE 9–18

Use of sutures to retract tissue edges. (Source: Hoppenfeld S, deBoer P: Surgical Exposures in Orthopaedics: The Anatomic Approach. Philadelphia, JB Lippincott, 1984, p 13.)

Sutures provide good retraction without the bulk of instruments or retractors. If fastened correctly, they will hold tissue in a continuous position.

Umbilical tapes, Penrose drains, and vessel loops can also be used to retract blood vessels, nerves, and gastrointestinal structures. These structures are fragile and slippery, which makes them difficult to retract; they are also easily traumatized, which can result in serious problems.

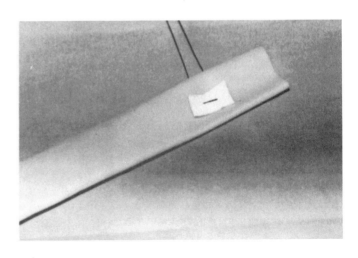

FIGURE 9–19

Teflon felt can be used with a suture for retracting delicate tissues.

Once the structure needing retraction is dissected free from surrounding tissues, an angled clamp is used to go under the structure. This clamp must be long enough and have a wide enough angle to slip around the structure easily. Various clamps are available; those used most commonly include kidney pedicle clamps, Semb ligature carriers, Rumel thoracic right-angle forceps, and lower gallbladder forceps.

Once the clamp is passed under the structure, it is opened, and the moistened tape (drain or loop) is inserted into the open jaws; the clamp is then closed and pulled back under the structure (Figure 9–20). This must be done carefully and gently so that the structure or surrounding tissues are not injured by the clamp. The tape (drain or loop) is moistened with warm saline solution to decrease the friction on the surrounding tissues. The RNFA usually uses two hands when placing a tape. One hand holds the clamp or forceps used to hold the end of the tape, while the other hand holds the tape taut. To prevent excessive drag through the tissue, only just enough tape to be grasped securely should be placed in the clamp's jaws.

Once the tape encircles the structure, it is clamped with a hemostat. The RNFA can provide traction by pulling on the hemostat, or the hemostat can be used to clamp the tape, preventing any possibility of injury to the structure itself.

Suctioning Devices

Suctioning devices remove blood or fluids from the operative area, which is essential for adequate visualization. Suction tips come in various shapes and sizes.

The Frazier suction tip is small and has an opening on the end. It is very useful for small incision sites with little blood loss. For operative procedures with larger incisions and increased fluid or blood loss, a Yankauer tonsil suction tip or

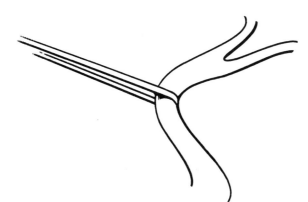

FIGURE 9–20
Vascular structure being retracted with a tape.

an abdominal suction tip may be used. The Yankauer suction tip's configuration makes it useful in retracting tissue as well as in suctioning blood or fluids.

Aspiration injury of tissue can occur with suction tips that have a single end opening. This can be prevented by protecting the tissue with a sponge so that the suction is not applied directly on the tissue. Should tissue be aspirated, the suction tip should not be pulled away forcibly. Instead, first the suction should be broken by bending off the suction tubing, then the tissue gently removed. Some suction tips have a finger hole. When the hole is covered, the suction force increases; when it is uncovered, suction force decreases.

When a suction tip is used, good visualization of the tip is important. Trauma to tissue can occur if the tip is used carelessly; a fine-pointed tip could puncture, tear, or abrade tissue.

The suction tip is used to remove blood or fluids in the area where the surgeon is working. It must never obstruct the surgeon's vision. The RNFA may need to use suction frequently and briefly in coordination with the surgeon's activities, observing the operative site continuously to anticipate the need for and timing of suctioning.

In cases involving trauma or anastomosis of a structure such as bowel, the RNFA should ensure no cross-contamination occurs via the suction tips. Once the dirty, contaminated area is closed, the contaminated suction tip should be replaced with a new one.

The RNFA also must be alert to the potential for losing removable parts of the suction tip. It is important to have a method of accounting for these parts. For example, the off/on controls may be held in place with screws that can back out and drop into the wound. Occasionally, the surgeon may find it necessary to unscrew the end of the suction tip, which is then given to the scrub nurse for safekeeping until needed again.

Retracting with Hands

The ideal retractor to provide exposure is frequently the RNFA's hands. The hand is gently padded, soft, and responsive to the texture of tissue being retracted through tactile sense. Fingers and hands can be repositioned or removed easily and quickly from the operative area. The amount of pressure or traction exerted on tissue can be readily adjusted.

After the initial incision, the RNFA uses the fingers to retract the skin edge while the subcutaneous layers are being cut. Fingers are usually used for retracting while the retractor is being positioned. By spreading the fingers, a broad area can be retracted with one hand. The RNFA should flatten the hand as much as possible. This causes less obstruction to the operative area and allows better visualization by the surgeon.

By placing a sponge under the fingers, the RNFA can grip the tissue more securely. However, with prolonged retracting, the fingers and hand may become fatigued. The RNFA must inform the surgeon when this is occurring to avoid untimely slipping of the retracted tissues. A brief rest or repositioning the hand will usually relieve the fatigue.

Plastic bags (sterile) have been designed for retracting small intestines during extensive abdominal operations. The bowel should be wrapped carefully in warm saline-soaked lap sponges and gently placed in the bag in an anatomically correct position. Once the RNFA is sure that the bowel has not accidentally twisted, it is secured properly within the bag to prevent it from inadvertently slipping out, into the operative area.

■ SUMMARY

The effects of the RNFA's retracting or providing exposure are apparent during the operative procedure. If exposure is poor, then the RNFA must find the first practical moment and method to improve it. By close observation, the RNFA determines the effectiveness of his or her actions. It is not uncommon for the surgeon to situate retractors or determine the method of providing exposure. In some situations, the surgeon determines how and what is retracted. The RNFA contributes significantly to the effectiveness, efficiency, and safety of the operative procedure by providing good exposure of the operative site for the surgeon.

Tissue injury resulting from carelessness while providing exposure will usually be apparent at the time of the surgical intervention. However, some injuries, such as nerve injury, may not be noticed until the postoperative period. Postoperative evaluation of the patient's status provides the RNFA with information that will be helpful in determining whether any injury related to providing exposure has occurred intraoperatively.

■ Review Questions

Fill in the blanks in the following questions.

1. A judgment made by the RNFA related to the patient's problems, needs, or health status is stated as a _____.

2. Surgery is the _____ risk factor for the perioperative patient with a high risk for injury.

3. Detailed guidelines for predictable care regimens may be developed as intraoperative _____.

4. A major consideration in selecting the appropriate method of providing exposure is the _____ of the operative procedure.

5. It is easier for the RNFA to vary the position of the retractor and force of retraction with _____ retractors.

6. Pronged retractors are usually selected for retraction of _____ tissue.

7. When retracting away from oneself, the retractor should be held in the hand with the palm _____ and the arm flexed at the elbow.

8. The longer the surgical procedure, the more _____ loss and tissue _____. For this reason, moist sponges are used under retractor blades.

9. Overexpansion of a self-retaining retractor can cause excessive pulling on tissue and subsequent _____.

10. Grasping pressure of tissue forceps is controlled by the _____.

11. A clamp with _____ allows more grasping power and tissue traction.

12. When a clamp is attached to tissue, it should be held by the _____ to prevent accidental unlocking.

13. When a sponge is used to absorb blood in the field, a _____ motion prevents tissue damage.

14. A gauze dissector should be inserted into a clamp with the end of the dissector _____ the end of the clamp.

15. A particularly useful way to fix a small, mobile structure is to use a _____ as a retraction method.

16. To keep a suture from cutting into fragile tissue, a _____ may be used with the suture.

17. If tissue is aspirated into the end of a suction tip, the RNFA should first _____, then gently remove the tissue.

18. The _____ is often the best retractor; it is softly padded and responsive through tactile sense.

19. Before repositioning any retracting device, the RNFA should _____.

20. During surgery, the best way to determine the effectiveness of retraction is by _____.

Answer Key

1. nursing diagnosis
2. situational
3. standards of care
4. stage
5. hand-held
6. shallow/subcutaneous
7. supine

8. fluid; dessication
9. tearing/laceration
10. thumb and fingers
11. teeth
12. shaft
13. blotting
14. beyond

15. suture
16. pledget of felt
17. break the suction
18. hand
19. inform the surgeon
20. observation

REFERENCES

1. Association of Operating Room Nurses: AORN official statement on RN first assistants. In: AORN Standards, Recommended Practices and Guidelines. Denver, Colo, Association of Operating Room Nurses, 1997, pp 23-24
2. Ibid, p 125

3. American Nurses Association: The Code of Ethics for Nursing. In: 1997 Field Review. Washington, DC, American Nurses Association, 1997, p 9
4. Association of Operating Room Nurses: AORN Recommended Education Standards for RN First Assistant Programs. In: AORN Standards, Recommended Practices and Guidelines. Denver, Colo, Association of Operating Room Nurses, 1997, pp 37–39
5. Residency programs downsizing. OR Manager 13(11):34, 1997
6. Fiesta J: Corporate liability update. Nurs Management 28(11):22–23, 1997
7. New study finds circulators in need of more protection. OR Manager 13(6):1, 10, 12, 1997

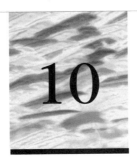

10

SUTURING MATERIALS
AND TECHNIQUES

NANCY B. DAVIS

∎

Suturing skills are required by the RN functioning as a first assistant during operative procedures. Suturing is one of the unique nursing behaviors identified for RNFAs in the Association of Operating Room Nurses (AORN) Official Statement on RN First Assistants (see Appendix I). The term suturing is broadly used; variations in practice environments and state nurse practice acts may further quantify and define parameters for what types of structures may be sutured. As with all skill acquisition, learning and performing the techniques of suturing progress from basic competency to excellence in skill performance.

Preparation and handling of suture materials, needles, and needleholders are basic functions of a scrub nurse. The nurse learns about the types of sutures and how and when they are used. By observing the surgeon, the scrub nurse becomes familiar with suturing techniques. These experiences as a scrub nurse are most helpful to the RNFA when learning to suture.

Learning to suture should first be undertaken in a simulated setting. Such laboratory experience facilitates educational assumptions about psychomotor skill learning. Skills are learned first by imitation; the skill is demonstrated, and the learner follows the example of the demonstrator. As the learner practices, skill in manipulation follows; the technique can be carried out without constant demonstration. As the RNFA learns to manipulate hand and arm movements in suturing, precision in the technique follows. Eventually the skill becomes naturalized; it is done with smooth, fluid motions, and the correct technique is selected for each application. Laboratory practice is especially helpful when learning more complex suturing techniques, such as those used in microsurgery. After practice and initial skill evaluation, suturing skills are refined in the operating room under the direction and supervision of the surgeon.

Although the choice of suture materials and techniques is often determined by the operating surgeon, the RNFA must consider the influence of the patient's condition and age, the presence of infection, and the type of tissue being sutured. Preoperative patient assessment provides data about the patient from which the RNFA identifies potential complications. Suture materials are foreign substances; in selecting the type of suture and suturing technique, the RNFA must consider patient risk factors and the potential for such problems as wound infection, inadequate wound healing, wound dehiscence, and excessive scarring. Taking these factors into consideration, the goal is to leave minimal foreign material in the wound. This is achieved, in part, by selecting the suture with the highest tensile strength and the smallest diameter and one that holds knots well, requiring fewer turns and throws during tying.

USES AND SELECTION OF SUTURES

The three common uses for sutures during operative procedures are as follows:

1. Strands of suture are used as ligatures to tie off blood vessels and control bleeding.
2. Sutures are used to sew tissue together (reapproximate) and to hold the tissue securely until it has healed.
3. When tension is applied to sutures placed through tissue, that tissue can be retracted, facilitating exposure of the operative site for the surgeon.

Sutures are considered to be medical devices and as such must meet certain standards established by the federal Food and Drug Administration (FDA). Since 1937, government regulations have established criteria for ensuring the safety and effectiveness of sutures. Sterility, tensile strength, size, dyes, needle attachments, coating or impregnation of suture material with other substances, packaging, and labeling are some of the areas addressed in these regulations.

A primary factor to consider when selecting a suture is the tissue being sutured. The suture must be as strong as the tissue it is holding, and the strength of the suture must last until the tissue is healed. Thus, the rate of suture absorption should correspond to the rate of healing. Tissues heal at different rates, and healing can additionally be affected by such factors as infection, obesity, the presence of malignancies or debilitating injuries, immunodeficiency, blood loss and fluid and electrolyte imbalances, debilitation, inadequate nutrition, chronic disease, and age.[1] The smallest diameter of suture is used to minimize tissue reaction and injury. The suture material should be pliable, strong, and hold knots securely; suture security depends on its intrinsic tensile strength and ability to hold a knot. Other considerations include location and length of the incision, desired cosmetic results, personal experiences, cost, and availability.

CLASSIFICATION OF SUTURES

Sutures are classified according to the effects of tissue enzymes and body fluids. A suture is a foreign body; the body reacts to it by attempting to dissolve or digest it. If this is possible, then the suture is absorbed. Nonabsorbable sutures, in contrast, cannot be dissolved or digested; rather, they become encapsulated by the body tissues.

Sutures are also classified according to the number of strands of material used. A suture with two or more strands of suture material twisted or braided together is termed a multifilament suture. Although the multifilament suture's higher coefficient of friction helps it hold knots, the multiple strands make it harder to drag through tissue, thus increasing tissue trauma and tissue reaction. This type of suture has a capillarity (transfer of body fluids along the suture strand) due to the interstices in the braided or twisted strands; capillary action can be reduced by coating the suture with silicone or paraffin. A monofilament suture consists of one strand of suture material that is noncapillary and causes very little tissue reaction.

Absorbable Sutures

Absorbable sutures are temporary; they will be digested or dissolved. Tensile strength, retention, and absorption rate vary among the absorbable sutures, and these factors must be considered separately. For example, a suture may lose its strength quickly and be absorbed slowly. These sutures can be treated to delay the absorption rate or coated with agents that have an antimicrobial action. Absorbable sutures vary in texture, structure, size, and color (Table 10–1).

Surgical Gut. Surgical gut (catgut) is used less frequently since the introduction of synthetic absorbable sutures. Gut is made from the submucosal layer of sheep intestine or the serosa layer of beef intestine; it is a highly purified collagen. Gut is processed by electronically spinning and polishing the strands into various sizes. The suture can be left "plain," or it may be dipped in chromium salt solution. "Chromicizing" the suture increases its resistance to the digestive action of the tissue enzymes, which delays suture absorption. This treated suture is called "chromic." Plain suture loses its tensile strength in 7 to 10 days and is absorbed in 70 days. Chromic suture's tensile strength lasts 10 to 14 days; it is usually not absorbed before 90 days. Chromic suture

TABLE 10–1. ABSORBABLE SUTURES COMMONLY USED IN SURGERY

Suture	Types	Frequent Uses	Tissue Reaction	Contraindications	Warnings	Tensile Strenth Retention in vivo	Absorption Rate
Surgical gut	Plain	Ligate superficial vessels; suture soft tissues that heal rapidly; not used in cardiovascular or neurological tissues Ophthalmology	Moderate	Should not be used in tissues that heal slowly, require support, or are under stress Should not be used in patients allergic or sensitive to collagen or chromium	Absorbs relatively quickly	Individual patient characteristics can affect rate of tensile strength loss	Digested by proteolytic enzymes
Surgical gut	Chromic	Suture or ligature for soft tissue Ophthalmology	Moderate	Being absorbable, should not be used where prolonged approximation of tissues under stress is required Should not be used in cardiovascular or neurosurgical tissues or in patients with allergy or sensitivity to collagen or chromium	Protein-based absorbable sutures have a tendency to fray when tied	Individual patient characteristics can affect rate of tensile strength loss	Digested by proteolytic enzymes

Material	Construction	Indications	Tissue Reaction	Contraindications	Contraindications (2)	Tensile Strength	Absorption
Polyglactin 910 Polyglycolic acid suture	Braided	Ligate or suture soft tissues	Minimal	Being absorbable, should not be used where prolonged approximation of tissues is required	Not for use in neural and cardiovascular tissue	Approximately 65% remains at 2 weeks; approximately 40% remains at 3 weeks	Essentially complete at 60–70 days; absorbed by slow hydrolysis
Polydioxanone	Monofilament	Soft tissue approximation, including pediatric cardiovascular and ophthalmic procedures	Slight	Being absorbable, should not be used where prolonged approximation of tissues under stress is required	Should not be used for placement of vascular prostheses or artificial heart valves	Approximately 70% remains at 2 weeks; approximately 50% remains at 4 weeks; approximately 25% remains at 6 weeks	Minimal until about 90th day; essentially complete within 210 days; absorbed by slow hydrolysis
Polyglecaprone	Monofilament	Soft tissue approximation and ligation	Slight	Being absorbable, should not be used where prolonged approximation of tissues under stress is required	Not for use in cardiovascular or neurological tissues, microsurgery, or ophthalmic procedures	Approximately 50%–60% remains at 1 week; 20%–30% at 2 weeks; lost at 3 weeks	Complete at 91–119 days; absorbed by hydrolysis

(Adapted from Ethicon: Wound Closure Manual. Somerville, NJ, Ethicon, Inc, a Johnson & Johnson Company, 1994, pp 22–23.)

causes less tissue reaction than does plain suture, which may elicit a marked foreign-body response.

Surgical gut suture must be handled as little as possible, because handling may cause the suture to fray. The suture material loses its pliability if allowed to dry. Pliability can be restored by moistening the suture with sterile water or saline. The suture must not be soaked any longer than a few seconds, because soaking decreases tensile strength and knot security.

Synthetic Absorbable Sutures. Polymers made from polyglycolic acid, polyglactin 910, polyglyconate, or polydioxanone, synthetic absorbable sutures are prepared as monofilament or multifilament sutures. Tissue reactions are mild and are decreased further when monofilament suture is used. This type of suture is stronger than surgical gut, and the tensile strength lasts longer. After 14 days, 60% or more of the suture's tensile strength remains. Absorption occurs through hydrolysis, and the suture will not be totally absorbed for 60 to 90 days. The polydioxanone suture will not be absorbed until after 90 days, and absorption may take as long as 180 days.

The braided polymers handle as silk sutures; because of their higher coefficient of friction, knot security is good. However, the monofilament or the coated sutures (polyglactin 910 and calcium stearate coating) are smoother and slicker, so they will require additional throws for knot security.

Nonabsorbable Sutures

Nonabsorbable sutures are not digested by tissue enzymes or hydrolyzed by body fluids. They are considered permanent sutures. Nonabsorbable sutures are used when the suture strength needs to be retained longer than two to three weeks. They are often used when it is necessary to minimize the tissue reaction or trauma that can occur with the absorbable sutures (Table 10–2).

With the exception of wire sutures, nonabsorbable sutures should not be used in the presence of infection. The suture itself could become a site for the infection, perhaps necessitating suture removal.

Surgical Silk. In the past, surgical silk was the most commonly used nonabsorbable suture because of its easy handling, its tensile strength, and the security of its knots with a minimal number of throws. All other sutures are compared with silk in relation to these handling properties. However, silk does cause a higher degree of tissue reaction than do the other nonabsorbable sutures. Silk is made from the silk of silkworms. After the silk filaments are processed, the strands are braided or twisted, treated to decrease capillary action, and usually dyed black. Silk loses up to 20% of its strength if moistened; therefore, it is used dry. The tensile strength of silk decreases after

TABLE 10–2. NONABSORBABLE SUTURES COMMONLY USED IN SURGERY

Suture	Types	Frequent Uses	Tissue Reaction	Contraindications	Warnings	Tensile Strength Retention in vivo	Absorption Rate
Surgical silk	Braided	Soft tissues for ligating and suturing; cardiovascular ophthalmology and neurological surgery	Acute inflammatory reaction	Should not be used for placement of vascular prostheses and artifical heart valves or where prolonged approximation is required	Slowly absorbs	Progressive degradation	Encapsulation by fibrous connective tissue
Surgical steel	Monofilament	Abdominal wall closure, sternal closure, hernia repair, orthopedic procedures	Low	Should not be used in patients with sensitivity/allergy to stainless steel or metals such as nickel and chromium	May break at points of bending, twisting, or knotting	Indefinite	Nonabsorbable
Nylon	Multifilament Monofilament	Soft tissue closure, cardiovascular surgery, ophthalmology, and neurosurgery	Minimal	Should not be used when permanent tensile strength retention is required	None	Progressive hydrolysis may result in gradual loss of tensile strength	Gradually encapsulated by fibrous connective tissue
	Braided	Most body tissues for ligating and suturing; general closure, neurosurgery					
Polyester fiber	Braided	Cardiovascular and neurosurgery, ophthalmology	Minimal	None	None	No significant change	Gradual encapsulation by fibrous connective tissue
Polypropylene	Monofilament	General and cardiovascular surgery, ophthalmology, and neurosurgical procedures	Minimal acute inflammatory reaction	None	None	No significant change	Nonabsorbable; remains encapsulated in body tissues

(Adapted from Ethicon: Wound Closure Manual. Somerville, NJ, Ethicon, Inc, a Johnson & Johnson Company, 1994, pp 22–23.)

90 to 120 days, and the silk usually is absorbed after two years. It is not a true nonabsorbable suture, but is classified as such because of the time that it remains in the tissues. Strict aseptic technique is necessary when using silk, and silk is never used in an infected wound.

Virgin Silk.   Virgin silk is processed differently than other silk. The sericin gum normally present on the silk filaments is not removed but rather is left on to hold the fine filaments together. The suture is very fine (8-0 or 9-0) and is used primarily for ophthalmic procedures.

Surgical Cotton.   Surgical cotton is made from natural cellulose cotton fibers. The fibers are twisted into strands, processed, and coated to provide a smoother surface. The weakest nonabsorbable suture, surgical cotton is used less frequently than silk. Cotton's tensile strength is increased 10% by moistening the suture immediately before use. Although 50% of tensile strength is lost in 6 months, 30% to 40% of tensile strength may remain after two years.

Linen.   Rarely used, linen is made from twisted flax fibers. The tensile strength of linen is inferior to that of the other nonabsorbable sutures.

Stainless Steel.   Surgical stainless steel wire sutures are made from a strong, flexible, and uniform steel alloy and can be used with stainless steel hardware or prostheses. (They should not be used in the presence of another alloy, because electrolytic reactions could occur.) Stainless steel wire is strong, minimally tissue reactive, and one of the most secure suture materials available. The suture is prepared as a monofilament wire or as braided multifilament wire. The monofilament wire kinks easily, but both types can be held securely in place by twisting or knotting the suture. However, knot security may be compromised when wire suture is twisted rather than tied. The major disadvantage is related to handling the suture; gloves can be punctured or tissue injured by the sharp ends of the wire. Wire's tensile strength is very high, and the tissue reaction is minimal. Wire cutters must be used, because the wire will damage suture scissors.

Nonabsorbable Synthetics.   Nylon is made from a synthetic polyamide polymer. Its tensile strength is high, and the tissue reaction is minimal. This monofilament suture is noncapillary and easy to handle. It does require additional throws for knot security, however. Moistening nylon suture makes it easier to handle and more pliable. Multifilament nylon is braided very tightly and treated for noncapillarity. It handles like silk but causes much less tissue reaction. Nylon suture loses 15% to 20% of its tensile strength per year in tissue and will not provide indefinite support.

Polyesters are made from polyethylene terephthalate fibers braided together. This suture is strong, and very little tissue reaction occurs. However, the uncoated polyesters can cause tissue trauma by friction as they are pulled through the tissues. They may be coated or impregnated with Teflon, polybutilate, or silicone to reduce the amount of friction produced when passing through tissue; but then additional throws are needed for knot security.

Polybutester is a monofilament that is more flexible and elastic than some of the other nonabsorbable monofilament sutures. Another new nonabsorbable suture, expanded polytetrafluoroethylene (PTFE), is strong relative to other monofilaments and has pliability and comparable knot security.

Polypropylene is made from a polyolefin of polymeric linear hydrocarbons. It is formed into a strong, smooth monofilament suture that does not weaken in tissues and causes very little tissue reaction. It is easy to handle, slides through tissue easily, and holds knots securely.

Polyethylene is a synthetic made from thermoplastic resins formed into monofilament sutures. It is easy to handle, passes smoothly through tissue, causes minimal tissue reaction, ties easily, and holds knots securely.

SURGICAL NEEDLES

The surgical needle transports the suture through the tissues during surgical operations with the least amount of trauma to the tissues. High-quality steel alloy is used in manufacturing surgical needles. The different sizes of needles are made from wire of various thicknesses. The wire is heat treated and tempered to provide the necessary strength and flexibility. A needle must be strong enough to penetrate the tissue without bending or becoming deformed. Because it is flexible, the needle can bend slightly without breaking. Bending alerts the user that the tissue is too tough for the needle.

Needles are carefully sharpened, finely polished, and smoothed for ease in tissue penetration. Silicone coatings are occasionally used. Because needles are noncorrosive, flaking of foreign material from needles into the surgical wound cannot occur. Before use, needles should be carefully inspected for any barbs, hooks, or rough areas.

Needle Designs

Basically, needles have three components: the eye, the shaft or body, and the point (Figure 10–1).

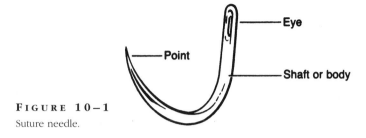

FIGURE 10–1
Suture needle.

Eye.   The eye of the needle is located at the end of the needle where the suture is attached. The three types of needle eyes are closed, French or split, and swaged.

The *closed-eye needle* has a round, square, or oblong hole through which the suture is threaded (Figure 10–2). The eye must be smooth to avoid cutting the suture. Eyed needles may be reusable or disposable.

Although eyed needles may be economical, the eye must be larger than the suture; the additional bulk of a double suture causes increased damage to the tissue that the needle penetrates (Figure 10–3).

The *French-eye* or *split-eye needle* has a spring opening (Figure 10–4) that allows the suture and needle to be almost the same size, which decreases tissue trauma. The double suture still must be pulled through the tissue, however. French-eye needles are quicker to thread but are usually finer needles that have limited use.

The *swaged* or *atraumatic needle* is actually an eyeless needle. The suture is attached to the end of the needle and is only as large as the needle itself. This type of needle provides the least amount of tissue trauma. Although expensive, swaged sutures are easier and quicker to use, and in some situations necessary to use. Many of the fine synthetic nonabsorbable sutures are used for delicate surgery, such as microsurgery or vascular surgery. This type of surgery necessitates minimal tissue injury, as results from using a swaged needle. Optimum sharpness is ensured because the swaged needle is used only with that suture and then discarded. Sutures are now available with swaged needles that can be removed from the suture with a slight tug. Generically called pop-off or breakaway sutures, "control release" is the trade name for this type of suture, manu-

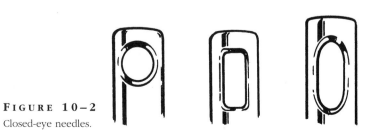

FIGURE 10–2
Closed-eye needles.

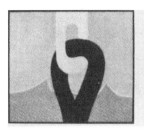
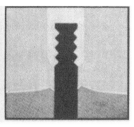

FIGURE 10–3

Left, Tissue disruption caused by double suture strand with eyed needle. *Right,* Tissue disruption minimized by single suture strand swaged to needle. (Source: Wound Closure Manual, 1985. Courtesy of Ethicon, Inc., a Johnson & Johnson Company, Somerville, NJ.)

factured by Ethicon. These needles are used for interrupted suturing techniques and allow several sutures to be placed rapidly.

The choice of needle eye is based on the location and type of tissue being sutured, the size of the suture being used, the availability of various needles, and considerations related to decreasing surgery time. The assistant must be familiar with the surgeon's preferences in all operative procedures with which he or she assists.

Shaft. The shaft, or body, determines the needle's shape, size, and diameter. This area of the needle is grasped or held as the needle is placed through tissue. The body may be straight, curved, or partially curved. The various needle sizes are determined by measuring the chord length, needle length, and needle radius (Figure 10–5).

A needle may be oval, round, triangular, side-flattened rectangular, or trapezoidal in design. Some needles are flat and ribbed in the area where they are grasped by the needleholder. This reduces slippage of the needle in the needleholder during suturing.

Needle shape, size, and thickness must all be considered when selecting a needle. The shape and size depend on the location and accessibility of the tissue being sutured. The thickness is determined by the type of tissue and size of the suture being used. The needle must be strong enough to penetrate the tissue without bending or breaking and be as close to the diameter of the suture as possible (Figure 10–6).

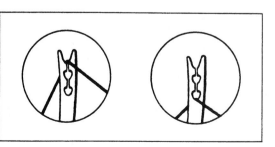

FIGURE 10–4

French-eye (split-eye) needle. (Source: Wound Closure Manual, 1985. Courtesy of Ethicon, Inc., a Johnson & Johnson Company, Somerville, NJ.)

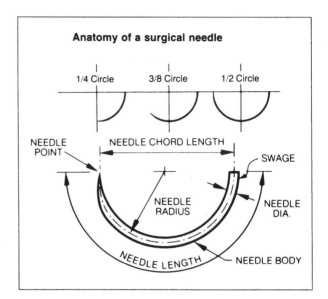

FIGURE 10–5

Methods of measuring the size of a suture needle. (Source: Wound Closure Manual, 1985. Courtesy of Ethicon, Inc., a Johnson & Johnson Company, Somerville, NJ.)

Point. The needle point is the end that first penetrates the tissue being sutured. The design of the point varies according to the type of tissue to be penetrated (Figure 10–7). The basic point types are cutting, taper, and blunt. Cutting needles are designed to penetrate tough tissue such as skin, tendons, fibrous or calcified tissue, and sternal bone. The variations in the cutting edges alter the direction of cutting and promote ease of tissue penetration.

Taper needles, usually called round needles, cause minimal tissue trauma but must be used on tissue that they can penetrate easily.

The blunt needle does not have a sharp point; it basically dissects the tissue as it is pushed through it. It can be used on a variety of tissues, and has been recommended as one mechanism to prevent percutaneous injury during suturing.[2] Injury prevention is discussed later in this chapter.

■ SUTURING

The RNFA needs skill in suturing and assisting during suturing. The application of this skill varies depending on the practice setting and legal constraints that may exist. In the scrub nurse role, the perioperative nurse has had the opportunity to observe suturing. Through this observation and by active inquiry, the nurse can learn how to handle tissues when suturing, principles for reapproximating tissues, different suturing techniques, and the criteria for selecting suture materials and suture needles. Suturing techniques should first

(text continues on page 238)

Shape	Comments
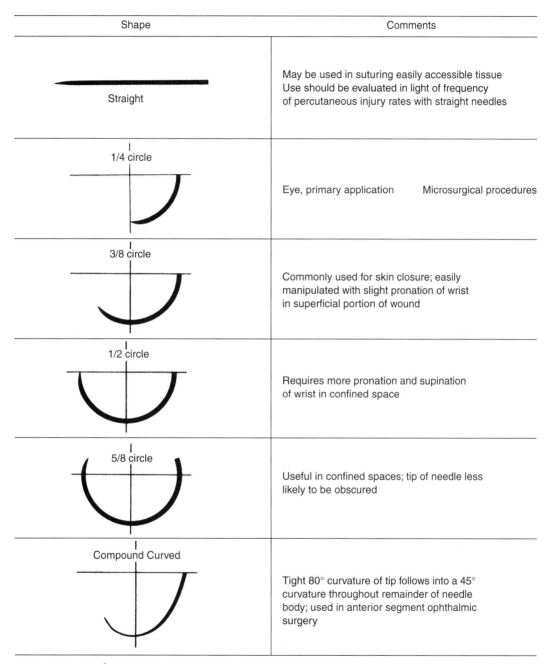 Straight	May be used in suturing easily accessible tissue. Use should be evaluated in light of frequency of percutaneous injury rates with straight needles
1/4 circle	Eye, primary application Microsurgical procedures
3/8 circle	Commonly used for skin closure; easily manipulated with slight pronation of wrist in superficial portion of wound
1/2 circle	Requires more pronation and supination of wrist in confined space
5/8 circle	Useful in confined spaces; tip of needle less likely to be obscured
Compound Curved	Tight 80° curvature of tip follows into a 45° curvature throughout remainder of needle body; used in anterior segment ophthalmic surgery

FIGURE 10–6

Needle shapes and uses. (Adapted from Wound Closure Manual, 1994. Courtesy of Ethicon, Inc., a Johnson & Johnson Company, Somerville, NJ.)

Needle Point and Body Shape	Applications	Comments
Conventional Cutting	Ligament Nasal cavity Oral cavity Pharynx Skin Tendon	Has three cutting edges—additional cutting edge on inside concave curvature Design modified from aesthetic plastic surgery (Precision Cosmetic) and sternotomy closure
Reverse Cutting	Fascia Ligament Nasal cavity Oral mucosa Skin Tendon sheath Pharynx	Has three cutting edges—additional cutting edge located on outside convex curvature Design modified for ophthalmology (MICRO-POINT), plastic surgery (Precision Point), and orthopedic surgery (OS)
MICRO-POINT Reverse Cutting Needle	Eye	Has smooth surface and extreme sharpness
Precision Point Cutting	Skin closure in plastic or cosmetic procedures	Bottom third cutting edge flattens out as it transitions to needle body to provide greater security in needleholder

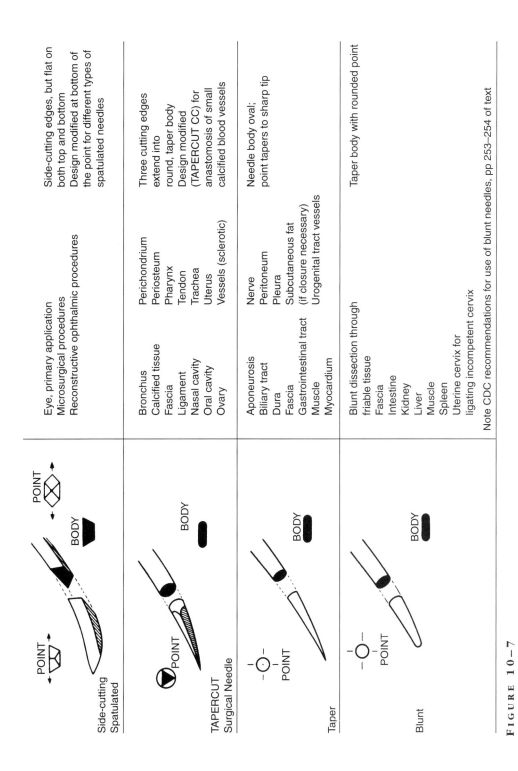

Side-cutting edges, but flat on both top and bottom
Design modified at bottom of the point for different types of spatulated needles

Eye, primary application
Microsurgical procedures
Reconstructive ophthalmic procedures

POINT
BODY
POINT

Side-cutting
Spatulated

Three cutting edges extend into round, taper body
Design modified (TAPERCUT CC) for anastomosis of small calcified blood vessels

Bronchus	Perichondrium
Calcified tissue	Periosteum
Fascia	Pharynx
Ligament	Tendon
Nasal cavity	Trachea
Oral cavity	Uterus
Ovary	Vessels (sclerotic)

POINT
BODY

TAPERCUT
Surgical Needle

Needle body oval; point tapers to sharp tip

Aponeurosis	Nerve
Biliary tract	Peritoneum
Dura	Pleura
Fascia	Subcutaneous fat
Gastrointestinal tract	(if closure necessary)
Muscle	Urogenital tract vessels
Myocardium	

POINT
BODY

Taper

Taper body with rounded point

Blunt dissection through friable tissue
Fascia
Intestine
Kidney
Liver
Muscle
Spleen
Uterine cervix for ligating incompetent cervix

POINT
BODY

Blunt

Note CDC recommendations for use of blunt needles, pp 253–254 of text

F I G U R E 1 0 – 7

Suture needle points and shapes. (Adapted from Wound Closure Manual, 1994. Courtesy of Ethicon, Inc., a Johnson & Johnson Company, Somerville, NJ.)

be practiced in a laboratory. Skill refinement occurs during the operative procedure, under the direction of the surgeon.

Assisting During Suturing

The RNFA can perform essential nursing behaviors to facilitate suturing. One of the first requirements is to know ahead of time the surgeon's preferences for suturing materials and techniques. As wound closure approaches, the field should be cleared of sponges and extraneous instruments to prepare for counts. The wound should be inspected for bleeders, and any found should be controlled. Overhead lights may need to be adjusted and retractors repositioned for better visibility. The RNFA and surgeon should have a synchronized plan for who will tie knots and who will cut sutures. When tying a suture that is being used only once, the RNFA will take the needle and its suture, tie the first knot with the correct tension, then rapidly throw on the additional knots. Both ends of the suture are then presented for cutting, the needle and remaining suture are returned to the scrub nurse, and the RNFA gets ready as the surgeon places the first bite of the next suture. When several stitches are to be made with the same suture, the RNFA grasps enough of the short end to tie rapidly and accurately. As the knot is being tied, the surgeon repositions the needle on the needleholder for the next stitch. The suture is cut, the short end discarded, and the long end retained as the process continues. When the suture becomes too short for convenient tying, another is requested.

At times, the RNFA may be required to assist in grasping a needle as it exits tissue. The RNFA may first use the tip of the unopened needleholder to provide a downward counterforce on the tissue (usually skin) where the needle is exiting. As the needle exits and the surgeon pauses to readjust, the RNFA should grasp the needle with the needleholder behind the point of the needle, rotating the needle 90 degrees through a natural curve. This will bring most of the needle above the skin surface. Some of the needle should remain below the skin surface; this provides a position of stability for the surgeon to regrasp it. As the surgeon pulls the needle through, the RNFA reaches for the suture as it emerges behind the needle and begins the first throw of the knot. This is known as the needle fixation and presentation technique.[3]

Suturing Instruments

Needleholders and tissue forceps are the basic instruments needed for suturing. Through years of experience, the perioperative nurse is familiar with the various needleholders and tissue forceps and their uses. Functioning as the scrub nurse is an excellent way of learning how and when these instruments are used during operative procedures. However, the actual use of instruments necessitates mastery of new technical skills.

Needleholders.   Needleholders are similar to hemostats. Most needleholders are designed with ring handles and ratchet locks. Some of the delicate needleholders are designed like tissue forceps and have spring locks (Figure 10–8). The tips of needleholders are usually short and blunt, but some are designed with very fine, pointed tips. Needleholders are available in various lengths and sizes (Figure 10–9).

Selection of a needleholder is based on the depth of the area where the sutures will be placed and on the size of the suture needle. Using a light, fine needleholder on a heavy suture needle could damage the instrument by springing the jaws or damaging the jaw inserts. Individual preference is another factor—understandable, considering the numerous needleholders available.

Needleholders must be inspected to ensure that they function correctly. The jaws must hold the needle securely so that it will not slip as it is passed through the tissue. The jaw insert should be inspected for worn areas, and the security of the needle should be tested by gently attempting to move it with the fingers. The needleholder must open and close easily; resistance might result in inadvertent needle displacement in the tissue.

Placement of the suture needle in the needleholder is important. The needle is grasped at a point approximately one-quarter to one-half the distance from the eye end (or swaged end). If the needle is grasped too close to the eye, it may bend as it is placed in the tissue. The needle may be placed at a right angle to the needleholder or at a slight angle. The needle is grasped in the tip of the needleholder jaws, and the needleholder is ratcheted one or two ratchets (Figure 10–10). If the needleholder tips are allowed to extend beyond the secured needle, they can interfere with suturing by pushing into tissue (Figure 10–11). The needle can be damaged, notched, or bent if it is clamped too tightly in the jaws of the needleholder. If the needle is placed in the holder in the direction of use, it will not have to be repositioned.

Needleholder Grips.   The grip used on a needleholder depends on the amount of exertion required, the amount of control needed (i.e., delicate), the location of the tissue being sutured, and the ease of suturing encountered.

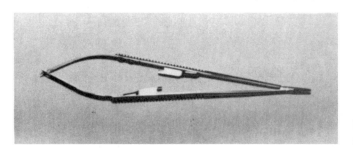

FIGURE 10–8
Castroviejo needleholder with spring lock.

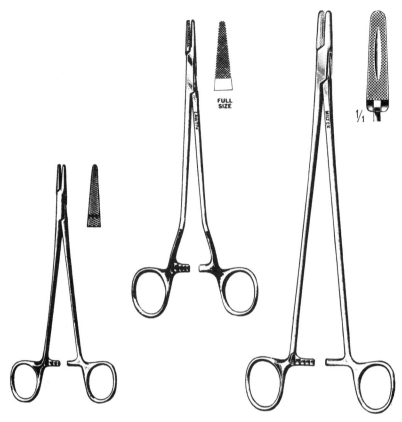

FIGURE 10–9

Examples of needleholders. *Left,* Crile-Wood; *center,* Sarot; *right,* Masson. (Source: Smith EJ, Smith YR: Smiths' Reference and Illustrated Guide to Surgical Instruments. Philadelphia, JB Lippincott, 1983, pp 510, 517, 541.)

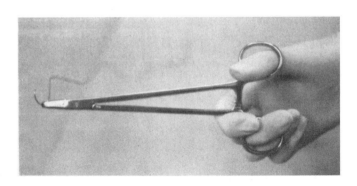

FIGURE 10–10

Needleholder with needle in correct position.

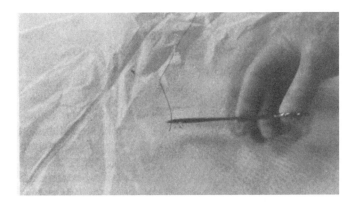

FIGURE 10–11
Needleholder with needle too far back in jaws.

The *palmed grip* is used when suturing very dense tissue that is difficult to penetrate (i.e., sternum). The needleholder is held in the palm of the hand and gripped on the shaft, close to the tip (Figure 10–12). This very secure grip is necessary when exerting a great deal of force on the needle. The direction of the needle is easily altered by rotating the needleholder in the hand. It is necessary to reposition the hand to release and reposition the needle.

The *thenar grip* is used for rapid, easy suturing. Precision is less exacting with this technique. The needleholder is grasped without inserting the thumb into the ring handle. The ball of the thumb (its metacarpal joint) is pressed against the thumb ring of the needleholder for control. This position puts the needleholder in a direct line with the axis of the forearm; the motion of rotating the needleholder is simple and natural. It also provides the necessary leverage for opening and closing the needleholder (Figure 10–13). However, the sudden opening of the needleholder can cause movement of the suture needle, a potential problem that must be considered when using this technique.

The *thumb-ring finger grip* is the most traditional method of using the needleholder. This technique is more precise and affords easier control of the

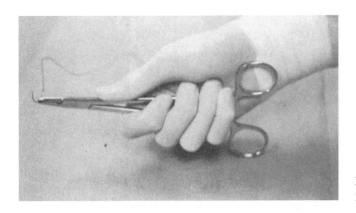

FIGURE 10–12
Palmed grip of needleholder.

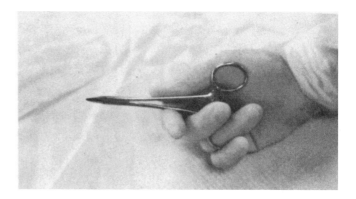

FIGURE 10–13
Thenar grip of needleholder.

needle. Hand position does not have to be changed when opening and closing the needleholder (Figure 10–14).

The *pencil grip* is used for very fine, delicate needleholders that operate with a spring latch or are latchless. The spring latch can be closed and released with finger pressure. The needleholder is controlled by rotating it between the index finger and the thumb (Figure 10–15). However, rotation of the needleholder on its axis may require more complex movement of the hand, wrist, and forearm.

Suture Scissors.   Suture scissors vary in length and size and may be straight or curved. The scissor is held in a position that provides stability and control. The "tripod" position provides the best control. The thumb and ring finger are placed in the ring handles and the index finger is extended along the shaft of the scissor. The palm of the hand faces down. The position can be easily changed by rotating the wrist (Figure 10–16).

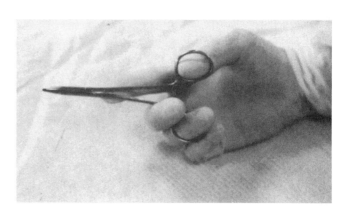

FIGURE 10–14
Thumb-ring finger grip of needleholder.

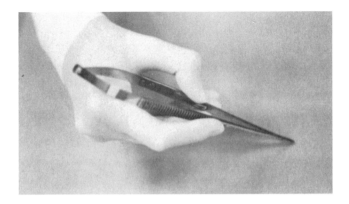

FIGURE 10–15
Pencil grip of needleholder.

Good visualization is essential when cutting sutures. The suture knot can be easily seen and the cutting distance estimated by looking through the opened scissor blades. Cutting with the tips of the scissor prevents inadvertent cutting of surrounding structures. Generally the suture is cut as close to the knot as possible, but the length of the suture "tail" that is left is determined by the type of suture. Cutting the knot too short may decrease knot security. If cutting sutures when there is motion, additional support can be provided by resting the scissors hand against the other hand. The suture is held taut as it is cut.

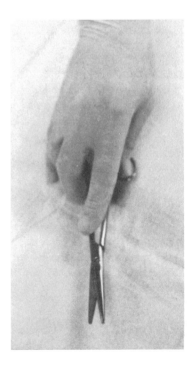

FIGURE 10–16
Position for using suture scissors.

Suture scissors must open and close smoothly. The blades should be sharp; dull or rough blades could snag the suture and cause it to be pulled loose, or possibly tear the tissue being sutured.

By anticipating the need to cut sutures, the RNFA can contribute to the efficiency of the operation. The RNFA should have the scissors ready and close to the area where the suture is being tied. By observing and counting the number of throws the surgeon has placed, the RNFA will know when the suture is to be cut.

Tissue Forceps.   Tissue forceps are used in conjunction with the needleholder. (For more information on forceps and their use, see Chapter 9, Providing Exposure: Retractors and Retraction, and Chapter 12, Using Grasping Instruments.) Using the forceps in the opposite hand allows the tissue to be stabilized and exposure to be provided before the suture needle penetrates the tissue. Tissue must be handled gently to avoid unnecessary injury or trauma, which may interfere with healing. The forceps brace the skin as the tip of the needle emerges on the exit side of the incision during closure. The teeth of the forceps should be set into the tissue only when necessary to avoid slipping. The tissue forceps can also be used to grasp and remove the suture needle after it has passed through the tissue. The forceps are then used to hold the needle while it is repositioned on the needleholder.

SUTURING TECHNIQUES

Suturing is the method of reapproximating tissues that have been cut during the operative procedure. The cut tissues should be sutured to resume as near normal a position as possible. It is important to correctly identify the different tissue layers being sutured to properly reposition them. The width and depth of the stitch will depend on the type of tissue being sutured. Suturing provides support to tissues while they heal, so that "gaps" or "dead space" will not delay healing (Figure 10–17). Dead space not only weakens the suture line, it is also a potential site for the collection of serum or blood, contributing to the subsequent risk of surgical site infection.

Whenever possible, the RNFA should sew toward himself or herself (Figure 10–18). This position is more comfortable and maximizes visibility. To begin suturing, the tissue is grasped with the forceps and, with the hand in the prone position, the needle tip is inserted. The needle should enter a structure at a right angle to its surface. The hand is rotated at the wrist so that the needle is arched through the tissue. The tip of the needle should be readily accessible after it goes through the tissue. To withdraw the tip of a curved needle, the hand starts in a pronated position. The needle tip is withdrawn with the forceps or the needleholder and pulled through the tissue in a small

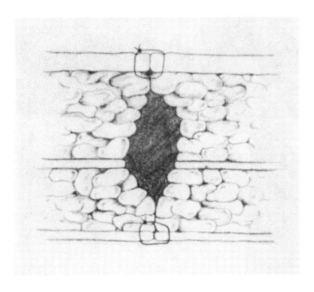

FIGURE 10–17

Dead space in tissue. (Soure: Wound Closure Manual, 1985. Courtesy of Ethicon, Inc., a Johnson & Johnson Company, Somerville, NJ.)

arc that follows its curve. While doing this, the hand turns 180 degrees to supination; this is a natural movement that involves only the forearm. Damage to the needle tip is avoided by grasping the needle on the body rather than on the tip itself. If the needle does not reach through the tissue, a larger needle is needed. The RNFA should not attempt to force the needle through, because it may break. If the tissue layers are close together, both sides may be sutured with one placement of the needle. In many instances the suture needle is passed through one side and then through the opposing side (Figure 10–19).

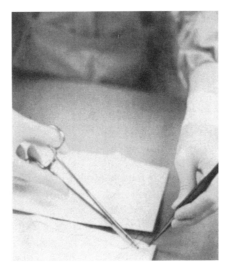

FIGURE 10–18

Suturing toward self.

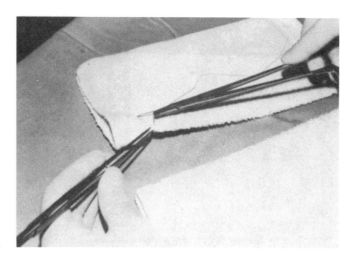

F IGURE 10–19

Placing suture in one side.

Interrupted Sutures

Interrupted sutures may be used when sutures will be under increased tension, such as for bowel and for fascial closure. Although this technique is somewhat slower than a continuous suture, it is safer if there is potential for suture breaking owing to tension or tissue fragility. When the fascia is closed with interrupted sutures, the extent of later fascial dehiscence is usually more limited (as opposed to using a continuous suturing technique).[4] Interrupted sutures also enable more precise approximation of tissues and thus are frequently used for plastic surgery, where minimal scarring is desired. When suturing with interrupted sutures, care must be taken to avoid excessive tension on the tissue and to leave an adequate amount of suture on both sides for tying.

Continuous Sutures

In this faster suturing method, the suture is pulled through the tissue in one continuous motion after the needle has been passed through both sides of the wound (Figure 10–20). Care must be taken not to pull the suture too tight; this will either strangulate tissue and cause possible necrosis, or cause the suture to cut through the tissue. When a long continuous suturing technique is used, the running suture may loosen, allowing the wound to gap in one area as the suture is being tightened at another. To avoid this, the RNFA may consider intermittently (approximately every 2 to 4 centimeters in a long, straight wound) locking a long running suture by wrapping the suture three times around the nearest limb of the previous pass and tightening it into place; the RNFA should provide traction on his or her end of the suture while

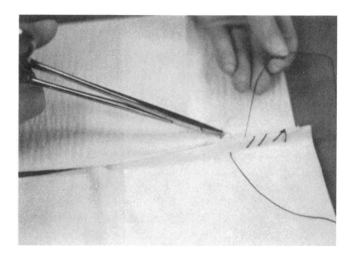

FIGURE 10–20
Technique for placing continuous sutures.

another assistant provides countertension on the other end. The lock is then squared or set as the RNFA pulls the suture toward the other assistant. This divides a long continuous running suture into multiple short segments without the need to tie multiple separate knots.[5]

Following a Suture

Following the suture for the surgeon using a continuous suture must be done carefully and correctly if it is to be effective. The RNFA holds adequate tension to keep the tissue layers together without distorting or strangulating the tissues. Whenever possible, the suture is held from the exited side of the wound, because there is less chance of tearing the tissue with the suture (see Figure 10–20). The suture should be held close enough to the wound to avoid shortening the suture length, but not so close as to obstruct the placement of the needleholder and sutures. When releasing the suture, it should not be allowed to become entangled in drapes, instruments, or other sutures. Timing between the RNFA and the surgeon is important in relation to releasing and grasping the suture. If tension is released prematurely, the suture line may loosen, resulting in poor approximation of the tissues, or the remaining suture may fall onto the suture site and obscure the surgeon's view before he or she moves the needle to reload it.

It may be necessary to grasp the suture with a forceps rather than with the fingers, as when the suture is too short to grasp with the fingers or when the operative site is deep or restricted. When grasping the suture with a forceps, the RNFA must be careful not to grasp too tightly or use a crushing type of forceps. Damage to the suture could cause the suture to break immediately or could weaken the suture, causing it to break later.

If necessary, it is possible to follow one's own suture when suturing. To do so, the suture is grasped with the little finger in the hand holding the tissue forceps (Figure 10–21). This technique can be most useful and is easily learned.

Subcutaneous Sutures

Suturing subcutaneous tissue is often unnecessary. Unless there is a strong line of Scarpa's fascia running through the subcutaneous layer, this layer has little holding power. If the fascia and skin are closely approximated, the subcutaneous tissue is unlikely to have dead space.[6] If it is necessary to close the subcutaneous layer, the suture is usually an absorbable type. Sutures are placed vertically through the tissue from one side of the wound to the other. Horizontal sutures should not be used; they can compromise the blood supply to the skin. Sutures must be placed close enough together to eliminate any gaps in the suture line. Tension on the sutures must be adequate to hold the tissue together but must not be excessive, or else the suture may pull through the tissue or strangulate the tissue itself. The suture needle must not be placed too deep into the tissue, because it is possible to inadvertently penetrate the skin, exposing the suture to the skin surface and providing a potential route of wound infection.

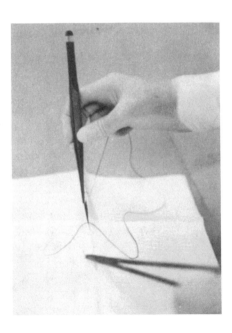

FIGURE 10–21
Following own suture. Note that suture is grasped by little finger.

Skin Sutures

The skin suturing technique depends on the type of incision, its location, the patient's condition, the desired result, and the surgeon's or RNFA's preference. Suture materials used for the skin are nonabsorbable and must be removed postoperatively. Monofilament sutures are more commonly used because they are less traumatic to the tissue. This type of suture is smooth and easier to remove. Braided materials may harbor infectious organisms and potentially cause superficial wound infection. More tissue reaction will occur with the braided sutures. The suture selected should be as fine a gauge as possible that still provides the necessary support to the skin edges as they are reapproximated.

Interrupted sutures provide a better cosmetic result as the wound heals. The *simple interrupted suture* is frequently used. Simple interrupted sutures are placed by entering the skin on one side of the wound edge and exiting on the other side. The entry and exit points are usually only a few millimeters from the incision site and should be approximately the same distance from the skin edges on each side, to avoid distortion of the incision line. After the suture is tied, the knot is pulled to one side of the wound, close to the skin. This technique will adjust the tension and equalize the skin edges. The result of the simple suture is a square-shaped suture that encloses an equal area of dermis on both sides and avoids inverting skin edges.

Interrupted mattress sutures may be needed in instances where increased accuracy is necessary. Mattress sutures also provide more support to the suture line, which may be needed in situations where there is increased strain on the suture line itself (Figure 10–22). The horizontal mattress suture is more commonly used in fascia than on skin. The interrupted mattress suture is placed by entering and exiting the skin edges at a slightly greater distance than with the simple interrupted stitch. Once the first stitch is placed, the needle is passed back through the skin very close to the edges (approximately 2 to 3 millimeters) and then tied in place. Again, gentle, loose tying approximation allows for the slight edema that occurs during wound healing.

Continuous suturing is frequently used on the skin because it can be done quickly, but the cosmetic result is not as good as with the interrupted techniques. To place the sutures, the assistant begins on one side of the incision and exits on the other side at approximately the same distance from the skin edges on each side. The suture is tied, and the short end of the suture is cut. The suture is then used in a "running" fashion or in an "over and over" looping fashion until the wound is closed. A continuous mattress suturing technique can be used if needed (Figure 10–23).

A *subcuticular suture* technique gives the best cosmetic result, with a scar that is very fine. Subcuticular sutures are most valuable for skin closure in parts of the body with a thick dermal layer or where skin is firmly attached to strong subdermal fascia. If the dermis is thin, subcuticular closure should be avoided. An absorbable suture is usually used; however, a nonabsorbable

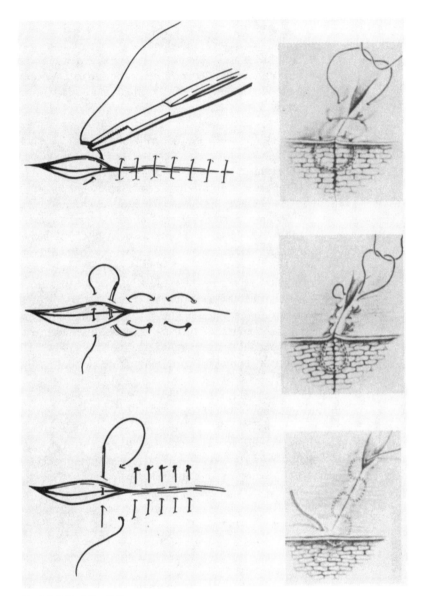

FIGURE 10–22

Examples of interrupted skin sutures. *Top,* simple interrupted suture; *center,* interrupted horizontal mattress suture; *bottom,* interrupted vertical mattress suture. (Source: Wound Closure Manual, 1985. Courtesy of Ethicon, Inc., a Johnson & Johnson Company, Somerville, NJ.)

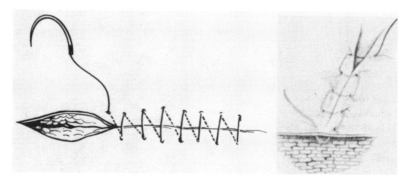

FIGURE 10–23

Examples of continuous skin suturing techniques. *Left,* continuous over-and-over suture; *right,* continuous horizontal mattress suture. (Source: Wound Closure Manual, 1985. Courtesy of Ethicon, Inc., a Johnson & Johnson Company, Somerville, NJ.)

suture can be used and removed later. To remove the nonabsorbable suture, it is necessary to secure the ends of the suture at the skin level, where they can be easily grasped for removal (Figure 10–24). Subcuticular stitches are placed in the lower part of the dermis. The first stitch is placed into the corner of the incision just below the dermal–epidermal junction. The stitches are placed in a horizontal fashion and alternated from one side to the other, with each stitch taking small epidermal bites. The stitches must be placed at the same depth on each side. If they are not, the wound will be uneven. When the suture line is completed, the suture is tightened by pulling the ends, and an instrument tie completed on each end at skin level.

Skin staples are being used with increasing frequency and are very versatile. The skin edges are everted and approximated with one or two tissue forceps as the staple is applied (Figure 10–25). Staples cause minimal tissue trauma or compression, and provide a superior cosmetic result to that produced by continuous or interrupted skin sutures.[7]

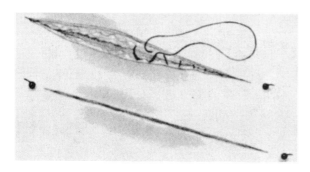

FIGURE 10–24

Continuous subcuticular closure anchored with lead shot. (Source: Wound Closure Manual, 1985. Courtesy of Ethicon, Inc., a Johnson & Johnson Company, Somerville, NJ.)

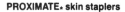

PROXIMATE® skin staplers

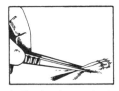 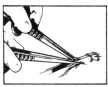

1. Evert and approximate skin edges as desired with one or two tissue forceps.

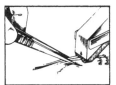 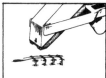

2. Position stapler very lightly over everted skin edges and squeeze trigger.

3. Back stapler off the staple.

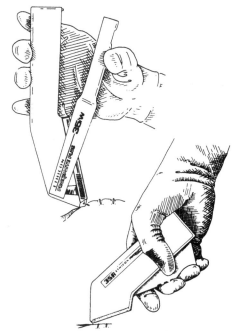

4. Both stapler configurations can be fired from any angle.

FIGURE 10–25

Skin stapling device. (Source: Wound Closure Manual, 1985. Courtesy of Ethicon, Inc., a Johnson & Johnson Company, Somerville, NJ.)

Regardless of the type of skin suturing technique used, some basic principles must be followed.

- Bleeding can distort the wound, disrupt the suture line, and create hematomas that could result in a potential site for infection.
- When the first bite of the needle is made, the wrist should be presupinated to cock the hand in a position that gives strength to drive the needle through the skin.
- Sutures are placed with as little trauma as possible.
- Tissue is handled carefully and gently, and crushing injury is avoided.
- Sutures are never pulled tight, because tissue can become strangulated and the blood supply compromised. Sutures should be only tight enough to hold the opposing tissues together. Tissue edema in the postoperative period can increase the pressure of tissue against the sutures, resulting in hatchmark scarring; this can be avoided by leaving sutures slightly loose when placed. To achieve this technique, the RNFA notes when the skin edges first make contact approximation during a closing stitch. The skin at the site rises just slightly above the surrounding skin surface. This is usually an indication of the right amount of tension at the suture line, and the knot can then be set.
- Skin edges are slightly everted as they are reapproximated, which results in better healing and a better looking scar. The skin edges are aligned as closely as possible to their original appearance.

PREVENTING PERCUTANEOUS INJURY

In 1994, the Centers for Disease Control and Prevention (CDC) reported more than 800,000 needle stick injuries to health care professionals in the United States.[8] Infections from exposures to bloodborne pathogens through percutaneous injury are an occupational hazard for RNFAs. Most reports of percutaneous injuries among health care workers focus on hollow-bore needle devices; suture needles, considered a "solid sharp," are one of the two most common devices causing non-hollow-bore percutaneous injury.[9] In a study of blood exposures in the operating room, suture needles accounted for 50% of the percutaneous injuries; almost half of these were used in suturing muscle or fascia.[10] These injuries usually occur during suturing and are most often self-inflicted (i.e., the injury occurs to the person doing the suturing). However, the assistant is also vulnerable to injury when someone else is suturing, as the hands are close to the suturing needle. Thus, RNFAs must utilize recommended strategies for safer technology during suturing to modify their exposure risk. Among these strategies is the use of blunt suture needles.[11]

The CDC has concluded that blunt needles are associated with a significant reduction in percutaneous injury rates, have minimal clinically important adverse effects on patient care (i.e., the technical difficulty of penetrating tissue or tearing tissue, while reported, was not considered clinically important by surgeons), and are generally accepted by surgeons.[12] Based on a study of gynecologic surgical procedures and an analysis of studies in other surgical specialties, the CDC has therefore suggested that blunt needles can probably be substituted for conventional curved needles in a variety of surgical interventions. During suturing in poorly visualized areas, blunt needles may be particularly useful, as the finger of the nondominant hand is often used to guide or palpate for the needle in these anatomical spaces. Additionally, the CDC study noted that the percutaneous injury rate when a straight needle was used was seven times the injury rate with conventional curved needles, and recommended that indications for the use of straight needles be reevaluated. Blunt needles are available in an improved design to be sharp enough to penetrate muscle and fascia and now come in a variety of sizes and combined with a variety of suture materials. The RNFA should consider using sharp needles only where necessary.

Other technology that RNFAs should participate in evaluating relate to puncture-proof and puncture-resistant gloves and pads. Earlier studies recommended double gloving to prevent punctures, tears, holes, and cuts.[13] Although tears and holes may be easier to detect, punctures from suture needles often go unrecognized.[14] Although double gloves should be worn when working in the operative site or when glove abrasion is anticipated, barrier products for hand protection should be considered when suturing in areas of poor visualization. These products need to be used selectively, as they diminish touch sensitivity. Cut-resistant pads might be selected for the nondominant hand so as not to interfere with the sensitivity and flexibility of the suturing hand. Additionally, the evaluation of breach detection devices has been recommended.[15] RNFAs should also implement safe work practices, including alternatives to sharps for incision and dissection, selecting retractors, scissors, and towel clips with blunt rather than sharp designs, using staples, adhesives, and skin closure tapes where possible, using a no-touch technique or neutral zone when passing instruments back to the scrub nurse, and using scalpels that are disposable or have a blade shield, or a blunt tip.

■ SUMMARY

Regardless of the suturing material and method used, the RNFA's goal during any suturing activity is to achieve a wound that heals without complications. To achieve this goal, the RNFA makes educated choices about the type of suture material, suturing instrument, and suturing technique. Coupled with these cognitive abilities, the RNFA must be proficient in the manipulative skills involved in suturing and use research findings in preventing percutaneous injury to self or another member of the surgical team. Such a combination of intellectual and manual dexterity results in effective and efficient patient care.

◪ Review Questions

1. One of the RNFA's goals during suturing is to leave minimal foreign material in the wound. To achieve this, suture should be selected that has
   a. A low coefficient of friction.
   b. Antimicrobial impregnated in it.
   c. High tensile strength and a small diameter.
   d. Tightly braided fibers with negligible interstices.

2. The rate of suture absorption should correspond to the
   a. Tensile strength of the tissue.
   b. Rate of healing of the tissue.
   c. USP designation as type A or B.
   d. Suture diameter.

3. Suture security depends both on knot-holding ability and
   a. Suture diameter.
   b. Incision location and length.
   c. Intrinsic pliability.
   d. Suture tensile strength.

4. An advantage of multifilament suture is its
   a. Ability to drag through tissue.
   b. Decreased tissue trauma.
   c. Knot-holding ability.
   d. Capillarity.

5. The most tissue-reactive absorbable suture is
   a. Plain catgut.
   b. Chromic catgut.
   c. Polydiaxanone.
   d. Polybutester.

6. In general, a monofilament suture requires _____ knot throws for security than a multifilament.
   a. Fewer
   b. More
   c. The same number of
   d. More, but only if it is coated with a lubricant,

7. The major disadvantage of wire suture is its
   a. Inertness.
   b. Need to be twisted for knot security.
   c. High tensile strength.
   d. Handling characteristics.

8. When assisting during wound closure with a suture that will be used for several interrupted stitches, the RNFA who is tying first grasps
   a. The short end of the suture.

    b. The needle.
    c. The long end of the suture.
    d. A pair of forceps.

9. To assist in grasping a needle as it exits tissue during skin closure, the RNFA grasps the needle with a needleholder and
    a. Brings most of the needle above the skin surface.
    b. Brings all of the needle out in a 90-degree arc.

10. A needle that is grasped in a needleholder too close to the eye may
    a. Break.
    b. Notch.
    c. Bend.
    d. Slip.

11. When suturing very dense tissue, the RNFA may select the _____ grip.
    a. Palmed
    b. Thenar
    c. Thumb-ring finger
    d. Pencil

12. The most traditional needleholder grip, and one that yields both precision and needle control, is the _____ grip.
    a. Palmed
    b. Thenar
    c. Thumb-ring finger
    d. Pencil

13. When using a very fine needleholder, the _____ grip is used.
    a. Palmed
    b. Thenar
    c. Thumb-ring finger
    d. Pencil

14. Although precision is less exacting with the _____ grip, it is used for rapid, easy suturing.
    a. Palmed
    b. Thenar
    c. Thumb-ring finger
    d. Pencil

15. When suturing, the hand begins in what position?
    a. Supine
    b. Prone
    c. Semisupine
    d. Right-angled

16. When following a suture for a surgeon, it is more desirable to hold the suture from which side of the wound?
    a. Exit
    b. Entry

17. When subcutaneous closure is necessary, _____ sutures should not be used because they may compromise blood supply to the skin.
    - a. Vertical
    - b. Horizontal

18. During skin closure, the RNFA uses a technique that _____ skin edges.
    - a. Everts
    - b. Inverts

19. During subcuticular closure, each stitch takes small _____ bites.
    - a. Dermal
    - b. Epidermal

20. The right amount of tension at the suture line takes into consideration the potential for
    - a. Dehiscence.
    - b. Suture sinus tract infection.
    - c. Hematoma formation.
    - d. Postoperative swelling.

Answer Key

1. c	8. a	15. b
2. b	9. a	16. a
3. d	10. c	17. b
4. c	11. a	18. a
5. a	12. c	19. b
6. b	13. d	20. d
7. d	14. b	

REFERENCES

1. Wound Closure Manual. Somerville, NJ, Ethicon, 1994
2. CDC finds using blunt needles prevents injury. OR Manager 13(3):15, 1997
3. Edgerton MT: The Art of Surgical Technique. Baltimore, Williams & Wilkins, 1988, pp 149–153
4. Thal ER, Eastridge BJ, Milhoan R: Operative exposure of abdominal injuries and closure of the abdomen. In: Care of the Surgical Patient, Section IV, Trauma. New York, Scientific American Medicine, 1997, pp 6-1–6-6
5. MacDougal BA: Locking a continuous running suture. J Am Coll Surg 181: 563–564, 1995
6. Ballard AG: Sutures: An overview of wound closure. Point of View 18:8–12, 1995
7. East SA: The registered nurse first assistant role in surgical wound closure: An integrated review. J Vasc Nurs 13(3):83–96, 1995
8. Health and safety on the job: Nurse, protect thyself. Am Nurse 29(5):1, 1997
9. Jagger J, Balon M: Suture needle and scalpel blade injuries. Infect Control Steril 2(9):12–17, 1996
10. New study finds circulators in need of more protection. OR Manager 13(6):1, 1997

11. Chiarello L: Sharps-related injuries in the health care setting: Impact and prevention strategies. Asepsis. Infect Prevent Forum 17(1):18–21, 1995
12. Evaluation of blunt suture needles in preventing percutaneous injuries among health-care workers during gynecologic surgical procedures: New York City, March 1993–June 1994. JAMA 277(6):451–452, 1997
13. Huss, M, Wong D, Lange K, Gasper P, Houghtaling C, Shearon N, Scott D, Stoeffler J: Risk of blood contamination in the operating room: A study of 9,795 cases. AORN Congress Resources, 1995, p 297
14. Korniewitz DM, Rabussay D: Surgical glove failures in clinical practice settings. AORN J 66(4):660–673, 1997
15. Beck WC: Barrier breach of surgical gloves. J Long-Term Effects Medi Implants 4(2, 3):127–132, 1994

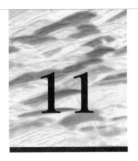

11

WOUND HEALING

JANE C. ROTHROCK

∎

By their very nature, surgical procedures disrupt the integrity of the skin and its underlying tissues. Wound healing focuses on the reestablishment of normal tissue physiology in reaction to surgical disruption. The surgeon and RN first assistant collaborate to augment the forces of repair and the patient's resistance to infection. Surgical wound management is based on knowledge of the physiology of wound healing and factors that interfere with the body's natural self-repair mechanisms. Although wound healing is accomplished through a cascade of complex mechanisms, the fundamental principles of wound healing are common to all types of surgical wounds. Understanding these principles is germane to the quality of care provided by the RNFA. This chapter focuses on the biology of wound healing in the subcutaneous tissues and considers issues of wound management in perioperative patients.

▧ TYPES OF WOUNDS

Wounds may be classified by etiology as either surgical or traumatic, and further subdivided on the basis of tissue loss as either closed or open. A closed wound heals by primary intention; it is a sharply made wound that is accurately reapproximated within hours of the incision and heals with minimal space between its edges (Figure 11–1). An open wound heals by secondary intention; the tissue defect decreases in size by contraction and is filled in by large amounts of newly formed connective tissue, vessels, and epithelium. The new tissue regenerated in this process is known as granulation tissue. Open wounds are usually external, but healing by secondary intention also

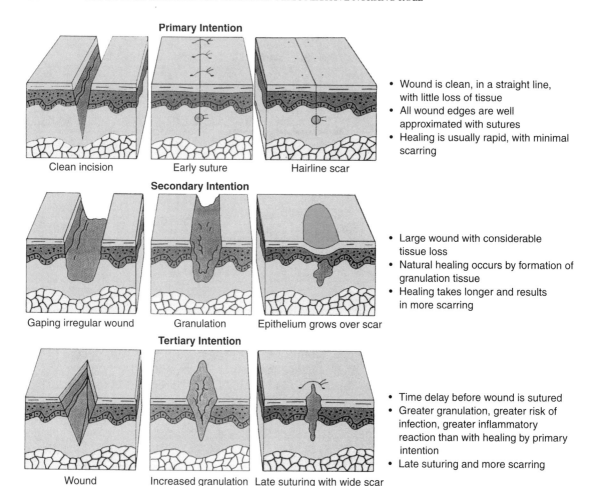

Primary Intention

Clean incision   Early suture   Hairline scar

- Wound is clean, in a straight line, with little loss of tissue
- All wound edges are well approximated with sutures
- Healing is usually rapid, with minimal scarring

Secondary Intention

Gaping irregular wound   Granulation   Epithelium grows over scar

- Large wound with considerable tissue loss
- Natural healing occurs by formation of granulation tissue
- Healing takes longer and results in more scarring

Tertiary Intention

Wound   Increased granulation   Late suturing with wide scar

- Time delay before wound is sutured
- Greater granulation, greater risk of infection, greater inflammatory reaction than with healing by primary intention
- Late suturing and more scarring

FIGURE 11-1

Types of wound healing: primary intention healing, secondary intention healing, and tertiary intention healing. (Source: Smeltzer SC, Bare BG: Brunner and Suddarth's Textbook of Medical-Surgical Nursing, 8th ed. Philadelphia, Lippincott-Raven Publishers, 1996, p 114.)

occurs in the healing of a closed space created after a pneumonectomy or a serum collection under a skin flap after mastectomy.

■ PHYSIOLOGY OF WOUND HEALING

Several biological properties are shared by both closed and open wounds. This discussion of wound healing examines the physiology of closed and open wounds and then focuses on events that are unique to wound healing.

Closed Wounds

Healing of closed wounds involves several phases (Table 11–1). Although they are discussed as separate entities, the phases frequently overlap chronologically, are interdependent, and may occur simultaneously. Following tissue injury, an *inflammatory* phase is initiated; vascular and cellular responses occur immediately when tissue is cut or injured. The length of the inflammatory phase is related to the degree of wound contamination; it may extend from several days to several weeks. The less contaminated the wound, the faster it will heal. In clean wounds, those created aseptically in surgery, few inflammatory cells are seen after five to seven days.

Injury disrupts tissue integrity. Blood vessels are damaged, cells are broken, and the complement cascade is initiated. Transient vasoconstriction occurs, during which platelets aggregate, promote the deposition of fibrin, and release growth factors. A fibrin clot forms, providing initial wound closure, localizing injury, and preventing further contamination and loss of blood and other body fluids. This is followed by blood vessel dilation. Capillaries become permeable to plasma proteins and plasma that leak into the site of injury. White blood cells stick to vascular endothelial surfaces and then move through vessel walls into the adjacent tissue. Within hours after the initial insult, the wound fills with a cellular inflammatory exudate containing white blood cells, red blood cells, plasma proteins, water, electrolytes, antibodies, complement factors, and fibrin. The duration and intensity of this phase depend on the amount of local tissue damage. Extensive injury or the presence of foreign material in the wound can prolong this phase for months. In the usual clean surgical incision, inflammation lasts a few days.

The white blood cells—mast cells, neutrophils, monocytes, and macrophages—are the key cells in the inflammatory response. Acting as the digestive tract of the wound, they engulf and remove injured tissue and cellular

T A B L E 1 1 – 1 . PHASES OF WOUND HEALING

Phase	Length of Time	Events
Inflammatory (also called lag or exudative phase)	1–4 days	Blood clot forms Wound becomes edematous Debris of damaged tissue and blood clot are phagocytized
Proliferative (also called fibroblastic or connective tissue phase)	5–20 days	Collagen produced Granulation tissue forms Wound tensile strength increases
Maturation (also called differentiation, resorptive, remodeling, or plateau phase)	21 days to months or even years	Fibroblasts leave wound Tensile strength increases Collagen fibers reorganize and tighten to reduce scar size

debris through phagocytosis and release chemicals, including enzymes to digest fibrin, oxygen radicals to kill bacteria, lysozymes to digest dead tissue, and growth factors to stimulate the next phase of healing.[1] Injured tissue and bacteria are believed to release chemotactic substances (chemoattractants) that draw leukocytes and other macrophages into the wound. This stimulates fibroblast activity and neovascularization in the wound space. If wound contamination is excessive, the white blood cells are overwhelmed. As these cells die, they release lysosomal enzymes such as proteases and collagenases, which contribute to tissue damage and prolong the inflammatory response.

The *proliferative* phase, also referred to as the connective tissue or fibroblastic phase of wound healing, begins next and may last for several weeks. By two or three days following injury, fibroblasts derived from locally injured or stimulated mesenchymal (perivascular) tissues invade the wound; these predominate by day 10. Fibroblasts are responsible for the synthesis and secretion of collagen, elastin, and the proteoglycans of ground substance. The fibrin strands that had filled the wound earlier now act as scaffolding for fibroblast movement. Collagen fibers appear soon after this cellular invasion.

Rapid capillary proliferation by budding of existing venules promotes neovascularization as the nutritional needs of the healing wound increase and a new vascular network is generated. New vessels develop from existing vessels as capillaries, a process called neoangiogenesis. Capillaries grow from the wound edges toward areas of inadequate perfusion. When they meet other developing capillaries, they join and establish new blood vessels. The lymphatic system is also reestablished at this time, facilitating local drainage of interstitial fluid. The epidermis adjacent to the wound edge thickens, and the basal cells enlarge, multiply, and migrate across the surface of the wound defect (reepithelialization). These cells migrate only over viable tissue; they are stopped by contact inhibition. By 48 hours, the wound surface may be completely reepithelialized. After the wound is bridged, specialized fibroblast action pulls the wound margins inward (contraction).

The *maturation* phase becomes evident by four to five weeks, when the fibroblasts decrease in number and collagen fibers fill the wound. These fibers initially appear as early as four to five days after injury in randomly oriented bundles. They gradually enlarge and produce a massive, dense, collagenous structure—the scar, which binds the severed tissues together. A phase of scar remodeling then ensues. During this phase, the collagen fibers in the scar are altered (cross-linked) and rewoven into different architectural patterns that affect the gross appearance of the "healed" wound. In reality, it is more accurate to think of scar physiology as a continuous dynamic process rather than an event that ceases at a given time. This process may last many years and is the reason an "old wound" may be affected by later events in particular patients. Although the cross-links between the collagen strands increase during the remodeling phase, scar tissue never reaches the tensile strength of unwounded tissue.

Open Wounds

Open wounds share many of the basic healing processes discussed for closed wounds; however, the need to repair a tissue defect in these injuries also involves wound contraction and granulation tissue formation. After the loss of tissue, an inflammatory exudate collects on the surface of the wound.

Cellular mitosis and migration from adjacent tissues give this wound bed a finely "granular" appearance. After a delay of two to three days, the wound undergoes contraction during the healing process. The wound margins move toward each other, stretching surrounding skin to make the surface defect smaller. Contraction is most rapid by five to ten days and slows by two weeks. The cells responsible for this phenomenon are known as myofibroblasts. In areas of loose, mobile skin, little deformity and acceptable cosmetic results may be obtained by wound contraction. Regions of the body with poor skin mobility (e.g., face, anterior lower leg, hands, neck, breasts) cannot heal by this mechanism, and severe contraction deformity, a nonhealing ulcer, or healing by epithelialization alone may result.

Epithelialization occurs beneath whatever nonliving covering (e.g., scab eschar) is on the wound. Epithelial cells migrate from the wound margins over the collagenous granulation tissue at the base of the wound bed. They usually cannot migrate more than a few centimeters from the wound edges, and the resulting junction of epithelium and underlying scar tissue is relatively weak. It is a poor substitute for skin, because minor shearing forces can disrupt this layer. It frequently deteriorates after traumatization. Epithelialization and contraction may be minimized by a combination of immediate skin coverage of the open wound and mechanical splinting of the adjacent tissues.

Examination of these wounds shows that heavily contaminated open wounds display markedly decreased bacterial counts during the three to six days after injury. Consequently, many of these wounds can safely be left open for healing by secondary intention or closed after several days (tertiary intention) with markedly decreased rates of wound infection. This latter technique is known as delayed primary closure (see Figure 11–1).

Skin Grafts

If a wound can be directly approximated without excessive tension or distortion, then this is most often the method of choice. Wounds deficient in surface covering may require closure by a skin graft or flap if secondary or delayed primary closure cannot be done. The skin graft is a segment of dermis and epidermis that has been separated from its blood supply and site of origin (donor site) before being transplanted to another area of the body (recipient site). It may consist of the epidermis and a portion of the dermis (split-thickness graft) or the epidermis and all of the dermis (full-thickness graft). It is usually used as a permanent wound covering and may be used to close any wound with a sufficient blood supply to produce granulation tissue.

A skin graft is placed in contact with its recipient bed, from which it initially absorbs a plasma-like fluid. A fibrin network forms between the graft and the bed, holding the graft in place. Vascular buds grow into this network and then into the graft during the first 48 hours after grafting. Lymphatics are also restored, so that drainage from the graft is established by the fourth or fifth postoperative day. The capillary buds that grow into the graft race to vascularize the graft before its cells undergo autolysis and death, as the plasmatic flow from the bed into the graft is insufficient to support indefinite survival. Improper tension on the graft, fluid (blood or serum) beneath the graft, and movement of the graft on its bed will delay or prevent revascularization and may result in graft failure. For these reasons, the RN first assistant will need to consider a patient care regimen that includes skin graft immobilization during the first five to seven days after placement; compression dressings may help with this. The risk of seromas and hematomas can be limited by elevating the part, if possible. In patients with flaps, the blood supply must not be impaired by pressure from a dressing, poor patient positioning, or hematoma formation. Drains are frequently placed to encourage tissue approximation and to prevent the collection of blood and serum under the flap.

Physical Events

Wounds begin to gain strength immediately after repair, irrespective of the type of closure. Initially, only relatively weak intercellular forces—that is, protein adhesion and fibrin polymerization—are responsible. After collagen fibers begin to appear, near the third day after injury, wound strength increases rapidly. The healing wound has its greatest mass approximately three weeks after injury, but the gain in strength continues at a rapid, constant rate for close to four months. After this the rate slows, but the wound continues to gain strength for about one year, reflecting prolonged collagen turnover. Wounds rarely if ever regain the strength and resilience of uninjured tissue; normal elasticity is lost in scars, which become relatively inelastic and brittle.

The scar undergoes a progressive change in appearance during this period of remodeling or maturation. It usually demonstrates a gradual loss of redness and firmness, becoming white, soft, and nonadherent to underlying structures. The healed wound may appear narrow or wide, raised or depressed, and delicate or thick. These varied end results reflect a combination of surgical technique, the activity of collagenase (which causes collagen turnover), and physical forces that act on the healing wound. Fibroblasts and collagen fibers tend to align along lines of tension; even minor stresses on the healing wound affect their activity. Incisions crossing lines of changing dimension (joints) produce large hypertrophic scars. Incisions within normal skin creases where tension is minimal tend to produce small, well-healed scars. For unknown reasons, scars exhibit more rapid wound maturation in older patients than in children.

Secondary Healing

A wound reopened within a week of primary repair will heal more rapidly than the original wound. This phenomenon, called secondary healing, is believed to be related to an immediate onset of fibroplasia without the usual four- to six-day lag period after injury. These wounds do not demonstrate increased rates of wound healing, and the ultimate strength of the healed wounds is the same as that of wounds that underwent primary repair. The sole difference is the absence of a lag phase in secondary healing wounds; the healing process already under way simply continues without alteration or delay.

Reopening an old, mature wound starts a different set of events than those that occurred when previously uninjured skin was incised. The scar that results from a second wound is different from the initial scar in both physical characteristics and appearance. The final secondary scar usually has less collagen and appears less hypertrophic than the initial scar.

■ METABOLIC REQUIREMENTS OF WOUND HEALING

All the steps involved in wound healing require numerous synthetic and energy-consuming reactions. The inflammatory response and the delicate balance between collagen synthesis and lysis are particularly dependent on the patient's metabolic status. The wound makes a nutritional demand; unless this demand is met by dietary sources, the body is forced to turn on itself, catabolizing certain of its own tissues to acquire the metabolites needed for repair. It should be noted, however, that patients undergoing major elective surgery who have no nutritional disturbances before the surgery are not apt to develop wound healing problems secondary to metabolic alterations induced by the operation unless a complication, such as serious shock, infection, renal failure, or liver failure, develops.

Proteins and amino acids must be available for cell multiplication and synthesis of the enzymes and substrates critically involved in the healing process. Protein deficiency—particularly deficits or imbalances in essential amino acids such as methionine, cystine, arginine, glutamine, and lysine—delays almost all aspects of healing, including neovascularization, fibroblast proliferation, collagen synthesis, and wound remodeling. If protein deficiency is prolonged or liver function is severely impaired, serum albumin levels decrease. Albumin is important for regenerating tissue for wound healing. Normal levels are 3.5 to 5.0 g/dL; low levels may indicate that cells are in a catabolic state, which can lead to tissue necrosis and infection.[2] Low values of total serum protein (normal is 6.0–8.0 g/dL) are associated with decreased colloid osmotic pressure. Fluids, especially plasma, do not flow into the cells, leading to poor cell nutrition and oxygenation and tissue edema that may impair wound healing. Protein-deficient patients also have a greater risk of postoperative wound dehiscence.[3]

Glucose is the body's major metabolic fuel. Short-term deficits may be supplemented by gluconeogenesis. Fibroblasts and leukocytes metabolize glucose, and glucose availability is vital during the first few days after injury. Glucose is of little value if a lack of insulin prevents its utilization, as in diabetes. Furthermore, hyperosmolarity resulting from hyperglycemia, another consequence of diabetes, also interferes with wound repair.

Certain unsaturated fatty acids (arachidonic, linoleic, and linolenic) are considered to be essential and must be supplied exogenously. They are important for the production of prostaglandins, which regulate cellular metabolism, inflammation, and circulation.

Vitamin A aids the entrance of macrophages into wounds. It is vital to the initiation of repair, required for maintenance of normal epithelium by aiding in glycoprotein synthesis, and is a co-factor for collagen synthesis and cross-linkage.[4] Vitamin C (ascorbic acid) is involved in collagen turnover and can alter the balance of collagen metabolism, thus affecting the wound's tensile strength. A deficiency of vitamin C (scurvy) can affect the function of macrophages, leukocytes, and immune responses, causing new wounds to heal poorly and old wounds to reopen. Vitamin K is required for synthesis of clotting factors. Lack of this vitamin may lead to clotting abnormalities and excessive bleeding into wounds.

Several minerals, particularly magnesium, are involved in many energy-producing cycles and protein synthesis. Of the trace elements necessary for wound repair, zinc (deficient in burned or highly stressed patients) affects epithelialization, wound strength, and collagen protein production. Iron is needed for the hydroxylation of collagen. Copper and manganese are important in the enzyme systems required for collagen cross-linking.

Patients with wounds healing by secondary intention are usually discharged from care before the wound is closed. A study of the adequacy of overall calorie, protein, vitamin C, and zinc intake in a small group of such patients indicated that most of the patients had inadequate caloric and zinc intake, over half had inadequate protein intake, and a third had inadequate vitamin C intake. This study suggests that RN first assistants should pay serious attention to patient education and postdischarge follow-up of nutritional intake with patients whose wounds are healing by secondary intention.[5]

■ WOUND MANAGEMENT

With the advent of modern wound management, the devastating consequences of wound infections, and their significant mortality, have decreased. In early attempts to control wound infections, the perioperative team's effort was primarily directed toward controlling infecting organisms through antiseptic and aseptic surgical technique. The epidemiology of wound infections has changed as the perioperative team has worked to control sources of bacterial contamination and focus on host defense mechanisms in a continuing effort to achieve improved results of wound healing.

Preoperative Considerations

Optimal wound healing requires careful attention to the details of preoperative, intraoperative, and postoperative management. The chief preoperative concern for all types of wounds is identifying and reducing risk factors that may lead to postoperative wound infection. For elective surgery, this includes skin antisepsis and judicious antibiotic administration so that an adequate tissue level of the appropriate antibiotic is attained before the operative procedure. In a recent study, the administration of prophylactic antibiotics more than two hours before surgery was associated with a greater than five-fold increase in the risk for infection.[6] A single preoperative dose administered within two hours before the surgical incision is usually sufficient for most surgical procedures, although patients undergoing lengthy procedures may benefit from additional intraoperative administration.[7] (See Chapter 4, Infection Control, for more information.) For traumatic wounds, major considerations include the time elapsed between injury and treatment and the strength and type of foreign inoculum in the wound. An absolutely "safe" number of hours between injury and treatment that permits closure of traumatic wounds without the risk of subsequent wound infection does not exist. Rather, the decision to primarily close a traumatic wound depends on the injury's clinical appearance, its location on the body, method of injury, and ultimately the surgeon's judgment.

In many cases, contaminated wounds may be converted to clean ones for closure soon after inoculation. This frequently requires anesthesia of the involved area to permit adequate surgical debridement of nonviable tissue and foreign material. But although local anesthetics containing vasoconstrictors may prolong the duration of anesthesia, they may damage wound defenses in contaminated wounds by restricting local blood flow. Antibiotics have limited usefulness in preventing wound infection in most traumatic injuries; a fibrinous coagulum frequently surrounds bacteria in these wounds and isolates them from contact with the antibiotic. Tetanus prophylaxis should not be neglected in these patients.

Intraoperative Factors

The determinants of an infectious process are the infecting organism, the environment in which the infection occurs, and host defense mechanisms. Controlling sources of infecting organisms—in surgery, most often bacteria—is vital. Endogenous bacteria play a significant role in wound infection. Remote infections, even those of the urinary tract, should be treated before elective surgery. The skin is a primary source of infection following clean operations (Table 11–2). The perioperative team and the environment are other potential sources of exogenous contamination. Basic principles of asepsis are predominant, controllable factors by the RN first assistant. Less controllable is expected duration of the surgical procedure. During lengthy procedures, the sources of bacteria represent increased time at risk for contamination. Abdominal surgery is another risk factor. Because major concentrations of endogenous bacteria are located in the abdomen, these operations are more likely to involve bacterial contamination. In all surgical procedures, the RNFA should work closely with the surgeon to carry out a procedure with minimal blood loss, avoidance of shock, and maintenance of blood volume, tissue perfusion, and tissue oxygenation. All of these efforts combine to minimize trauma and the secondary, unintended immunological effects of major surgery.

The many intraoperative factors that affect wound healing are discussed in detail in other chapters of this book. The driving force in the prevention of wound infection is knowledge and expertise in the fundamentals of aseptic technique.[8] An understanding of the microbiological principles of asepsis (see Chapter 4, Infection Control) assists the RNFA in breaking the chain of infection. The importance of preoperative skin antisepsis and the use of microbial barriers in creating and maintaining the sterile field (see Chapter 6, Perioperative Patient Preparation) guides the RNFA in initiating preventive patient care measures. Ensuring proper tissue handling (see Chapter 8, Principles of Tissue Handling), providing adequate exposure (see Chapter 9, Providing Exposure: Retractors and Retraction), judiciously selecting suture materials and suturing techniques (see Chapter 10, Suturing Materials and Techniques), skillfully handling clamps (see Chapter 12, Using Grasping Instruments), and achieving meticulous hemostasis (see Chapter 13, Providing Hemostasis) are

TABLE 11–2. CLASSIFICATION OF SURGICAL WOUNDS

Classification	Description
Clean	Nontraumatic
	No inflammation
	No break in technique
	Respiratory, GI, GU tracts not entered
	Primary closure
	Drainage by closed system
Clean-contaminated	Respiratory, GI, GU tracts entered under control (no spillage)
Contaminated	Fresh, traumatic wound
	Gross spillage
Dirty/infected	Acute inflammation
	Traumatic wound with retained, devitalized tissue
	Perforated viscera

all intraoperative maneuvers with which the RNFA is intimately involved. The critical role played by the RNFA during the intraoperative period contributes significantly to satisfactory wound healing. For this reason, much of this book explores in detail these critical elements of RNFA functions. Tables 11–3 and 11–4 provide a brief, not inclusive, review of important RNFA nursing behaviors to facilitate wound healing and reduce the risk of surgical site infection.

Postoperative Wound Care

Initially applied under sterile conditions in the operating room, dressings prevent wound and suture line contamination, protect wounds from additional trauma, and immobilize surrounding skin. A wound's susceptibility to surface contamination is greatest during the first postoperative day. After this period a coagulum seals the wound, and the wound rapidly gains resistance to infection. Consequently, the dressings on elective surgical wounds are generally left intact until the wound is inspected one to two days after surgery. Exceptions may be made for dressings that become saturated with blood or serous drainage and thus effectively disrupt the sterile barrier created by the dressing. Traumatic wounds are at higher risk for wound infection and are generally examined within 24 hours after treatment. (See Chapter 8 for a more thorough discussion of dressings.)

T A B L E 1 1 – 3 . RNFA OBSERVATIONS/INTERVENTIONS

Inspect wound to verify hemostasis
Assess wound for classic signs of inflammation:

- Erythema
- Warmth
- Edema
- Pain/tenderness

Note any exudate; document color, consistency, odor; obtain/review culture results as appropriate
Monitor vital signs
Elevate part (as appropriate)
Utilize proper technique for dressing changes
Monitor drainage system for function/volume and characterisics of drainage collection (as applicable)
Keep wound edges approximated
Provide written instructions for home care of incision, dressings, drains; clarify, verify patient's understanding
Maintain moist environment (appropriate dressings to promote formation of granulation tissue and reepithelialization)
Protect wound from trauma (chemical/mechanical)
Review nutritional instructions prior to discharge; make referrals if indicated

T A B L E   1 1 – 4 . NURSING DIAGNOSIS: HIGH RISK FOR INFECTION

Definition: Patient at risk to be invaded by opportunistic or pathogenic agent at surgical site

Risk Factors:

Host factors: ASA class, disease severity index, prolonged preoperative stay, presence of remote infections, morbid obesity, old age

Surgery-related factors: Wound classification, prolonged duration of surgery, specific type of surgery (i.e., abdominal organs), intraoperative microbial contamination

Related Factors: Chronic, concomitant diseases; immunosuppression or deficiency; impaired circulation, tissue perfusion; diabetes; medications (steroids, immunosuppressants, antimicrobials); presence of invasive lines; trauma, presence of foreign body; malnutrition; cancer; low serum albumin, prolonged hospitalization; multiple procedures

RNFA Care Regimen:

1. Assess for risk and related factors.
2. Use nursing diagnosis, High Risk for Infection, when one or more factors are present.
3. Initiate preventive strategies:
   a. Collaborate in treatment of remote infection site
   b. Implement preoperative patient education (prepare patient and family/significant other for postoperative routines/care regimens):
      - early ambulation
      - techniques to promote coughing and deep breathing
      - nutrition
      - wound care
      - reportable signs and symptoms; how to contact RN first assistant/surgeon
      - medication regimen (postoperative, as appropriate)
      - home care referral, as necessary
   c. Collaborate in:
      - preoperative shower or scrub; patient skin preparation in operating room
      - selection of appropriate surgical barriers (gowns/drapes)
      - controlling perioperative environment
      - initiating principles of surgical technique to facilitate wound healing (duration of operation; cautious tissue handling; judicious use of electrosurgery, sutures, drains; careful hemostasis; maintenance of tissue perfusion; correct use of instruments; meticulous attention to surgical asepsis; obliteration of dead space during wound closure; appropriate selection and application of dressings).

Many skin irritations are mistakenly attributed to a problem with a wound or to an allergic reaction to tape. They may be caused by taping techniques or tape effects on skin. Tape should be applied without tension. It should be applied from the center of the incision outward, with gentle rubbing of the ends to improve adherence (Figure 11–2). Stripping the skin of its superficial layer interferes with the skin's ability to control water metabolism and can interfere with wound healing.

Sutures and staples in skin are usually removed when their purpose has been achieved. Too early removal invites wound dehiscence and scar widen-

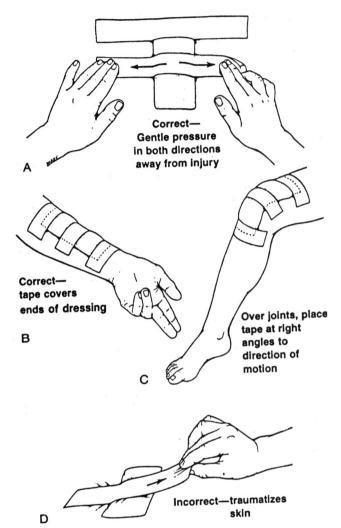

Correct—
Gentle pressure
in both directions
away from injury

A

Correct—
tape covers
ends of dressing

B

Over joints, place
tape at right
angles to
direction of
motion

C

Incorrect—traumatizes
skin

D

FIGURE 11–2

Application of tape. Views **A, B,** and **C** illustrate the correct method of application. The method shown in **D** is incorrect. (**A**) Pressure is applied evenly and directed away from the incision. (**D**) In the incorrect method, the tape is pulling against the skin and exerting pressure over the wound. (**B**) The proper way to cover the ends of a dressing for additional protection of the wound. (**C**) The correct way to position a dressing over a joint for maximum comfort and effectiveness. (Source: Smeltzer SC, Bare BG, eds: Brunner and Suddarth's Textbook of Medical-Surgical Nursing, 8th ed. Philadelphia, Lippincott-Raven Publishers, 1996, p 417.)

ing; on the other hand, leaving them in place too long leads to the development of epithelium-lined suture tracts, infection, and unsightly scars. As healing rates vary according to the patient's age and overall condition and the type of wound, an absolute rule for removing all types of sutures does not exist. Generally, in an uncomplicated wound, skin sutures are removed 5 to 15 days postoperatively. Retention sutures in the abdomen are usually removed after the third postoperative week. Nonetheless, the RN first assistant should understand that such factors as the amount of tension on the wound edges, the presence of any risk factors that would prolong wound healing, and cosmetic concerns are better guidelines than postoperative day counts for the timing of suture or clip removal. While removing sutures or skin sta-

T A B L E   1 1 – 5 . PATIENT EDUCATION: WOUND CARE

Until Sutures Are Removed:
1. Keep the wound dry and clean.
    a. If there is no dressing, ask your nurse or physician if you can bathe or shower.
    b. If a dressing or splint is in place, do not remove it unless it is wet or soiled.
    c. If wet or soiled, change dressing yourself if you have been taught to do so; otherwise, call your nurse or physician for guidance.
    d. If you have been taught, instruction might be as follows:
        (1) Cleanse area *gently* with 70% isopropyl alcohol once or twice daily.
        (2) Cover with a sterile Telfa pad or gauze square—sufficiently large to cover wound.
        (3) Apply hypoallergenic Dermacel or paper tape (adhesive is not recommended because it is difficult to remove without possible injury to incision site).
2. Report immediatley if any of these signs of infection occur:
    a. Redness, marked swelling (beyond 2.5 cm [½ inch] from incision site), tenderness, increased warmth around wound
    b. Red streaks in skin near wound
    c. Pus or discharge, foul odor
    d. Chills or fever (over 37.7 °C [100 °F])
3. If soreness or pain is causing discomfort, apply a dry cool pack (containing ice or cold water) or take prescribed acetaminophen tablets (2) every 4–6 hours. Avoid aspirin without direction or instruction because bleeding may be enhanced with its use.
4. Swelling following surgery is common. To help reduce swelling, elevate the affected part to the level of the heart.
    a. Hand or am
        (1) Sleep—elevate arm on pillow at side.
        (2) Sitting—place arm on pillow on adjacent table.
        (3) Standing—rest affected hand on opposite shoulder; support elbow with unaffected hand.
    b. Leg or foot
        (1) Sitting—place a pillow on a facing chair; provide support underneath the knee.
        (2) Lying—place a pillow under affected leg.

After Sutures Are Removed:
Although the wound appears to be healed when sutures are removed, it is still tender and will continue to heal and strengthen for several weeks.
1. Follow directives of physician or nurse as to extent of activity.
2. Keep suture line clean: do not rub vigorously; pat dry. Wound edges may look red and may be slightly raised. This is normal.
3. Massage around wound gently using a bland baby oil, petrolatum, or moisturizing cream (twice a day)
4. Report to the health care provider if after 8 weeks the site continues to be red, thick, painful to pressure. (This may be due to excessive collagen formation and should be checked.)

ples, the RNFA should take the opportunity to teach the patient (and family, significant other, or caregiver) how to care for the incision and change dressings at home (Table 11–5).

Wound drains and tubes are generally removed before the risk of induced infection or interference with healing outweighs their benefit—usually within five days, because most fluid collections will have been decompressed by that time. Changing wound wicks and packing daily helps keep wounds clean by gentle debridement and removal of wound debris, and also facilitates delayed primary closure; most of these wounds may be closed safely five days after surgery.

Skin graft survival requires adequate continuous contact with the recipient bed. Grafts are usually immobilized with stents or splints to prevent shearing when the patient moves. These wounds are usually inspected two to three days postoperatively for fluid collection beneath the graft. Such collection frequently gives the overlying area of the graft a translucent appearance and can prevent successful grafting. Needle aspiration or an incision in the graft can evacuate the fluid while the graft is still viable and prevent potentially devastating complications. Skin grafts on extremities (particularly the lower extremities) are elevated after surgery to decrease dependent edema in the wound until adequate lymphatic drainage is restored.

■ EARLY WOUND COMPLICATIONS

Problems encountered in healing wounds may be broadly classified into those that occur early in the postoperative period and those that develop late. Infection, the most frequent complication, usually manifests several days after surgery. Local signs may be occult, but patients often develop systemic signs of distress, with fever, tachycardia, and elevated white blood cell counts that suggest an ongoing infectious process.

Infections

The nature, diagnosis, and treatment of wound infections are multifaceted. Subcutaneous abscesses, cellulitis, necrotizing soft tissue infection, and intra-abdominal and retroperitoneal infections and their etiological agents must be diagnosed correctly and treated quickly. Wound surveillance, close patient assessment and evaluation, laboratory confirmation, and balancing the risks and inherent benefits of antibiotic therapy are all major considerations in infection control.

Cellulitis. A bacterial infection that spreads in tissue planes, cellulitis usually causes intense inflammation manifested locally as tenderness, pain, swelling, erythema, and warmth. The responsible organism is frequently a streptococcus. Treatment involves adequate rest to decrease muscle contractions, which may force bacteria into lymphatics and veins. Elevation of limbs reduces dependent edema, and heat enhances local blood flow in the affected area. Drainage is rarely used and is indicated only to relieve pressure-induced ischemia. Appropriate systemic antibiotics are indicated.

Abscess.   Localized bacterial infection marked by a circumscribed area of pus (necrotic tissue, bacteria, and white blood cells) constitutes an abscess. Abscesses tend to develop point tenderness and fluctuate on palpation. They are often under high pressure and tend to seed bacteria, causing bacteremia or sepsis by invasion of vascular spaces, or cellulitis from involvement of adjacent tissues. They should be surgically drained or excised, with the resulting wound packed open to prevent recurrence of a closed-space infection. Rest, heat, and elevation are helpful. Antibiotics may not be indicated unless regional or systemic involvement is evident.

Lymphangitis.   Bacterial spread through the lymphatic system, usually arising from a local area of cellulitis or abscess, is known as lymphangitis. Antibiotics, local heat, and rest, along with proper treatment of the infectious source, are appropriate therapy.

Tetanus.   A complication of traumatic wounds rarely seen today, tetanus is caused by a toxin from *Clostridium tetani* bacteria that usually manifests after an incubation period of seven to ten days after inoculation. Tetanus should be suspected in a patient with insomnia, irritability, tremors, spasms, and rigidity of muscles adjacent to a traumatic wound. Treatment involves administering tetanus immune globulin and sedation. Occasionally, mechanical ventilation and surgical debridement of necrotic tissues with wide excision of the affected area are indicated.

Gas Gangrene.   Clostridial myositis, also known as gas or invasive gangrene, is a rapidly progressive infection that causes extensive local and regional tissue destruction and systemic toxemia. It arises from injuries associated with devitalized muscle and decreased local oxygen tension. Swelling and pain occur early (within 24 hours) after injury and may be associated with crepitus from gas formation in the muscles. Often, the wound produces a thin, watery, brown, foul-smelling discharge that may contain gas bubbles and bacteria. Skin overlying the affected area may appear bronze-colored and dusky; dark red muscle may protrude through the wound. The patient rapidly develops systemic signs of pallor, weakness, apathy, profuse diaphoresis, dyspnea, and tachycardia that seem out of proportion to the low-grade fever.

Such a patient faces impending septic shock. Treatment consists of immediate surgical exploration of the wound with decompression of the involved muscle compartment, wide excision and muscle debridement, antibiotics (usually penicillin), hyperbaric oxygen, and supportive therapy.

Meleney's Ulcer.   Progressive bacterial synergistic gangrene, also called Meleney's ulcer, is a necrotic process involving large areas of skin that may ulcerate one to two weeks after the placement of stay sutures or drainage of abdominal or thoracic abscesses. It may also follow operative procedures in poorly vascularized tissues. The lesions are caused by a mixed infection from *Staphylococcus aureus* and a streptococcus. They are characterized by a tender, centrally brown, shaggy area of necrosis and ulceration surrounded by a purple zone and a red cutaneous flare. These wounds are treated by radical excision and antibiotics.

Actinomycosis.   *Actinomyces* is frequently responsible for chronic suppurative infections with multiple draining cutaneous sinuses complicating recent wounds. The purulent exudate characteristically contains yellow sulfur granules. In addition, local granulomatous tissue proliferates, forming parallel cutaneous ridges in the wound. Treatment consists of incision and drainage with prolonged antibiotic therapy.

Dehiscence.   Dehiscence, or the breakdown and separation of tissue layers in a wound, usually occurs five to eight days postoperatively. Although half of all cases are associated with infection, dehiscence may also occur in many patients who did not demonstrate a cutaneous "healing ridge" of tissue in their incisions. Poorly managed ischemic wounds and wound closure under extreme tension are other common causes of dehiscence. If dehiscence is noted within six hours and is caused by premature suture removal, the wound is immediately resutured. Otherwise, the wound is usually managed with open packing and secondary or delayed primary closure. When there is serosanguinous drainage from an abdominal wound five to eight days after surgery and the healing ridge is absent, then the wound should be explored to define the extent of fascial dehiscence. If fascial dehiscence is significant, it may lead to evisceration. If immediate operative reclosure is not possible, then evisceration is prevented with abdominal binders and bed rest.

Serum or Blood Collections.   Seromas frequently complicate wounds involving undermined tissues, such as mastectomy flaps or large incisions in obese patients. Although these collections are initially sterile and resistant to infection, they quickly become susceptible to contamination and should be

T A B L E   1 1 – 6 .   CAUSES OF NONHEALING WOUNDS

Cancer	Drug therapy
Basal cell carcinoma	Infections
Leukemia	Nutrition
Melanoma	Starvation (protein depletion)
Squamous cell carcinoma	Inflammatory bowel disease (malabsorption)
Chronic trauma	Radiation
Factitious ulcer	Locally irradiated tissues
Hyperactivity	Radiation enteritis
Peripheral neuropathy	Vascular disorders
Poor hygiene	Arterial ischemia and atherosclerosis
Proximal nerve injury	Diabetes
Pruritus	Pressure sores

drained. Hemorrhage within a wound may be related to hypertension, coagulopathy, or excessive postoperative motion. However, most wound hematomas are the result of surgically controllable bleeding, such as an unligated vessel; these should be evacuated under sterile conditions, as they predispose wounds to infection and may take months to organize and resorb. They can be resutured unless infection or ongoing bleeding is present. If a seroma develops after a drain is removed, it should be aspirated intermittently. If it does not resolve, then the closed suction drains should be reinserted or the wound allowed to heal by secondary intention. Antibiotics and graded compression dressings may be indicated.

Nonhealing Wound.   This phenomenon is usually the manifestation of a local complication in the wound healing process, such as undue tension on tissue edges with ischemia and necrosis of tissues, hematoma, infection, or retention of foreign material. Occasionally, other causes or underlying systemic diseases may need to be ruled out (Table 11–6).

■ LATE WOUND COMPLICATIONS

Certain wound complications have catastrophic implications. One often focuses on such factors as wound dehiscence, its related factors, prevention, and nursing intervention. Yet in the broad sense of potential morbidity of wound complications, the RN first assistant must consider an array of complicating events that are not as emergent as dehiscence but nonetheless are consequential to the patient.

Incisional Hernia

Incisional hernia is considered to be iatrogenic in origin. It usually occurs after abdominal wounds and is rare in chest or flank incisions. These hernias are frequently multiple and represent a failure of healing. The most common cause of incisional hernia is wound infection, but technical errors in closing wounds, severe obesity, and prior dehiscence all predispose to this complication.

Epithelial Cyst

Cysts are occasionally seen along suture lines. The needle and suture used to approximate skin edges create a microwound that epithelial cells migrate into and line when sutures are left in skin for an excessive time. Cysts may be prevented by properly timed skin suture removal (usually within five days).

Suture Sinus

Developing from small abscesses in or near a wound associated with localized infection around a suture, suture sinuses persist as long as the suture remains in the tissue and may resolve spontaneously after several weeks as the suture is ejected from the wound. Suture sinuses occur most frequently with silk, cotton, or heavy multifilament sutures.

Hypertrophic Scars and Keloids

Large, firm masses of scarlike collagenous tissue may arise in healing wounds for unknown reasons. Certain ethnic types (blacks and Asians) and younger patients may be more susceptible to these lesions; however, the lesions also may be seen in patients with normal scar formation and may even occur interspersed between areas of normal scar formation in the same healing wound. Hypertrophic scars usually stay within the boundary of the wound and tend to occur around joints, where areas of varying motion and tension exist. Keloids characteristically grow beyond the original incision. The management of these lesions is extremely varied and beyond the scope of this discussion.

Contracture

Contracture is occasionally an end result of wound contraction involving shortening of skin and soft tissues adjacent to an area of injury. Motion around joints may be severely limited, and distortion of adjoining tissue structures may result.

Wound Pain

Irritating nonabsorbable sutures or traumatic neuromas are frequent causes of late postoperative wound pain. Although most of these complaints usually remit spontaneously, some may require surgical intervention. Hyperesthesia around a wound is usually due to local sensory nerve injury and frequently diminishes or becomes well tolerated.

Cancer

Any chronic ulcer in a wound that has not healed after several months should be investigated for malignant changes. Ulcerated keloids and chronic sinus tracts may be prone to malignancy. Squamous cell carcinomas have been known to develop in old burn wounds (Marjolin's ulcer).

■ HIGH-RISK PATIENTS

Certain groups of patients are predisposed to developing wound complications postoperatively. Patients at high risk for these problems usually have local or systemic conditions that make them more susceptible to wound infections, affect the inflammatory response to injury, or alter collagen synthesis and maturation.

Local Factors

A wound's general condition significantly influences its final result. Well-made and well-tended wounds resist infection, whereas ischemic tissues dessicated by electrosurgery, strangulated by haphazardly placed ligatures, approximated by excessive tension, or sustaining prolonged exposure to air all heal poorly. Grossly contaminated wounds that have been inadequately debrided or closed primarily tend to become infected.

Previous therapy at the injury site will also affect tissue repair. Radiation delivered to a wound site frequently leaves a wasteland of relatively hypoxic and poorly vascularized tissues. The replication of vascular endothelial cells is often suppressed and contraction is retarded, but this situation is usually more deleterious to open wounds healing by secondary intention.

Systemic Factors

Malnutrition has been demonstrated to cause poor wound healing through both delayed repair and increased susceptibility to infection.[9] Patients who are significantly malnourished, such as from ethanol abuse, prolonged starvation, eating disorders, chronic illness, or malabsorption, should have their nutritional abnormalities corrected before major surgery is performed. Healthy patients will generally not encounter these problems if they are allowed to resume nutritional intake within one week. If a patient cannot be expected to begin adequate nourishment by oral or nasogastric tube routes after this time, then nutritional support via total parenteral nutrition may be considered.

Victims of multiple trauma are included in the high-risk group. Massive injury alters the body's metabolic steady state markedly by increased heat production and gluconeogenesis; negative nitrogen, potassium, sulfur, and phosphorus balances; early hyperglycemia; and altered carbohydrate utilization.[10] The body's reaction to acute injury or illness appears to involve almost all its metabolic pathways. At no time are the body's nutritional demands as great as they are following serious injury, especially when the injury is complicated by infection. Wound repair is influenced by the nutritional disorders stemming from altered metabolic processes associated with severe injury, as well as by the patient's previous nutritional status. Persistent imbalances, frequently seen after major multiple injury, can produce serious malnutrition and impair wound healing. Superimposed on these disturbances are problems posed by contaminating microorganisms, foreign bodies, and compromised blood supply to the injured tissues.

Poor nutrient and oxygen delivery to wounds related to anemia or hypotension retards repair. Oxygen is essential to white blood cell and fibroblast functions, which are depressed by hypoxia. Oxygen is also needed for energy production in the healing wound through hydroxylation and oxidative metabolism. Both functioning systems are required for collagen synthesis.

Several diseases are associated with poor wound healing. Patients with Cushing's syndrome exhibit delayed repair secondary to a glucocorticoid excess, which can depress the inflammatory response. Diabetic patients are highly susceptible to wound infections secondary to an impaired inflammatory response with hyperglycemia-induced impaired collagen synthesis and dysfunctional white blood cells. In addition, these patients frequently manifest microvascular disease, which creates local wound hypoxia. Peripheral neuropathy in this illness may lead to repeated accidental trauma to a healing wound. Vasculitis and atherosclerosis also have been implicated in delayed healing due to poor circulation. Disorders of the immune system, especially in leukopenic patients, may lead to a decrease in the natural immunity of the wound and higher infection rates.

Extreme age and obesity have been associated with a higher incidence of wound complications. Both elderly and obese patients tend to heal poorly, suffer infection, and experience dehiscence more often than do their younger and leaner counterparts. Other patient populations at high risk for surgical wound infection include those with multiple diagnoses (more than three), those whose surgery involved a number of organs, those with contaminated or dirty tissues, and patients who received a large number of units of blood or blood products.[11] In patients with wounds classified as contaminated or dirty (see Table 11–2), wound infection rates increase to 5% to 10% and 10%

to 40%, respectively.[12] However, wound classification alone is not an adequate predictor of infection rates and is only one essential element in surveillance programs. The Centers for Disease Control and Prevention (CDC) operate the major surveillance system for surgical site infections as part of the National Nosocomial Infections Surveillance (NNIS). This system uses a risk-stratified approach wherein the wound classification, along with duration of the surgery and the American Society of Anesthesiologists (ASA) physical status classification, are used to estimate range of risk. Thus, clean surgical procedure infection rates may fall into a range of 1% to 2% for patients who have no risk factors or may be as high as 13% to 14% if all three risk factors are present.[13] RNFAs can access current CDC data and statistics on the Internet

---

BOX 11-1

Sample Information Obtained from the CDC Web Site

NATIONAL NOSOCOMIAL INFECTIONS SURVEILLANCE (NNIS) SYSTEM

The NNIS system is conducted by the Hospital Infections Program to collect high quality nosocomial infection surveillance data that can be aggregated into a national database. The database is used to describe the epidemiology of nosocomial infections in hospitals in the United States and to produce nosocomial infection rates that can be used for comparison purposes by hospitals following NNIS methodology.

Approximately 245 hospitals voluntarily report their nosocomial infection data to the NNIS system. By law, CDC assures NNIS hospitals that any information that would permit identification of any individual or institution will be held in strict confidence. The NNIS data include infections from acute care general hospital patients only and exclude those from rehabilitation, mental health, nursing home, and other extended care services. To our knowledge, there are no national surveillance systems that collect nosocomial infection data for these types of patients. There are also no national data on infections in outpatient surgery or home care.

The most current report of NNIS rates is found in the following article: *National Nosocomial Infections Surveillance (NNIS) report, Data summary from Oct 1986–April 1996, issued May 1996.* AJIC Am J Infect Control 1996 volume 24, pages 380–388. The same report can be found on the Internet by accessing CDC's home page, then selecting About CDC, then National Center for Infectious Diseases (NCID), then Hospital Infections, then Surveillance, then NNIS. From here, choose the NNIS report. The report will be updated annually in the AJIC and on the Internet.

Hospital Infections Program
National Center for Infectious Diseases
Centers for Disease Control and Prevention
Atlanta, GA
Updated: August 4, 1997

T A B L E   1 1 – 7 . DRUGS THAT DELAY WOUND REPAIR

Anticoagulants	Methysergide
Hematoma formation	Causes excess scarring
Anti-inflammatory agents	Penicillin
Suppress inflammation	Liberates penicillamine
Suppress protein synthesis	Pentazocine
Suppress contraction	May cause extreme fibrosis
Suppress epithelialization	Radiation
Chemotherapeutic agents	Suppresses cell replication
Arrest cell replication	Destroys blood supply by endarteritis
Suppress inflammation	
Suppress protein synthesis	
Colchicine	
Arrests cell replication	
Suppresses collagen transport	
Diphenylhydantoin	
Causes hypertrophic scars	

(http://www.cdc.gov). In general, all information presented at this web site and all items available for downloading are for public use. The information is recent and regularly updated, and there is no cost for access (Box 11–1).

Concomitant drug therapy has been proven deleterious to wound repair in several instances (Table 11–7). In general, any agent that interferes with the inflammatory process or cell proliferation retards healing. Corticosteroids and other anti-inflammatory agents are notorious for this side effect. They suppress repair if administered within two to three days after injury; healing will continue, but very slowly. The inflammatory response is decreased as macrophages do not migrate into the wound, fibroblastic proliferation and collagen synthesis are depressed, epithelial migration is hindered, and wound contraction is delayed. Open wounds, by their dependence on all these factors, are particularly vulnerable to these effects. Several chemotherapeutic agents are cytotoxic (e.g., methotrexate and nitrogen mustard) or antimitotic (e.g., vinblastine). Their activity against cell division does not differentiate between malignant cells or those involved in wound healing. Occasionally, these drugs are combined with corticosteroids and may be devastating to wound repair. Anticoagulant therapy (coumadin and heparin) may lead to wound complication from excessive bleeding into wounds.

◪ SUMMARY

RN first assistants are involved in all phases of wound healing, from perioperative patient assessment through intraoperative dimensions of tissue handling and suturing to postoperative wound evaluation and patient education.

Wound healing is a complex process that involves many facets of human physiology. Because all patients are to some degree individual and variable in biological behavior, one cannot impose rigid guidelines for their care. Rather, the RNFA focuses on optimizing the conditions for the repair of injury based on sound surgical experience and knowledgeable attention to details of proper treatment tailored to each particular situation and patient. The RNFA, along with other members of the patient care team, must identify the physiological processes that are occurring in the wound, the needs of the wound as it progresses through the various phases of healing, and the optimum treatment regimens available to manage both the health status of the patient and the microenvironment of the wound.

■ Review Questions

1. Sharply made wounds that are reapproximated and heal with minimal space between their edges are classified as
   a. Open wounds.
   b. Closed wounds.
   c. Aseptic wounds.
   d. Primary wounds.

2. When a tissue defect decreases in size by wound contraction, it is designated as healing by
   a. Primary intention.
   b. Secondary intention.
   c. Tertiary intention.
   d. Delayed intention.

3. After tissue injury, the initial vascular and cellular response is the
   a. Inflammatory phase.
   b. Phagocytic phase.
   c. Injury phase.
   d. Epithelial phase.

4. This initial phase lasts
   a. A few days.
   b. 24 hours.
   c. 5 to 7 days.
   d. A few days to a few weeks.

5. Key to the effectiveness of the cellular response during the inflammatory phase of wound healing is the activity of
   a. Vasoconstriction.
   b. Chemotaxis.
   c. Leukocytes.
   d. Fibroblasts.

6. During the proliferative phase of wound healing, epithelial cells travel over viable tissue to bridge the wound. They cease migration through
   a. The effects of fibroblast growth factor.
   b. Mitosis.
   c. The healing cascade.
   d. Contact inhibition.

7. What cells are responsible for the synthesis and secretion of collagen and elastin?
   a. Proteoglycans
   b. Ground substance
   c. Fibroblasts
   d. Collagenases and elastinases

8. Scar remodeling is the effect of
   a. Plastic surgery.
   b. Collagen reweaving.
   c. Capillary cross-links.
   d. Lymphatic drainage of interstitial fluid.

9. If a skin flap is required to cover a tissue defect, the RNFA will most likely assist in
   a. Drain insertion.
   b. Splint application.
   c. Compression dressing changes.
   d. Seroma evacuation.

10. One reason that diabetic patients may have compromised wound healing is the presence of
   a. Protein deficiency.
   b. Amino acid deficits.
   c. Hyperglycemia.
   d. Impaired serum albumin.

11. Dietary sources of _____ are important for collagen turnover and metabolism in healing wounds.
   a. Unsaturated fatty acids
   b. Vitamin C
   c. Calories
   d. Lysine

12. Preoperative patient considerations in preventing wound complications are focused on
   a. Providing antimicrobial prophylaxis.
   b. Identifying and reducing risk factors.
   c. Performing wound classification.
   d. Correcting host defenses.

13. When taping dressings in place, the RN first assistant applies tape without tension, working from

    a. The center of the incision outward.

    b. The edge of the incision toward the center.

14. Nursing research indicates that

    a. Skin irritation and skin stripping may be lower when elastoplast is used.

    b. RNFAs should focus on nutritional education for patients whose wounds are healing by secondary intention.

    c. Low serum albumin levels are an indication for total parenteral nutrition.

    d. Prophylactic antibiotics should be administered within two hours of the start of surgery and two hours post-incision time.

15. Cellulitis may be treated by

    a. Needle aspiration.

    b. Heat and elevation.

    c. Surgical debridement.

    d. Drain insertion.

16. When palpating an area that may be an abscess, the RN first assistant will note that the area usually _____ on palpation.

    a. Has crepitus

    b. Sounds hollow

    c. Fluctuates

    d. Resonates

17. Gas gangrene, a rapidly progressive infection, is accompanied by swelling, pain, and

    a. High fever.

    b. Low-grade fever.

    c. Septic shock.

    d. Dark, red muscle.

18. A wound that is closed under extreme tension may exhibit what wound complication?

    a. Dehiscence

    b. Myositis

    c. Cutaneous healing ridges

    d. Shaggy necrosis

19. Locally irradiated tissue may cause

    a. Meleney's ulcer.

    b. Draining cutaneous sinuses.

    c. Nonhealing wounds.

    d. Pruritus.

20. Among those patients classified as at high risk for wound infection are those with

    a. Alcoholism.

    b. Malnutrition.

  c. Hypoxia.

  d. Hypoglycemia.

21. Common practice allows a maximum of _____ days of severely limited nutrient intake before initiating nutritional support.

  a. 3

  b. 7

  c. 10

  d. 15

22. Normal laboratory values for serum total protein, a necessary parameter of patient nutrition, are

  a. 6.0 to 8.0 g/dL.

  b. 3.5 to 5.0 g/dL.

  c. 180 to 260 mg/dL.

  d. 50% greater than the individual patient's serum albumin level.

23. In a risk-stratified approach to surgical wound surveillance, the three risks identified in the CDC's NNIS are

  a. Nutritional status, age, co-morbidity.

  b. ASA class, disease severity index, low albumin.

  c. Surgical wound class, duration of procedure, ASA class.

  d. Prolonged surgery, surgical wound class, multiple procedures.

24. Impaired leukocyte function can be a result of

  a. Hyperglycemia.

  b. Hypophosphatemia.

  c. Thrombocytopenia.

  d. Insulin administration.

25. Of the many factors which may contribute to impaired wound healing, one which the RNFA has direct control over is

  a. The patient's nutritional status.

  b. Length of preoperative hospitalization.

  c. Surgical wound classification.

  d. Suturing technique.

Answer Key

1. b	10. c	18. a
2. b	11. b	19. c
3. a	12. b	20. b
4. d	13. a	21. b
5. c	14. b	22. a
6. d	15. b	23. c
7. c	16. c	24. a
8. b	17. b	25. d
9. a		

REFERENCES

1. Barr JE: Physiology of healing: The basis for the principles of wound management. Medsurg Nurs 4(5):387–392, 1995
2. Hahn JF, Olsen CL: Wounds: Nursing care and product selection. Nurs Spectrum 3(21):12–14, 1994
3. Pontieri-Lewis V: Utilizing a team approach to wound management. Medsurg Nurs 5(6):427–429, 1996
4. George S, Bugwadia N: Nutrition and wound healing. Medsurg Nurs 5(4):272–275, 1996
5. Stotts NA, Whitney JD: Nutritional intake and status of clients in the home with open surgical wounds. Res Rev Studies Nurs Practice 7(2):1, 1990
6. Infection control: Timing prophylaxis of surgical wound infection. Am J Nurs 97(7):11, 1997
7. Butts JD, Wolford ET: Timing of perioperative antibiotic administration. AORN J 65(1):109–114, 1997
8. Patterson P: What infection rates do—and don't—mean. OR Manager 13(7):22–23, 1997
9. Sweed MR, Guenter P, Jones S: Nursing implications for the adult patient receiving nutritional support. Medsurg Nurs 4(2):99–108, 1995
10. Ritchie WP, Steele G, Dean RH: General Surgery. Philadelphia, JB Lippincott, 1995
11. Schumann D: Reducing post critical care infection. Medsurg Nurs 5(3):169–176, 1996
12. Butts and Wolford, 112
13. Patterson P: What's your role in a surveillance system? OR Manager 13(7):20–21, 1997

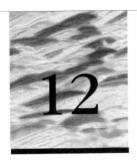

12

Using Grasping Instruments

Sergius Pechin

■

Grasping instruments are used for clamping or holding tissues for hemostasis, for retraction, for dissection, and in tissue approximation. This chapter will not attempt to catalog all the numerous types of grasping instruments. The operating surgeon will have an individual preference based on personal experience and technique. The experienced RN first assistant will develop preferences as well, but should have no difficulty in adapting to a particular technique when the fundamental principles are understood.

Both the American Nurses Association Standards of Clinical Nursing Practice and the Association of Operating Room Nurses Standards of Professional Performance set forth the expectation that a nurse will acquire and maintain current nursing practice knowledge and evaluate her or his own nursing practice. The RNFA, as an accountable professional, should actively identify self-learning needs, including critical thinking, interpersonal, and technical skills, and be self-directed and purposeful in seeking the knowledge and skills necessary to meet those self-learning needs.[1] Constructive feedback, peer review, and self-evaluation should be part of the RNFA's regular performance appraisal to establish areas for practice improvement.[2]

■ HEMOSTASIS

Applying a hemostat is one way to achieve hemostasis. The clamped vessel may be secured either with a tie or by application of a desiccating current. (Refer to Chapter 13 for a thorough discussion of the use of the ESU when "buzzing" a hemostat.) One of the RN first assistant's primary roles is to provide hemostasis and a dry field. Control of both superficial and deep bleeding can be challenging for even the most experienced RNFA. Superficial bleeders, depending on anatomical location, may be clamped quickly and independently. Deep bleeders and large amounts of bleeding require a team effort for efficient control of blood loss. Collaboration with the surgeon is essential.

Hemostats

Hemostatic clamps come in a variety of sizes, ranging from the delicate mosquito clamp to large Kelly and Kocher clamps. Small, short hemostats are used for superficial vessels. Deeper vessels may need a clamp designed for specific purposes. These may be long and curved or long and straight. The curve may be gentle or angled 45 to 90 degrees. Each clamp design provides, by its length and contour, the best aid for each particular anatomical structure. Vascular clamps are designed to provide hemostatic control by shutting off arterial flow without injuring the layers of the vessel wall, particularly the delicate intima. Vascular clamps also come in a variety of sizes, curves, and lengths to accommodate the special requirements of vascular structures.

There are two criteria that should be considered when the hemostat is placed in the RNFA's hand. First, the length of the hemostat should be sufficient to (1) reach comfortably into the area where you are working and (2) allow the handles to be left outside the surgical site, making it easier for the RNFA to manipulate the clamp.[3]

Hemostat Technique

The RN first assistant should develop a comfortable, efficient technique in handling and using the hemostat (Figure 12–1). As the assistant develops this technique, certain important general principles become part of the RNFA's skill repertoire in all instrument handling techniques. The assistant should first become familiar and comfortable with the feel of the hemostat and its balance in the hand. As this familiarity is established, the instrument gradually becomes an extension of the assistant's hand. As awkwardness decreases, the assistant positions the hemostat naturally and comfortably. Soon, the assistant becomes adept at holding it with a light grip to allow the best feel of the tissue to which the hemostat is applied.

Securing a bleeding vessel with a hemostat can be accomplished with either the tip or jaw technique. A correct clamp should be selected for the technique that is used. Fully serrated clamps, where the serrations extend all the way to the hinge, will securely grasp tissue all the way to the hinge (jaw technique). A tip technique is used with a partially serrated clamp. Tissue will be securely held within the serrated area. When using the tip technique, the principal objective is to grasp only the open vessel, with little or no surround-

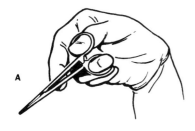

FIGURE 12–1A

Hemostat technique. In grasping a bleeder, the method shown in **A** is the most sure. Only the very tip of the instrument is used to capture the smallest amount of tissue containing the bleeder. Consequently, the smallest amount of tissue is devitalized by ligature or electrical current.

FIGURE 12–1B

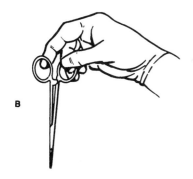

Once the hemostat is placed, however, the fingers should be withdrawn from the rings, and the hemostat should be grasped as in **B.** The ring closest to the assistant is grasped between thumb and middle finger; the index finger is kept mobile enough to release the ratchet of the instrument by pressure against the ring. In this maneuver, the whole instrument is firmly stabilized with the ring that is held between the thumb and third finger. This technique allows the assistant to manipulate the point of the instrument through an almost 360-degree arc, which would not be possible if the fingers were still placed through the rings, as shown in the original position in **A.** Performing the recommended technique will require practice and expertise to develop smooth manual dexterity.

FIGURE 12–1C

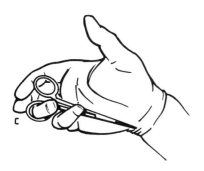

Once the hemostat has performed its function, it may be carried for immediate reuse as indicated in **C.** The lower ring is hooked by the distal end of the fourth finger and the body of the instrument is then held to the palm of the hand by the fifth finger. This allows the thumb, middle, and third fingers to be mobile. The assistant's ability to continue to assist is not limited, inasmuch as an entire operative procedure can be expertly handled with just these three digits. Any time the hemostat is to be used again, it can be flipped out to the attitude shown in **A** and then returned to the position shown in **C** again when its duty is accomplished. This maneuver is not limited to the use of the hemostat. It can be used with scissors or any comparable ringed instrument that is not too long.

ing tissue. This reduces or eliminates tissue devitalization. In the tip technique, the hemostat tip is pointed toward the vessel. In contrast, the jaw technique grasps the vessel in the greater curvature of the clamp; the tip points away from the vessel. This technique allows the hemostat tip to extend beyond the exposed vessel, trapping a ligature more easily as it is passed during tying. This technique includes more tissue in the hemostat jaw, and therefore more tissue is devitalized. The jaw technique is used only when it is most useful, for example, when clamping across uncut tissue before transection. When transecting vascular pedicles, omentum, or other structures between clamps, knot tying is easier if the clamp jaws are applied with tips pointed toward the intended cut (and away from the vessel).

The RNFA should hold the hemostat without fingers in the finger rings when the vessel is ready to be tied. This permits optimal rotation for tie placement without twisting the vessel. The handles of the hemostat are held away from the wound to facilitate placement of the hands of the person tying the knot. Once the first loop of the ligature is placed, the hemostat tip is exposed without pulling. As the first knot is thrown, the hemostat is gradually removed. The fingers do not need to be in the rings to remove the clamp. The finger ring is grasped on the left by the thumb, then the ring is pinched between the thumb and the ring finger. The lock is disengaged by pressing the index finger on the finger ring. Then the clamp is gently removed.

The RNFA may use the three-point grasp, with the thumb and index fingers in the instrument rings to facilitate controlled release of the clamp. To release the hemostat from this grip, the tip is rested on a firm surface as the index finger presses on the closed shanks, "pushing" the clamp from the hand.

▨ RETRACTION

Grasping instruments may be used for retraction, either to facilitate visibility or to help with dissection by providing countertraction on the appropriate tissue. The instrument is applied carefully and deliberately to avoid trauma to friable tissue. Although certain clamps may not have been originally designed as retracting instruments, surgeons have adapted their use to specific situations. The most common of these are described in the following sections.

Kocher Instrument

The Kocher instrument is used when retraction is needed to dissect heavily scarred or fibrotic areas, such as the opening or closing of an old incision. The Kocher clamp holds such heavy, dense tissue better than a tissue forceps, lessening hand fatigue for the RNFA or surgeon. During blunt or sharp dissection of adhesions, the Kocher clamp is well suited to lift and hold peritoneum, allowing abdominal contents to fall away as underlying structures are exposed. Kocher clamps are also useful during midline closure of the abdomen. The dense fascia is grasped with a Kocher clamp immediately adjacent to the site where the suture will be placed. A scrub nurse may inadvertently hand the RNFA a curved or straight Kocher clamp instead of a Kelly or other type of clamp. The assistant should always note the kind of clamp passed before applying it to tissue. The Kocher clamp is considered a crushing instrument; its small jaws apply great pressure to a small area. When a Kocher clamp is used to clamp across tissue, such as bowel, before cutting it, a cuff of tissue should be left distal to the clamp. Tissue is less likely to slip between the jaws this way.

Allis Clamp

The fine-toothed Allis clamp is used for retracting more delicate tissue, such as a transected bowel lumen. The numbers and fineness of the teeth on an Allis clamp dictate the type of tissue on which it may be used. Like a Kocher clamp, this clamp also applies great pressure to a small area. The RN first assistant may hold it with minimal pressure, knowing that the jaws will not slip.

Babcock Clamp

This broad but thin-bladed, untoothed clamp is used to lift and retract bowel and other delicate structures. Considered a nontraumatic clamp, the Babcock clamp is commonly used to encircle tubular structures, such as the appendix or fallopian tube, and gently hold soft tissue. The ratchet on the Babcock clamp should be tightened only enough to hold the tissue.

Tenaculum

A more heavily toothed instrument than the Allis clamp, the tenaculum is used particularly for clamping and retracting heavier tissue. A prime example is the tenaculum forceps used for retraction during thyroid gland dissection or to grasp the uterine cervix. Smooth instruments can crush tissue, and toothed instruments sometimes can cause less trauma, because less metal comes in contact with tissue and less pressure needs to be exerted to lift tissue when gently biting. Tissues should always be handled gently with any instrument.

▓ THUMB FORCEPS

The thumb forceps provides an extension of the surgeon's and RN first assistant's fingers to allow for more precise handling of tissue. Forceps are commonly used by the nondominant hand to assist maneuvers undertaken by the dominant hand. Thus, they are commonly used as an adjunct to the needle-holder to stabilize tissue while suturing, as an adjunct to the scalpel and scissors to hold tissue while cutting, and as an adjunct to the hemostat to retract tissue for exposure before clamping. Forceps are also used to grasp vessels for electrosurgical coagulation, to pack sponges, to grasp objects for extraction, and to grasp the end of needles. Because of their versatility, a large variety of thumb forceps are available, each adapted to a particular anatomical structure.

Here, as with other grasping instruments, the question of smooth opposed to toothed instruments must be considered. The RNFA will likely be asked to provide countertraction in dissection, so the choice of forceps must be based on knowledge of tissue type and the requirement of the traction. In general, fibrotic, scar-type tissue warrants the use of a toothed forceps. Bowel and peritoneum, on the other hand, require a nonpuncturing forceps. The anatomical proximity of tissue guides the RNFA in selecting a long forceps or a shorter forceps, such as the Adson. This small-toothed forceps has variation with longitudinal rows of teeth, which distribute the force and allow firm fixation without trauma. An Adson forceps is well suited to grasp moderately dense tissue such as the skin. The fine points on the teeth give more holding power by concentrating force in a small area; they cause less tissue destruction than smooth forceps when holding skin.

Using an instrument such as a tissue forceps correctly is a highly valuable clinical skill that makes the RNFA an asset to both the surgeon and patient. Consider the following simple routine in using tissue forceps to lift the peritoneum during abdominal surgery. The surgeon first picks up peritoneum with tissue forceps; the RNFA remains still during this move. The surgeon then remains still while the assistant picks up peritoneum a few millimeters away. The assistant gently holds the tissue forceps while the surgeon readjusts the forceps to ensure that only a single layer of peritoneum is grasped. Then, both the surgeon and RNFA hold the forceps still while the surgeon incises the peritoneum between the two sets of forceps. This kind of clinical skill becomes intuitive for the experienced RNFA. Smooth, synchronized moves and countermoves between surgeon and RNFA produce a flowing, dynamic continuity throughout the surgical intervention.

Tissue forceps should be held so that one blade acts as an extension of the thumb and the other acts as an extension of the opposing fingers. The grip should be gentle and balanced. If the RNFA's fingers or hand become fatigued, or if the forceps fails to hold the tissue or structure, the assistant should consider changing the type of tissue forceps or using a clamp. Holding the forceps in the pencil position, or in a modified pencil grip, gives the assistant the greatest maneuverability. When not in active use, the forceps may be palmed and supported by extending the ring and little finger. The unflexed middle finger remains free for use. Palming an unused instrument, when alternately grasping with forceps and fingers, saves time. If the little finger and ring finger are required for completing a one-handed tie, the forceps can be temporarily pinched in the web between the thumb and index finger. To move forceps back to a position of use, the palm is turned down and the thumb and index finger are used to grasp the forceps in the desired place.

■ SUMMARY

Gentleness in handling tissue, experience based on appropriate education, good manual skills, knowledge of surgical anatomy and procedural aspects of the intervention, and familiarity with instruments are fundamental to providing assistance to the surgeon and to achieving quality patient outcomes. Peri-

operative nurses, functioning in the expanded role of intraoperative first assistant, are well positioned to gain clinical experience, enhance their knowledge of surgical interventions, and augment role function while providing
quality patient care.

◧ Review Questions

Indicate whether each of the following statements is true (T) or false (F):

_____ 1. The American Nurses Association Standards of Professional Performance require that the nurse systematically evaluate the quality and effectiveness of medical practice.

_____ 2. Hemostasis can be secured with a clamp either by applying the
tip to the bleeding vessel or by trapping the bleeding vessel in
the convexity of the clamp's jaws.

_____ 3. Crushing clamps, such as a Kocher clamp, used during transection are more secure from having tissue slip between their jaws
if a cuff of tissue is left distal to the clamp.

_____ 4. The objective of the jaw technique of applying a curved hemostat is to include a minimum of surrounding tissue.

_____ 5. Tip clamping makes it easier to pass a ligature around a vessel.

_____ 6. Speed should be the primary goal of surgical technique.

_____ 7. An accurate and secure hemostat grip is the tripod grip, in which
the thumb and ring finger are inserted into the instrument rings
and the index finger is placed on the shaft.

_____ 8. To manipulate a hemostat during vessel ligation, the hemostat
should be held for encirclement by the ligature with the fingers
in the rings.

_____ 9. In a deep wound, the RN first assistant should trap the ligature
beneath the tip by gently pressing the clamp deeper in the
wound and rotating the tip away from the person tying the knot.

_____ 10. While the knot tier tightens the first half-hitch, the RN first assistant should quickly snap the hemostat off the wound.

_____ 11. The three-point grasp is the most secure and accurate grip for a
clamp in a critical situation.

_____ 12. A left-handed assistant removes a clamp by grasping the left ring
between the thumb and index finger and disengaging the lock
by applying pressure of the middle, ring, and little fingers on the
right finger ring.

_____ 13. Atraumatic clamps are designed to hold tissue while exerting the
least possible crushing force.

_____ 14. The palm position of holding forceps gives the widest range of maneuverability.

_____ 15. When sewing, then tying, palming the forceps can save time.

_____ 16. To change from "hold" to "use" with the forceps, the palm should be turned up.

_____ 17. Forceps are a principal instrument for fine retraction during dissection.

_____ 18. When elevating a clamp for vessel ligation, the RN first assistant pulls gently on the vessel while showing the tip.

_____ 19. When holding soft viscera with a Babcock clamp, the RN first assistant tightens down to the third ratchet.

_____ 20. When smooth-jawed forceps are used, more force or tissue compression is required to lift tissue against resistance without slipping.

Answer Key

1. F (Nursing practice, not medical practice, is what should be evaluated. Evaluation should be in relation to professional nursing practice standards as well as relevant statutes and guidelines.)
2. T
3. T
4. F (The tip technique of applying a curved hemostat clamps the open vessel while including the minimum surrounding tissue.)
5. F (Jaw clamping leaves the tip exposed beyond the tissue; this traps the ligature as it is placed around the vessel.)
6. F (Speed is the by-product of expert surgical technique rather than its primary goal; speed should not take the place of technique.)
7. T
8. F (To allow optimal rotation for placing the tie, hemostat handles should be held without fingers in the rings.)
9. T
10. F (Clamps are always removed gradually to prevent the tissue from escaping while the first half-hitch is tightened.)
11. T
12. T
13. T
14. F (The pencil grip, with the forceps' shanks against the index finger metacarpal-phalangeal joint, gives the widest range of maneuverability. The palm grip requires too much wrist flexion.)
15. T
16. F (With the palm up, gravity makes the grasp too far from the tips; turning the palm down allows gravity to assist the RN first assistant by moving the forceps from the palm. The index finger and thumb can then grasp the forceps in the desired place without extreme flexion.)
17. T
18. F (The clamp is elevated without pulling on the clamped structure.)

19. F (The ratchet should be tightened only enough to hold the tissue.)
20. T

REFERENCES

1. American Nurses Association: Standards of Clinical Nursing Practice (field draft review). Washington, DC, American Nurses Association, 1997, p 3
2. Association of Operating Room Nurses: Standards of Perioperative Professional Performance. In: AORN Standards, Recommended Practices and Guidelines. Denver, Colo, Association of Operating Room Nurses, 1997, pp 112–114
3. Scott-Conner CE, Dawson DL: Operative Anatomy. Philadelphia, JB Lippincott, 1993

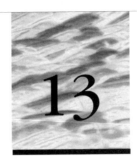

PROVIDING HEMOSTASIS

NANCY B. DAVIS
BRENDA C. ULMER

■

Hemostasis occurs when blood stops flowing from an injured blood vessel. The achievement of hemostasis during surgical procedures is fundamental to surgical intervention as a form of treatment. Excessive or uncontrolled bleeding is life-threatening. Controlling bleeding not only is important in relation to the patient's prognosis, it is also necessary for adequate visualization of the operative site. Moreover, prolonged bleeding interferes with healing of the surgical wound.

The natural defense mechanism of blood clotting is not adequate to control bleeding during surgery (Figure 13–1). The surgeon and RNFA depend on this defense mechanism as an important factor but also use mechanical, thermal, or chemical hemostasis techniques.

Bleeding during or after surgical intervention is influenced by several factors, among them the type of surgical intervention, the patient's physical condition, coagulation mechanisms, and fibrinolytic activity. During surgery, the most frequent cause of bleeding is injury to blood vessels. The amount of bleeding depends on the amount of injury to blood vessels, the type of vessels injured, and the anatomical site of the injury to vessels. These factors, related to the vessel injury and the technical skills of the surgeon and RNFA, influence the achievement of hemostasis during surgery.

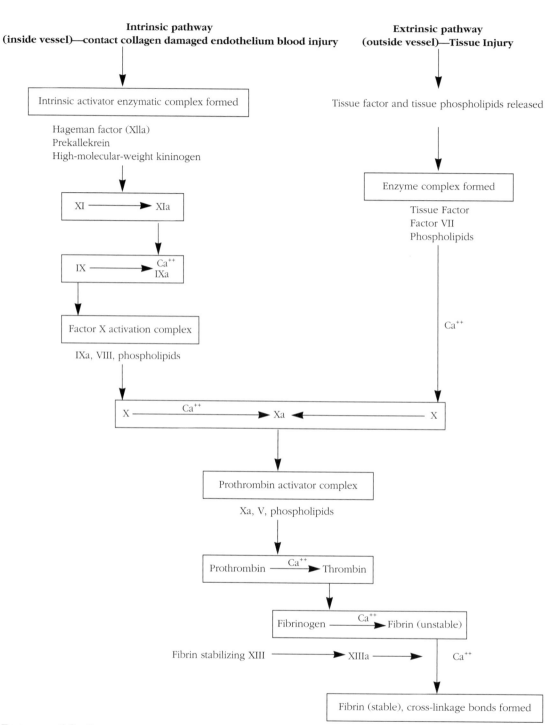

FIGURE 13–1

In the coagulation sequence, the intrinsic pathway is initiated by surface contact, whereas the extrinsic pathway is initiated by the release of tissue factor from injured tissues. The pathways are interrelated and operate in tandem to achieve hemostasis. a, activated enzyme; Ca^{++}, calcium, neccessary in several reactions. Final common pathway begins with the activation of factor X.

PATIENT ASSESSMENT

The RNFA collaborates in obtaining information related to the patient's health status and increased risk of intraoperative bleeding. All patients undergoing invasive surgical procedures face the risk of bleeding because of the traumatic nature of surgery.

Sepsis, deficiencies in blood clotting mechanisms, anticoagulant drugs, allergies, or diseases such as leukemia, thrombocytopenia, lymphoma, or multiple myeloma increase a patient's risk of bleeding. The history and physical examination provide information related to the patient's present condition, past history, and medication use. The patient should be queried about hemostatic responses to previous surgical interventions, as well as about easy bruising, epistaxis, gingival bleeding, and menorrhagia. Medication history should be reviewed for such drugs as anticoagulants, aspirin (and aspirin-containing drugs), or other nonsteroidal anti-inflammatory medications, including over-the-counter medications. Laboratory tests related to clotting factors must be reviewed for any abnormality; these may include tests of coagulation mechanisms (i.e., activated coagulation time, partial thromboplastin time [PTT], prothrombin time [PT]), tests of platelet function (i.e., platelet count, Ivy bleeding time, clot retraction time), and tests of fibrinolysis (i.e., fibrinogen level). Any clotting defects must be communicated to the surgeon before surgery. Any needed clotting factors can then be prepared.

The operative procedure must be considered in relation to increasing the patient's risk of bleeding. The more extensive the operation, the greater the involvement of vascular structures. Also considered are the type of surgery, the ability to control bleeding in the planned procedure, and anticipated bleeding. The need for blood transfusions, the use of cardiopulmonary bypass procedures, and the need to use heparin intraoperatively all increase this bleeding risk.

Preoperative assessment should also consider fluid balance. Fluid balance depends on normal volume and osmotic pressure in the intracellular, interstitial, and intravascular compartments; adequate fluid intake and output; normal renal function; a responsive endocrine system; and good nutritional status. The patient's general physiological status should be assessed to establish outcome criteria. Specific data to be reviewed include the patient's normal intake and output of serum sodium, potassium, hemoglobin, hematocrit, total protein, albumin, and glucose levels. The urinalysis should be reviewed to determine urine specific gravity. Body weight should be documented. The history should be investigated for evidence of preexisting illnesses involving the liver, pancreas, renal system, thyroid gland, adrenal gland, or respiratory system. The patient's use of diuretics or laxatives should also be noted.

Protein levels are important in relation to fluid volume. The liver manufactures albumin from amino acids, and albumin aids in the maintenance of colloidal osmotic pressure. Decreases in total protein cause fluids to shift from the vascular system to the tissues. It will be of concern to the RNFA if total plasma protein falls below 6 g/dL and if albumin falls below 4 g/dL. Careful preoperative assessment can identify treatable problems and assist in predicting the body's fluid preservation response to surgical stress.

The assessment phase concludes with the formulation of nursing diagnoses. One nursing diagnosis related to the possibility of bleeding during or after surgical intervention might be stated as High Risk for Fluid Volume Deficit related to intraoperative or postoperative bleeding. Assessment of bleeding is ongoing during the intraoperative phase, and the RNFA must recognize abnormal or excessive bleeding during this phase. Also, the RNFA must not inadvertently contribute to increased intraoperative bleeding through unnecessary tissue trauma or improper application of hemostatic techniques.

▨ GENERAL CONSIDERATIONS IN HEMOSTASIS

Invasive operative procedures always injure tissue and interrupt the integrity of vascular structures to some extent. The RNFA must be knowledgeable about the normal blood supply to various tissues. Whenever possible, injury to blood vessels is avoided; the assistant must recognize vascular structures and be skilled in handling the structures without causing trauma. Some anatomical areas are more vascular than others; the scalp, face, and tongue are examples of highly vascular areas.

Excessive intraoperative blood loss is usually obvious. Arterial bleeding occurs more rapidly than venous bleeding because of the higher pressure in the arterial system. Arterial bleeding is bright red in the well-oxygenated patient, whereas venous blood is darker. Subtle blood loss can occur when there is a slow but continuous oozing of blood.

Shock

With sudden or rapid blood loss, the patient may develop signs of shock. Shock is defined as the inefficient or inadequate cardiac generation of both pressure and power for tissue perfusion.[1] There are a number of physiological classifications of shock, one of which is hypovolemic (which includes hemorrhagic) shock. When uncompensated, hypotension, oliguria, metabolic acidemia, hypoxemia, myocardial ischemia, dysrhythmias, and sinus tachycardia are significant findings. Regional cutaneous vasoconstriction decreases tissue perfusion, and the patient's extremities may be cold, pale, or cyanotic.

Blood loss can be determined by weighing sponges that are soaked with blood (1 gram = 1 cubic millimeter) and by noting the amount of blood that has accumulated in the suction canister (minus any irrigating fluids or other body fluids). Blood lost on the drapes must also be estimated.

Fluid Replacement Therapy

If hemorrhagic shock develops, it usually can be reversed by restoring the blood volume. Initially, this is done through rapid administration of intravenous fluids. The American Society of Anesthesiologists (ASA) has developed guidelines for blood component therapy in perioperative settings.[2] While transfusion of blood components has the potential of improving clinical outcomes, it is not without risks. Potential adverse effects of blood component therapy include nonhemolytic and hemolytic transfusion reactions and infectious disease transmission. Appropriate transfusion guidelines can help to obviate these, as well as control costs related to inappropriate transfusions.

Red blood cells (RBCs) are administered to improve inadequate oxygen delivery; RBCs contain hemoglobin, which binds with oxygen for transport to the tissues. RBC volume is monitored via the hematocrit and hemoglobin (normal ranges can be found in Appendix III). The transfusion of one unit of whole blood or RBCs increases the hematocrit by approximately 3% and increases the hemoglobin by approximately 1 g/dL. The ASA guidelines state that transfusion is rarely recommended with a hemoglobin value greater than 10 g/dL and almost always indicated when it is less than 6 g/dL. Intermediate ranges require an assessment of the patient's risk of developing complications of inadequate oxygenation that would necessitate RBC transfusion.

Excessive bleeding with the use of multiple blood transfusions, damage to the platelets through prolonged use of cardiopulmonary bypass, or quantitative (as in thrombocytopenia) or qualitative platelet defects can cause coagulation problems. Administration of platelets, according to the ASA guidelines, is usually indicated in patients with microvascular bleeding if the platelet count is less than 50×10^9/L; intermediate platelet counts require a determination of the patient's risk of developing more significant bleeding. In patients with an apparently adequate platelet count, platelet transfusion may still be indicated if there is a known platelet dysfunction and microvascular bleeding.

Plasma component therapy (fresh frozen plasma, FFP) may be necessary in patients at risk of adverse effects from inadequate coagulation factors. Fresh frozen plasma may be administered to reverse the effects of warfarin therapy, to correct known coagulation factor deficiencies when the specific concentrate is unavailable, or when there is microvascular bleeding secondary to coagulation deficiency in transfused patients. The ASA guidelines recommend administering FFP in doses calculated to achieve a minimum of 30% of plasma factor concentration; this is usually achieved with 10 to 15 mL/kg of FFP. For patients with inherited or acquired coagulopathies, cryoprecipitate, which contains factors VIII and XIII, fibrinogen, fibronectin, and von Willebrand's factor, is used. Cryoprecipitate may also be indicated to correct microvascular bleeding in massively transfused patients; the ASA recommends that the trigger of fibrinogen concentrations less than 80 to 100 mg/dL be used for component therapy.

Whole blood is used to correct massive blood loss that necessitates immediate replacement of RBCs and volume expansion via the colloid plasma proteins it contains.[3] Whole blood must be ABO identical and Rh compatible. With the recognition of the risks associated with blood transfusions, as well as religious beliefs that forbid such transfusions, the surgical community has developed interventions that reduce or eliminate the need for blood transfusion in the surgical patient. Referred to as "bloodless" surgery, perioperative strategies incorporate various technological advances throughout the patient's continuum of care.

Bloodless Surgery

Preoperatively, bloodless surgery programs focus on minimizing blood loss, using techniques such as microsampling for withdrawing blood, discontinuing medications that interfere with clotting times, and providing pharmacological therapy with epoetin alpha (EPO), which increases RBC production.[4] Other pharmacological therapy to stimulate erythropoiesis includes ferrous sulfate or iron dextran, folic acid, and vitamins C and B_{12}.[5] Intraoperative measures aimed at conserving blood include autologous transfusion, platelet sequestration, use of gamma-knife radiosurgery, laser beam coagulation, electrosurgery, the harmonic scalpel, administration of hetastarch (a non-blood volume expander), and anesthetic techniques to reduce blood loss. Prior to participation in a bloodless surgery program, patients complete an informed consent form, advance directive, and release from liability. A "do not administer blood products" wristband is often used to identify these patients.

▓ MECHANICAL MEANS OF ACHIEVING HEMOSTASIS

To minimize intraoperative bleeding, the RNFA must know how hemostasis is achieved during surgery. Controlling bleeding and preventing hemorrhage are priorities, and the RNFA facilitates this process by having the technical skills necessary to assist the surgeon in providing hemostasis. A priority is anticipatory control of any vessels before they are ligated. The RNFA then selects the most appropriate and efficient method to quickly control any bleeding that does occur.

Direct Pressure

Direct pressure can be the simplest and fastest way to control bleeding. During the skin incision, the RNFA should instinctively place his or her fingers or a moistened sponge against the ends of any transected and bleeding vessels. When this pressure is maintained for 15 to 20 seconds, small clots will usually form in the ends of small vessels. Digital pressure can be applied with a gauze sponge directly over the site of bleeding; however, care must be taken that the adherent surface of a gauze sponge does not dislodge fresh clots when the sponge is removed. The tip of an instrument, such as a suction tip, may also be used to initially cover and compress a bleeding point.

Indirect pressure might be applied to an area proximal to the bleeding area of the blood vessel, with the fingers or with a sponge on a sponge stick. Especially useful in a deep recess, the sponge stick should be held gently in position until lights and retractors are positioned for good visualization and the suction has cleared away any free blood. Once a clamp is ready, the sponge stick is slowly rolled off the vessel to expose the end to be clamped. Packing can be used to exert pressure on bleeding surfaces, thereby achieving hemostasis.

In diffuse bleeding, pressure may be required for an extended time. When this is the case, a cool saline moist pack is pressed against the bleeding surface for 10 to 20 minutes while another aspect of the surgical procedure is undertaken.

When bleeding is extensive, it may be impossible to visualize the bleeding point by suctioning or sponging. In such a case, the bleeding can be slowed or stopped using pressure. With better visualization, the bleeding point can be identified and hemostasis achieved. The use of pressure to control bleeding has the advantage of being least traumatic to the vascular structures. The major disadvantage is that it is often only a temporary measure. When removing any sponge or pack, the RNFA should be ready to immediately control any renewed bleeding from larger vessels that have been controlled by pressure.

Hemostats

Hemostats are clamping instruments designed for temporary control of bleeding from small blood vessels. They are available in various sizes, lengths, and shapes. The tips may be straight, angled, or curved, and the jaws may be fine, pointed, or heavy, or blunt. Hemostats that are lighter in weight and construction are less damaging to tissue. Hemostats with fine and pointed jaws can be applied with more precision and less damage to the vessel or surrounding tissues. Hemostats with heavy, broad jaws can be used to clamp across larger amounts of tissue that may contain several small blood vessels (Figure 13–2). The serrations in the jaws also vary. Serrations may cover only the lower portion of the jaws, or may cover the total jaw surface (Figure 13–3). The extensiveness of serrations affects the security of the jaw's grip on the tissues when clamped. Hemostats should be clamped tightly enough to stop blood flow while maintaining the security of the clamp on the vessel, but without exerting excessive pressure, which can cause unnecessary tissue damage. The RNFA must be knowledgeable about the types of hemostatic clamps available and skilled in applying them to bleeding vessels.

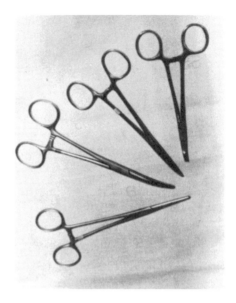

FIGURE 13–2

Examples of hemostats. *Right to left, top to bottom:* Curved Crile hemostat; tonsil hemostat; curved-pean and straight-pean hemostats.

To apply a hemostat, the open end of the bleeding vessel is grasped in the tip of the clamp. Only the minimal amount of the vessel is clamped. If the open end of the vessel cannot be held securely with the tip of the hemostat, it should be cross-clamped with the hemostat jaws (Figure 13–4).

Whenever possible, blood vessels are clamped before being cut to decrease blood loss. Either the tips or the jaws may be used, depending on vessel size and location and on the content of surrounding tissues. The vessel is usually clamped with two hemostats, with space left between the clamps for cutting the vessel. The amount of vessel between the clamps must be sufficient to prevent the clamps from slipping off the vessel once it is severed. When placing a hemostat on a branch of a blood vessel, the assistant should allow space on the branch between the clamp and the major vessel; this facilitates placing a ligature around the cut branch and prevents fracturing (or in-

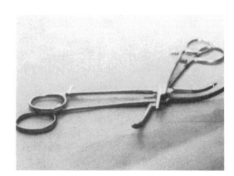

FIGURE 13–3

Top, Kelly hemostat (partial serrations), and *bottom,* Crile hemostat (fully serrated).

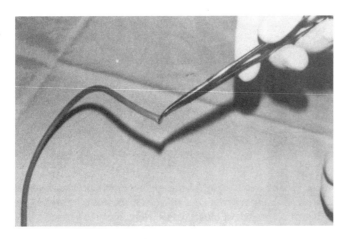

FIGURE 13-4

Method of clamping blood vessel (represented by rubber tubing) with hemostat.

juring) the major vessel (Figure 13–5). If curved hemostats are used, the tips of the two clamps should point toward each other. This facilitates cutting between the clamps and the subsequent placement of ligatures (Figure 13–6).

Removing a hemostat during vessel ligation requires coordination between the person holding the clamp and the one tying the ligature. The hemostat handle is lifted so that the ligature can be placed behind the clamp (Figure 13–7). This must be done carefully, so that the hemostat is not pulled off the vessel. The hemostat is then lowered or flattened to hold the ligature behind the clamp and elevate the point (tip) of the hemostat. The ligature is then brought around the tip of the hemostat, encircling the vessel to be ligated (Figure 13–8). As the first throw of the ligature knot is being tightened, the hemostat is slowly and carefully opened, thereby releasing the end of the vessel. The hemostat should be removed in a direction that will not interfere with the placement of the ligature or obstruct the vision of the person doing

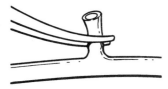

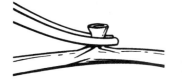

FIGURE 13-5

Top, proper application of clamp to branch of blood vessel allows room for ligating without injuring vessel. *Bottom,* improper placement of clamp on branch of blood vessel. Note injury to vessel.

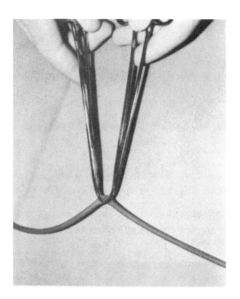

FIGURE 13–6
Method of clamping vessel (represented by rubber tubing) with hemostats curved toward each other.

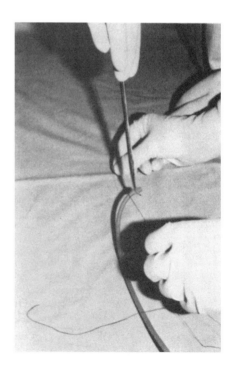

FIGURE 13–7
Lifting handle of hemostat for ease in placing ligature.

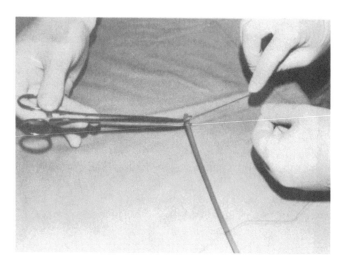

FIGURE 13–8
Flattening handle of hemostat and tying
ligature.

the tying. The hemostat can be opened and removed with precise control by placing the third finger and thumb into the ring handles, although in many instances the hemostat can be removed with the use of leverage on the handle (Figure 13–9). Although the release of the hemostat is not as precise, it is acceptable when ligature placement and tying are easy. The leverage method is quicker and easier once the skill is developed.

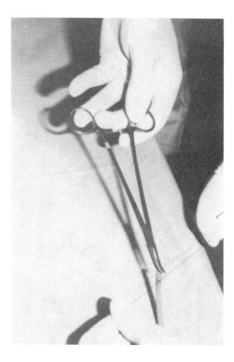

FIGURE 13–9
Releasing hemostat by leverage on handle.

There are three basic techniques for clamping and ligating blood vessels deep within a wound. The method used is usually related to the accessibility, size, and fragility of the vessel or surrounding tissue structures. In one technique, the vessel is clamped with longer, fine hemostats and divided with a scissor or knife. The ligature is held at one end with a tissue forceps or a tonsil hemostat, and the free end of the ligature is passed around the handle of the clamp and held taut with the free hand. The clamped end of the ligature is then placed under the tip of the hemostat. The RNFA, holding the hemostat, then tilts the hemostat tip downward and holds the ligature.

The hemostat's position must be changed very cautiously to prevent it from slipping off the end of the vessel. After the ligature is passed under the tip of the hemostat holding the vessel, the ligature is pulled until enough length is available for ease in tying (Figure 13–10). The ligature is released from the clamp or tissue forceps, and the first throw of the knot is slipped down behind or to the side of the hemostat clamped to the vessel as the hemostat is slowly removed by the RNFA.

In another method, the blood vessel is clamped and cut in the same manner. Instead of using a free ligature, however, the surgeon uses a ligature on a needle (stick tie). The surgeon holds the hemostat clamped to the vessel as the suture needle is placed through the blood vessel behind the hemostat. The ligature is pulled through the vessel, leaving enough length on the free

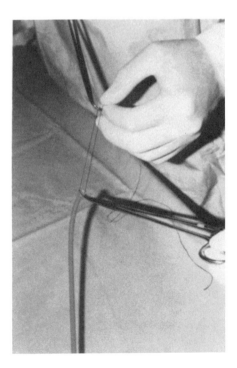

FIGURE 13–10
Using a hemostat to pass ligature around vessel (represented by rubber tubing).

end for easy tying. The ligature is then tied behind and around the vessel as the RNFA slowly removes the hemostat.

In the third technique, the ligatures are placed before the vessel is cut. The vessel is dissected free of surrounding tissue so that it can be visualized. An angled clamp of the appropriate length is used. The tip of the clamp is placed under the vessel and opened. The assistant then passes the ligature into the open tip of the angled clamp. It will be necessary for the RNFA to hold the ligature with both hands; one hand to keep the ligature taut and the other hand to hold the end of the ligature that will be placed in the angled clamp. In deep wounds, a tonsil hemostat or tissue forceps can be used to hold the end of the ligature to be placed in the open clamp tip (Figure 13–11). The angled clamp is closed so that the ligature is gripped securely between its jaws as the RNFA releases the ligature. Care must be taken not to close surrounding tissue in the clamp jaws. The angled clamp is then withdrawn and the ligature passed under the vessel. Enough ligature is pulled under the vessel to allow it to be tied easily. The ligature is released from the angled clamp and tied securely around the vessel. The procedure is then repeated. Before the second ligature is tied, it is positioned such that space on the vessel is allowed between the two ligatures. The vessel is cut between the two ligatures. The amount of vessel between the cut ends and the ligatures must be long enough so that the tie will not slip off. It is easier to cut the vessel if both ligatures are held taut, thereby pulling on the vessel. The ligatures are then cut (Figure 13–12).

Hemostatic Clips and Staples

In deep, narrow areas, where tying may be difficult or use of the electrosurgical unit inadvisable owing to the potential for damage to adjacent structures, hemostatic clips may be used.

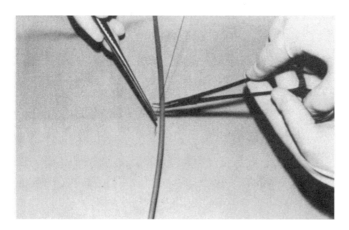

FIGURE 13–11

Using a forceps to pass a ligature into an angled clamp.

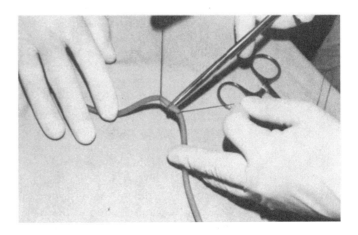

FIGURE 13–12
Cutting blood vessel between tied ligatures.

Clips.   Clips for ligating vessels vary in size and are made from tantalum or stainless steel wire. Serrations across the inside keep the clip from slipping off the vessel after it is applied. Absorbable clips made of polydiaxanone are absorbed in approximately 210 days. Ligating clips are useful for ligating vessels that are difficult to clamp with a hemostat. They are easy and quick to use and decrease the risk of foreign body reaction that may occur with sutures.

Although using ligating vessel clips is relatively easy, it must be done correctly. The correct clip size must be selected to ensure that the vessel is completely obliterated. Clip applicators are available in different lengths and are angled at the tip for ease in visualizing the vessel while the clip is being applied. Once the clip is in position around the vessel, the applicator handle is firmly squeezed and released. The applicator must be completely released before it is removed from around the clip, to avoid pulling on the clip. If the clip is accidentally pulled, it may come off the vessel or the vessel could be torn. The clip must be far enough back from the open end of the vessel to avoid slipping off the vessel later.

Scalp clips (e.g., Adson, Raney) may be reusable or disposable. Designed to provide hemostasis of the scalp incision edges, these clips are applied with special applicators after the scalp incision has been made. They are left in place during the surgery and removed as the incision is closed.

Staples.   Stapling devices provide hemostasis and closure of a transected organ such as the lung, bowel, or stomach. Staples are also available for vascular structures. Staples are available in various lengths and types and are selected according to the surgeon's preference. It is important to inspect the edges of stapled tissues to ensure adequate closure and hemostasis.

Vascular Clamps

Vascular clamps are designed to completely or partially occlude blood vessels with minimal injury to the vessel. The jaws have single or multiple rows of teeth, serrations, or cushioned inserts. Numerous variations in vascular clamp size, length, and configuration provide for adequate hemostasis in many different anatomical locations (Figure 13–13). The RNFA can facilitate clamp placement by retracting surrounding tissues so that they do not interfere with the clamp's occlusion.

Once the surgeon has placed the vascular clamp, the RNFA usually holds it in position. This must be done in a manner that does not interfere with clamp position or cause vessel injury. By holding the clamp by the shaft rather than by the ring handles, the RNFA is less likely to accidentally unlock the clamp ratchet. Excessive pulling or twisting of the clamp must be avoided, as the clamp may slip off the vessel or fracture the intimal wall of the vessel.

The vascular clamp provides a temporary means of hemostasis until the vessel opening is sutured. Before the clamp is removed, it must be opened completely free from the vessel, to prevent accidental tearing of the vessel. Partial occluding clamps are usually removed by placing the fingers and thumb through the ring handles from behind the clamp (Figure 13–14). This position is more comfortable for the RNFA's hand, and it allows the clamp to be opened more easily and with less chance of it turning or twisting on the vessel. The clamp can also be released by unlocking it from above (Figure 13–15).

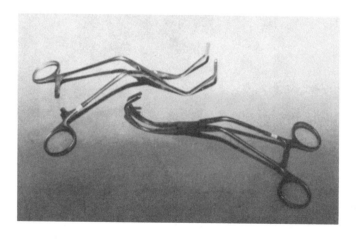

FIGURE 13–13

Examples of vascular clamps for aorta. Note different angles and curves of clamp jaws and handles.

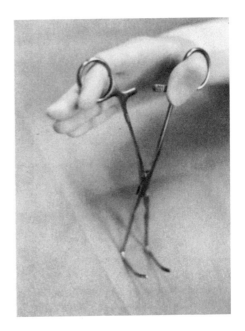

FIGURE 13–14
Removing a vascular clamp by opening from behind.

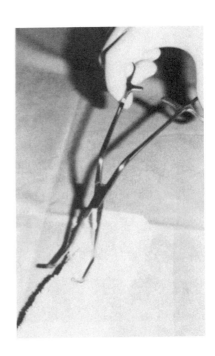

FIGURE 13–15
Removing a vascular clamp by opening from above.

Sutures, Knots, and Knot Tying

Sutures provide hemostasis by permanently holding tissues or vessel walls to-gether while they heal. Once the suture is placed and tied securely, the bleeding is stopped.

Sutures can be used as free ties to ligate vessels that have been clamped with a hemostat. Sutures are also used with needles to place single or multi-ple stitches. Stitches are indicated when there is a chance that the ligature will slip off the vessel or when the open area in the vessel is too large to ligate.

Regardless of how the suture is used to provide hemostasis, the RNFA must be skilled in tying secure knots. To develop this skill, the RNFA must become familiar with the various types of knots and must practice the tech-niques until dexterity is achieved.

Three basic types of knots are used in surgery: the square knot, the sur-geon's knot (Figure 13–16), and the granny knot. The square knot is used most frequently and is the most secure. The surgeon's knot is helpful when tying under a moderate amount of tension. If the first throw is doubled, the suture will not slip while the second knot is being placed. The granny knot, or slip knot, is made by placing two identical throws of the suture. This knot can be slipped or cinched tighter and is especially useful in wounds with lim-ited access. A square knot is tied on the granny knot to keep it from slipping.

The three techniques for tying knots are two-handed, one-handed, and instrument ties. The two-handed technique is usually the first one the assis-tant learns because it is easy to learn, provides control of the knot, and ties easily under tension (Figure 13–17). The one-handed technique is a little more difficult to learn, but it ties quickly (Figure 13–18). An instrument tie is necessary when the free end of the suture is too short to tie by hand. It is also very useful for economizing on sutures (Figure 13–19).

Regardless of the technique used, some basic principles guide knot tying. The free end of the suture must be of sufficient length to allow easy grasping; excessive length, however, is clumsy and interfering. The amount of tension exerted on the suture while the knot is being secured depends on the suture type and size. The knot should be tied tightly enough to hold securely with-out cutting through the tissue or breaking the suture. The knot is usually se-cured with three throws if the vessels are small or the tissues are not under tension. Four throws are advised for larger vessels or tissues under tension.

(text continues on page 326)

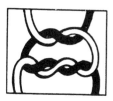 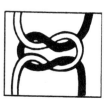

FIGURE 13–16

Types of surgical knots: *right,* square knot; *left,* surgeon's knot. (Source: Ethicon Knot Tying Manual, 1983. Courtesy of Ethicon, Inc., a Johnson & Johnson Company, Somerville, NJ.)

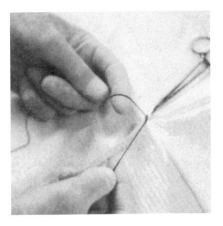

1. Grasp the short end of the suture with the right hand. Hold the long end of the suture in the left hand with the suture over the index finger.

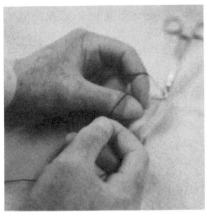

2. Bring the short end of the suture held in the right hand under the left index finger and over the left thumb.

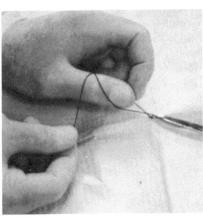

3. Slip the suture from the left index finger over the left thumb so that the thumb is through the loop.

FIGURE 13–17

TWO-HANDED TIE. Step-by-step instructions for completing the two-handed tie.

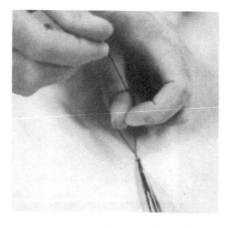

4. Bring the short end of the suture held in the right hand toward the left thumb and index finger.

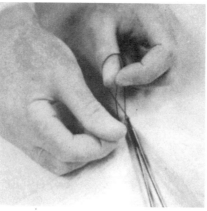

5. Grasp the suture in the right hand with the left thumb and the index finger.

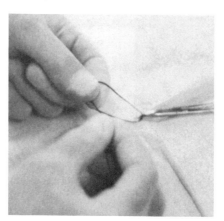

FIGURE 13-17 *(continued)*

6. Rotate the wrist and push the short end of the suture through the loop while releasing the suture end from the right hand.

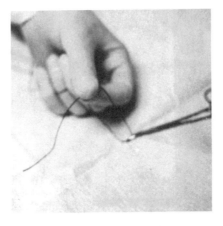

7. Short end of the suture passes through the loop and can be grasped by the right hand.

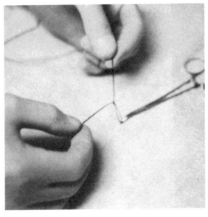

8. Secure the knot.

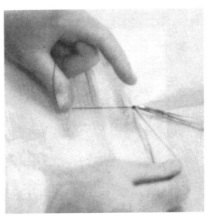

9. While holding the long end of the suture in the left hand, place the left thumb on the suture.

FIGURE 13–17 *(continued)*

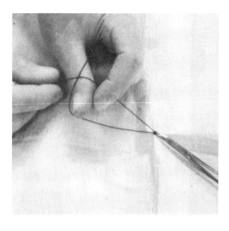

10. Bring the short end of the suture in the right hand over the thumb, and place the left index finger over the suture, touching the thumb.

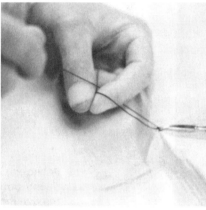

11. Rotate the left hand so that the suture slips off the thumb and the index finger is through the loop.

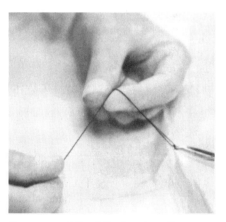

12. Place the short end of the suture that is held by the right hand between the thumb and index finger of the left hand.

FIGURE 13–17 *(continued)*

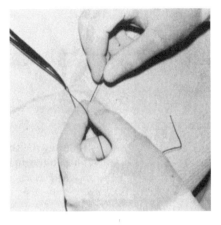

13. Hold the short suture with the thumb and finger while performing step 14.

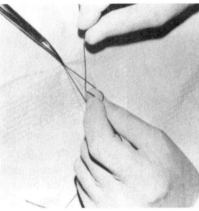

14. Rotate the left hand so that the thumb pushes the short suture through the loop.

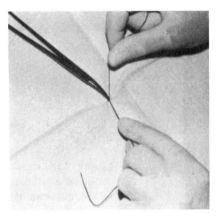

15. Regrasp the suture with the right hand after it passes through the loop, and secure the knot.

FIGURE 13–17 *(continued)*

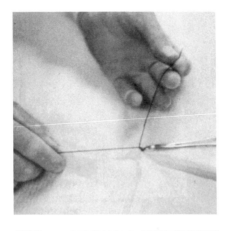

1. Grasp the short end of the suture with the thumb and index finger of the left hand.

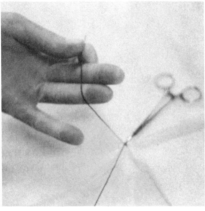

2. Rotate the left hand so that the suture rests across palmar surface of the long finger and the ring finger.

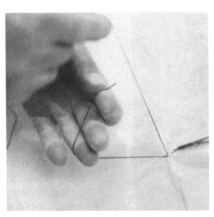

3. Bring the suture in the right hand over the left hand.

FIGURE 13–18

ONE-HANDED TIE. Step-by-step instructions for completing the one-handed tie.

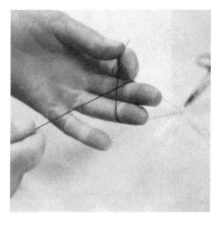

4. Place the suture in the right hand onto the long finger of the left hand, and across the suture being held in the left hand.

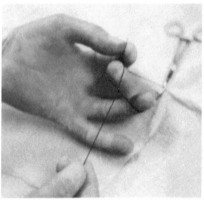

5. Flex the long finger of the left hand so that the tip goes under the short suture that is being held by the left thumb and index finger.

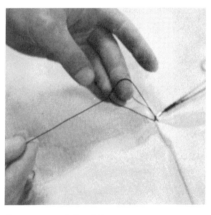

6. Release the short suture from the left thumb and index finger while extending the long finger and rotating the left hand. This flips the suture through the loop.

FIGURE 13–18 *(continued)*

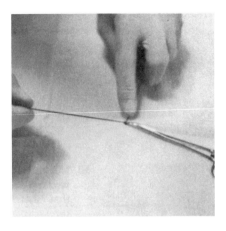

7. Secure the knot.

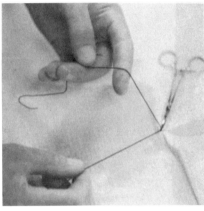

8. The short end of the suture is held in the left hand and over the extended index finger. The right hand holds the long part of the suture taut.

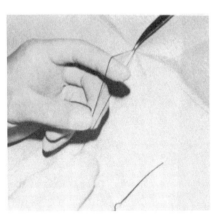

9. Bring the suture in the right hand under the extended left index finger.

FIGURE 13-18 *(continued)*

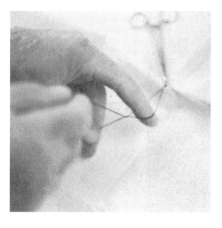

10. Lift the suture in the right hand while rotating the left hand so that the index finger passes through the loop.

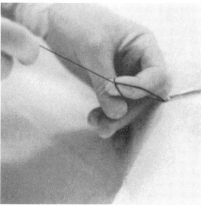

11. Flex the left index finger under the suture held in the left hand.

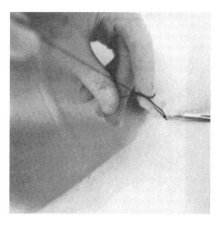

12. Extend the left index finger and release the suture from the left hand.

FIGURE 13–18 *(continued)*

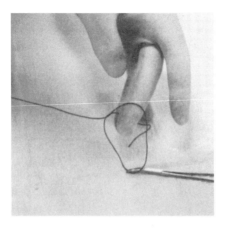

13. This flips the suture through the loop.

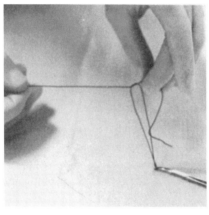

14. The suture is held in the left hand between the tips of the middle finger and long finger after it passes through the loop.

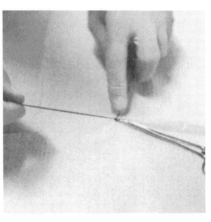

15. Secure the knot.

FIGURE 13–18 *(continued)*

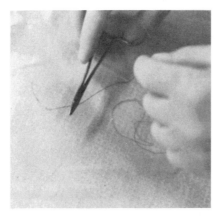

1. After the suture is placed through the tissue, pull the suture and leave a short end. Place the needleholder against the suture.

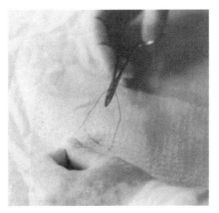

2. Wrap the suture around the needleholder (once or twice).

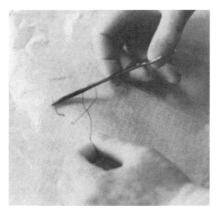

3. Grasp the short end of the suture with the needleholder and pull it through the suture wrapped around the needleholder.

FIGURE 13–19

INSTRUMENT TIE. Step-by-step instructions for completing the instrument tie.

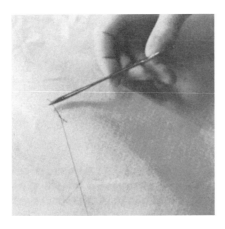

4. Secure the knot.

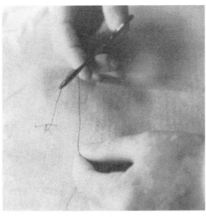

5. Wrap the suture over the needle-holder in the direction opposite that of the initial wrap.

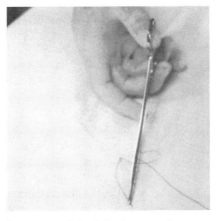

6. Again, grasp the short end of the suture with the needleholder and pull it through the suture wrapped around the needleholder. Secure the second half of the knot.

F I G U R E 1 3 – 1 9 *(continued)*

Slippery or very smooth sutures (e.g., nylon) require five to ten throws for security. Fine, braided wire can be tied like suture, but heavier wire must be twisted for at least three complete turns. Suture material will weaken if strands are "sawed" against each other during tying. Care must also be taken to ensure that the suture is not partially cut with instruments.

Bonewax

Made from refined beeswax, bonewax is used to control bleeding from bone marrow. It is gently pushed and rubbed into the edge of the bone where the marrow is exposed and bleeding. Foreign body reactions can occur from excessive bonewax application. Only just enough wax should be used to control the bleeding; excess wax must be removed.

Tourniquets

Pneumatic Tourniquets. Used to control bleeding during extremity surgeries, a pneumatic tourniquet restricts both venous and arterial blood flow. It is inadvisable to use a tourniquet on patients who have vascular disease or problems with peripheral circulation.

A pneumatic tourniquet can cause neurological or vascular injury if used incorrectly. Cuff selection is based on the size of the extremity. The cuff is placed around the largest circumference of the extremity, overlapping itself by three to six inches. It should not be placed around an elbow or knee, as injury may occur to the nerves and vascular structures. The skin under the cuff is padded with a stockinette. The padding should not have wrinkles, which could cause skin or nerve damage.

Venous blood is removed from the elevated extremity by wrapping it with a rubber bandage (e.g., Esmark), starting at the toes or fingers. Once the venous blood is removed, the tourniquet cuff is inflated. The optimum pressure in the cuff depends on the patient's age, size, and blood pressure and is determined by the physician. Usually, the pressure is 50 to 75 mm Hg above the patient's systolic blood pressure for the arm and 100 to 150 mm Hg above the systolic pressure for the leg. The inflated cuff should be left in place for only brief periods—a maximum of one and one-half hours for the leg and one hour for the arm. If the operation is not yet completed, the cuff can be deflated for 10 minutes and then reinflated. The periods of cuff inflation should be accurately documented, with the surgeon kept informed at 30-minute intervals.

Once the tourniquet is deflated, bleeding in the operative area will need to be controlled. Postoperative evaluation of the patient's extremity will be necessary to determine whether any injury occurred related to the use of the pneumatic tourniquet.

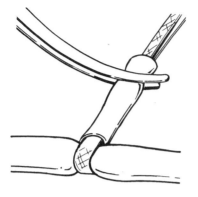

FIGURE 13–20

Umbilical tape is used to obstruct blood flow through the blood vessel. A rubber tubing tourniquet is slid down the tape toward the blood vessel and held in place with a hemostat clamp.

Vascular Tourniquets.   Vascular tourniquets are used to control bleeding from vascular structures. The Rummel tourniquet is used to control the tightness of a purse-string suture in a blood vessel or heart chamber. Umbilical tapes are commonly placed around major arteries and veins to be used as tourniquets. The tourniquet effect may be accomplished by passing the umbilical tape around the vessel, tightening the tape until blood flow stops, and holding it secure with a hemostat. The umbilical tape can also be threaded through a piece of catheter tubing (using a stylet), then pulled tight and held with a hemostat clamp above the tubing that holds both the tape and the tubing (Figure 13–20). A vessel loop, pulled tightly around the vessel and secured with a hemostat, may be used instead of umbilical tape.

◼ THERMAL MEANS OF ACHIEVING HEMOSTASIS

Wound hemostasis can be achieved quickly by applying electrical current to vessels. However, damage to adjacent tissue may be extensive if the correct technique is not used. Although the electrosurgical unit (ESU) is the most frequently used electrical unit for hemostasis, the argon beam coagulator may also be used to control hemorrhage from vascular structures. This unit uses argon gas, which flows through a handpiece, to clear fluid from the target site and then create a superficial eschar. The argon beam coagulator may produce less necrotic tissue than is caused by high-current electrosurgery.

Electrosurgical Principles

By understanding the basics of electricity and electrosurgery, clinical applications, and available technologies, the RNFA can collaborate in preventing patient injury and maximize the capabilities of the ESU.

Basics of Electricity.   Electricity arises from the existence of positively and negatively charged particles. As particles move, like charges repel each other and unlike charges attract each other. Electron movement is termed *electricity*. There are two properties of electricity that affect patient care in surgical and other invasive procedures. As electricity moves at nearly the speed of light, it always follows the path of least resistance and always seeks to return to ground. Electron movement through a conductor (electricity) and back to ground is known as the *electrical circuit*. The variables associated with the electrical circuit must be considered when using it during patient care. There are two types of current used in the operating room, direct current (DC) and alternating current (AC). *Direct current* follows a simple circuit as the electricity flows in one direction. For example, batteries contain a simple circuit. Energy flows from one terminal on the battery and must return to the other terminal to complete the circuit.

Alternating currents switch, or alternate, direction of electron flow. The frequency of these alterations is measured in cycles per second, or Hertz (Hz), with 1 Hertz being equal to 1 cycle per second. Household current alternates at 60 cycles per second, as does much of the equipment in the operating room. Alternating current at 60 Hertz can cause tissue reaction and damage. Neuromuscular stimulation ceases at about 100,000 Hertz, as the alternating currents move into the radiofrequency (RF) range.[7] Electron flow is measured in *amperes*, or amps.

Resistance (or impedance) is the opposition to the flow of current; it is measured in ohms. In the operating room, one source of resistance or impedance is the patient. A push is needed to overcome this resistance, and that push is *voltage*. Voltage is the force that will cause 1 amp to flow through 1 ohm of resistance. It is measured in volts, and it is the voltage in an ESU generator that provides the electromotive force that pushes electrons through the circuit. *Power*, measured in watts, is the energy produced. The power setting used by the RNFA or surgeon either is printed on an LED screen in watts, or a percentage of the wattage is demonstrated on a numerical dial setting.

Modes of Electrosurgical Current.   There are three different modes (cut, fulgeration, and desiccation) of producing electrosurgical current from generators, and each has a distinct tissue effect. The *cutting current* from an electrosurgical generator is a continuous waveform. Since the delivery of current is continuous, much lower voltages are required to achieve the desired effect, which is tissue vaporization. To achieve the cutting effect, the RNFA should hold the active electrode (ESU pencil tip) just over the target tissue (Figure 13–21). The current vaporizes cells in such a way that a clean tissue cut is achieved.

Tissue *fulgeration* is achieved using the coagulation mode on the ESU generator. The *coagulation mode* produces an interrupted or dampened waveform with a duty cycle that is activated approximately 6% of the time,

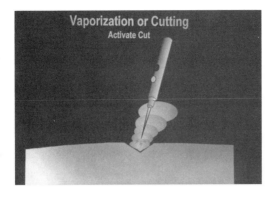

FIGURE 13–21

To achieve electrosurgical cutting, the RNFA should hold the electrode tip just above the tissue and let the spark divide the tissue by vaporization.

producing spikes of current of as much as 5,000 volts at 50 watts. The tissue is heated as the wave spikes and cools down during the 94% off cycle, thus coagulating the cell. To achieve fulgeration when using the coagulation mode, the RNFA should hold the active electrode (ESU pencil tip) slightly above the target tissue (Figure 13–22).

Electrosurgical *desiccation* can be produced using either the cut or coagulate mode. The difference is that the active electrode tip (ESU pencil tip) must contact the target tissues in order to desiccate it. Desiccation is the method used when the RNFA grasps a bleeding vessel with a clamp and then touches the clamp (or the vessel) with the active electrode tip.

The *blended mode* on an ESU generator is a function of cut. Blended currents produce voltage higher than that of the pure cut mode. The current is modified to a dampened waveform that produces some hemostasis during cutting.[8] There are several blend settings that provide different ratios of coagulation with the cutting current (these may vary among manufacturers):

- Blend 1: 80% cut/20% coagulation
- Blend 2: 60% cut/40% coagulation
- Blend 3: 50% cut/50% coagulation

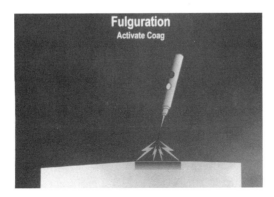

FIGURE 13–22

Fulgeration or coagulation, like electrosurgical cutting, is a noncontact use of the electrosurgery active electrode.

The electrosurgical mode selected has a definite impact on patient tissue. There are also additional variables that can alter the outcome of electrosurgical tissue effect:

- Time—The length of time the active electrode is on determines the extent of tissue effect. Activating the electrode too long produces wider and deeper tissue damage. Too short an activation will not produce the desired tissue effect.
- Power—The power setting alters tissue effect. The RNFA should always use the lowest setting that achieves the desired tissue effect. That time varies from patient to patient.
- Electrode—The size of the active electrode (pencil tip) influences the tissue effect. A large electrode requires a higher power setting than a smaller one. The RNFA should also remember that a clean electrode will conduct current more effectively than a dirty one; using a clean electrode requires lower power settings.
- Tissue—Patient tissue can determine the effectiveness of the generator. A lean, muscular patient will conduct the electrical current better than an obese or emaciated patient. The physical condition of the patient determines the amount of impedance encountered as the current attempts to return to the generator to complete the circuit.

Types of Electrosurgical Units.   There are multiple types and models of ESUs in operating rooms. The RNFA should be familiar with each type to maximize the use of its associated technology while also avoiding any potential hazards. The simplest unit is the *electrocautery pencil.* It uses a simple direct current generated from a battery within the system. The term "electrocautery" or "cautery" is often used to describe all types of electrosurgical devices. This is an inappropriate term unless one is referring to the simple, direct-current cautery device. The small, hand-held eye cautery is an example of this device. The battery heats a wire loop at the end of the cautery pencil; the current never leaves the device to travel through patient tissue. Thus, a patient return electrode (dispersive pad) is not required. In ophthalmic surgery and other minor procedures where minimal bleeding is encountered, an electrocautery pencil is useful. However, it is limited in that it cannot cut tissue or coagulate large bleeders, and because the target tissue has a tendency to stick to the electrode.

Bipolar electrosurgery is the use of electrical current where the circuit is completed by using two parallel poles located close to one another. One pole is positive, the other is negative. The flow of current is restricted between these two poles, which are most often the tines of the bipolar forceps. Because the poles are in such close proximity, low voltages are used to achieve tissue effect. Because electrical current does not flow through the patient, a return electrode (dispersive pad) is not necessary. This makes bipolar electrosurgery very safe, but not without disadvantages. The RNFA using the bipolar ESU will find it cannot spark to tissue, and the low voltage renders it less effective on large bleeding vessels. Bipolar electrosurgery is widely used in neurosurgery and gynecological surgery, and is a safe unit to use when the RNFA has a question about the efficacy of using more powerful monopolar ESUs in certain patients with devices such as pacemakers or implantable cardioverter defibrillators.

The first generation of ESUs, developed in the early 1900s, were ground-referenced, meaning that the ground completed the electrosurgical circuit. They were spark-gap systems that had high output and high performance, making them a favorite with surgeons. However, in a grounded system, a major hazard is that current division can occur. If the electrical current finds an easier and quicker way to return to ground, the patient can be burned at any point where the current exits the body, such as a hand touching the metal side of the operating room bed, a knee in contact with a metal stirrup, or any number of other alternative exit sites.

In 1968, solid state generators were introduced. These were much smaller and used isolated circuitry. Isolated units reference the electrical current to the generator and ignore all grounded objects that may come in contact with the patient. Current division cannot occur with an isolated generator, which eliminates the possibility of alternative site burns. During use, an isolated generator will not work if the patient return electrode (dispersive pad) is not on the patient. However, the generator cannot determine how *well* the dispersive pad is on the patient. Should the return be compromised in any way, a return electrode burn can occur. The RNFA must be certain that the patient electrode is in good contact with the patient's body surface throughout the surgical procedure.

By 1981, patient return electrodes employing a quality contact monitoring system had been introduced. Return electrode monitoring (REM) uses a split pad system whereby an interrogation current constantly monitors the quality of the contact between the patient and the return electrode. If a condition develops at the return electrode site that could result in a patient injury, the REM system inactivates the generator. This represented a major safety device for patients and RNFAs, since return electrode burns account for a majority of patient burns during surgery.[9]

In the late 1980s, an argon delivery system, combined with electrosurgery, created *argon-enhanced electrosurgery*. This is not a laser. The argon gas shrouds the electrosurgery current in a stream of gas that delivers the spark to tissue in a beamlike fashion. Argon is an inert, nonreactive gas that is heavier than air and easily ionizes. Because the beam concentrates the electrosurgical current while displacing blood and oxygen, a smoother, more pliable eschar is produced. And because some of the oxygen is displaced at the surgical site by the heavier argon, less smoke is produced. Argon-enhanced electrosurgery can reduce blood loss and surgical time.

The most recent technology available on ESU generators is a *tissue density feedback system*. Tissue density ESU generators use a computer-controlled instant response system that senses tissue resistance and automatically adjusts the output voltage to maintain a consistent tissue effect. The feedback mode reduces the need to adjust power settings for different types of tissue. It also yields improved performance at lower voltages, helping to reduce the potential for patient injury.

Electrosurgery During Endoscopic Procedures

With the explosion of endoscopic procedures being performed in the 1990s, there has been a concomitant concern about the safe use of monopolar electrosurgery. There have been reports of illness and death following endoscopic procedures, in which electrosurgery has contributed to an adverse outcome. The primary associated hazards are direct coupling, insulation failure, and capacitative coupling, which may result in injury outside the field of vision of the surgical team. *Direct coupling* can occur when the active electrode is activated close to another object inside the abdomen. Care must be taken to prevent activation of the active electrode when it is in contact with, or close to, other clamps or clips in the operative area. *Insulation failure* occurs when the material used to coat the active electrode is compromised in some way. This can result from rough handling, repeated uses, or because of high voltages used during electrosurgery. Current can escape from the active electrode anywhere a break in the insulation occurs. RNFAs should keep in mind that using the coagulation mode instead of the cut mode results in the use of higher voltages, which is undesirable. They should also consider checking with the manufacturer of the active electrodes purchased by the surgery department to verify that they meet the standards for electrosurgical devices set by the Association for the Advancement of Medical Instrumentation (AAMI) or the American National Standards Institute (ANSI).

Capacitative coupling is the least understood of the hazards that can occur endoscopically. A capacitor is two conductors separated by an insulator. Inserting an active electrode down a metal cannula creates a capacitor. Capacitatively coupled electrical current can be transferred from the active electrode, through intact insulation and into the conductive metal cannula. Should the cannula then come in contact with body structures, the energy can be discharged, damaging those structures. A metal cannula does provide a pathway for any energy stored in the cannula to disperse along the patient's conductive abdominal wall. For this reason, it is unwise to use plastic anchors to secure the cannula; this isolates the current from the abdominal wall. Some institutions use plastic trocar cannula systems, believing them to be safer. The plastic systems can be just as hazardous because the patient's own conductive tissue within the abdomen can form the second conductor, creating a capacitor. Omentum or bowel draped over the plastic cannula could discharge stored energy to adjacent body structures.

An active electrode monitoring system can be used in conjunction with the ESU to protect the patient from insulation failure and capacitative coupling. When in place, this system continuously monitors and actively shields against stray electrosurgical current. This is the most effective means of minimizing the potential for patient injuries related to insulation failure and capacitative coupling. Additional methods the RNFA should use to prevent accidental injury during endoscopic electrosurgery are presented in Table 13–1.

Safety Considerations

Since 1994, the Association of Operating Room Nurses (AORN) recommended practices for the use of electrosurgery have noted that patients and perioperative personnel should be protected from inhaling the surgical smoke generated during electrosurgery.[11] Toxic fumes and carcinogens have been isolated from surgical smoke.[12] Smoke evacuation should occur whenever surgical smoke or plume-generating equipment is used. The simplest way for the RNFA to ensure that smoke plume is evacuated and filtered is by using a small carriage that attaches to the ESU pencil.

Active electrodes should be placed in holsters when not in use. They should be easily accessible and visible to the surgical team. Holsters should be of the type recommended by the manufacturer of the active electrode and should meet standards for heat and fire resistance. Pouches or other makeshift holsters that are not designed for use with an ESU active electrode could pose a threat to patient safety.

Placement of the dispersive pad is an important consideration. The manufacturer's specific recommendations for the pad being used should be implemented. In general, the pad should be placed as close to the surgical site as possible and over a large muscle mass; muscle is a better conductor than fatty tissue. Scar tissue and any bony prominence should be avoided; they are more resistant to current flow and impedance may therefore be increased at these sites. Dispersive pads should not be placed over metal prostheses; the scar tissue surrounding the implant increases resistance to the electrical cur-

---

TABLE 13–1. TECHNIQUES FOR PREVENTING ACCIDENTAL PATIENT INJURY DURING ENDOSCOPIC ELECTROSURGERY

- Always use the lowest possible power setting
- Use the lower voltage cut waveform
- Inspect insulation on the active electrode carefully
- Do not activate the electrode if in contact with other metal objects in the abdomen
- Do not open circuit activate the active electrode
- Use bipolar electrosurgery whenever possible
- Do not combine metal and plastic cannula systems for use with the active electrode

TABLE 13–2. TECHNIQUES FOR AVOIDING HEMOSTAT BURNS

- Use lowest power setting possible
- Key cut (less voltage)
- Avoid touching the patient
- Hold the hemostat with a full grip
- No open circuit activation (avoid metal-to-metal sparking)
- Remember that surgical gloves do not insulate against radio-frequency current

rent flow. The pad site should be clean, dry, without excessive hair, and not where fluids are likely to pool. If the patient has a pacemaker, the manufacturer should be consulted to determine if the pacemaker is susceptible to electrical interference.

It is not uncommon for RNFAs or surgeons to report receiving a shock during ESU use (Table 13–2). Holes in gloves have been implicated as the cause; holes may be present as a manufacturing defect or may occur during the surgical procedure. To avoid being shocked by the ESU, the RNFA should not lean on the patient; leaning on a patient inadvertently includes the RNFA in the electrosurgical circuit (Figure 13–23). When preparing to "buzz" a hemostat that is attached to target tissue, hold it with a full grip; this disperses the current over a wider surface area. Touch the clamp before activating the ESU pencil. Open-circuit activation of the ESU pencil causes current to jump the air to reach conductive metal. Current demodulation can occur and shock the person holding the clamp and blow a hole in the glove. The cut waveform should be used because the voltage is much lower. Use brief, intermittent activations and avoid overheating the target tissue; as tissue becomes charred, the ESU current will seek a more conductive path back to the dispersive pad. That path can be the clamp and the hand of the RNFA (or other operator), creating a shock and subsequent hole in the glove.

FIGURE 13–23

To avoid a "hemostat burn," hold the hemostat with a full grip and do not lean on the patient. Leaning on the patient puts the RNFA in the electrosurgical circuit.

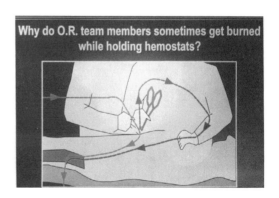

Why do O.R. team members sometimes get burned while holding hemostats?

Hypothermia

Hypothermia causes vasoconstriction and decreases bleeding. However, generalized hypothermia is not effective unless the temperature is lowered to 35 °C, and shivering and ventricular fibrillation may occur at this temperature, making hypothermia a poor choice as a method for hemostasis. Localized cooling has been effective for controlling esophageal or gastric bleeding, but this is not usually done intraoperatively. Cryogenic surgical procedures affect bleeding by causing necrosis of the vascular structures at extremely cold temperatures (–20 °C).

■ CHEMICAL MEANS OF ACHIEVING HEMOSTASIS

Chemical methods useful in achieving hemostasis include blood pressure regulation with medication or anesthetic agents, the use of topical agents, and appropriate treatment of coagulation defects.

Blood Pressure Regulation

Regulating blood pressure can be very effective in controlling bleeding. This is considered a chemical method of providing hemostasis, because medications or anesthetic agents are used.

Hypertension. Hypertension is controlled medically whenever possible. Intraoperative and postoperative bleeding can increase when blood pressure is elevated. Blood pressure is monitored frequently, and hypertension is treated with appropriate medications. Pain can cause hypertension and is controlled as much as possible postoperatively. Intraoperatively, pain occurs when the anesthesia is inadequate. A rise in blood pressure may be one of the first signs that the patient is experiencing pain.

Hypotension. Hypotension during the intraoperative period may be induced to decrease bleeding. The hypotensive state is closely monitored and controlled by the anesthesiologist. Medications and anesthetic agents are used intraoperatively to induce hypotension for procedures that are highly vascular (e.g., hip surgery) or when surgery involves vascular structures (e.g., cerebral aneurysms). Complications from hypotension can arise when the perfusion of vital organs is inadequate.

Topical Agents

Thrombin.   Thrombin is used topically to promote hemostasis by directly clotting the fibrinogen in the blood. It is useful in controlling bleeding or oozing from small blood vessels or capillaries.

Thrombin most commonly comes in solution but may come as a dry powder, to which isotonic saline or sterile distilled water is added to make a solution. The speed with which the thrombin acts to coagulate blood depends on solution concentration. Solutions should be prepared immediately before use.

When absorbable gelatin sponges soaked in thrombin are used, it is important to squeeze the sponge gently to remove any trapped air so that the sponge is completely saturated with thrombin and more effective in promoting hemostasis.

Thrombin must never be injected into the bloodstream or allowed to gain access through opened, large blood vessels. Extensive intravascular clotting and possible death may ensue.

Excess blood should be removed by sponging or suctioning the operative area before applying thrombin. Once the area has been treated, it should not be sponged, as the clots will be removed.

Gelatin Sponges.   Absorbable gelatin sponges (trade name, Gelfoam) are prepared from a purified gelatin solution that has been whipped into a foam, dried, and sterilized. Gelatin sponges can be applied to the bleeding surface either dry or moist. The sponge can be moistened by dipping it in normal saline solution that may have thrombin or epinephrine added to it. The sponge absorbs many times its own weight in blood, which then clots within the sponge. The blood is drawn into the sponge by capillary action, but it can be suctioned into the sponge if the sponge is protected with a gauze sponge or cotton pledget.

The gelatin sponge liquefies in two to five days following application to bleeding mucosal areas and is absorbed completely in four to six weeks. A gelatin sponge should not be used in the presence of an infection that could localize in the sponge. When used in cavities or closed tissue spaces, care must be taken not to overpack; swelling of the sponge could cause pressure, injuring surrounding tissues, nerves, and vascular structures. The sponge is often cut into the desired size and, if used moist, immersed in the solution, squeezed to remove air, and stored in the solution until used.

Microfibrillar Collagen.   A hemostatic agent derived from bovine dermis, microfibrillar collagen (trade name, Avitene) can help provide hemostasis when other methods are ineffective or impractical. Collagen promotes hemostasis by causing platelets to aggregate and activate by releasing substances that initiate the coagulation mechanisms. Collagen is available in a loose fibrous form and in a compacted, "nonwoven" web form. Collagen adheres to wet surfaces and therefore is applied with dry, smooth forceps to the bleeding site. The bleeding site is compressed with a dry sponge, the collagen is applied, and pressure is then applied with a sponge placed over the collagen. Pressure should be continued for one to ten minutes, depending on the severity of the bleeding. If bleeding continues through the collagen, the application can be repeated. Any excess collagen should be removed by gently teasing it away, because excess collagenous material could later cause complications such as bowel adhesions or mechanical pressure on ureters.

Absorbable Collagen Sponges.

Absorbable collagen sponges (trade name, Collastat) are made from collagen derived from bovine flexor tendon. The sponge can be cut to size and applied directly to the bleeding area. It will not disperse as the microfibrillar collagen does and is easier to handle and place. It, too, is handled with dry, smooth, tissue forceps. After placement on tissue, the sponge controls bleeding in two to four minutes by causing platelet aggregation and clot formation.

Oxidized Cellulose.

Oxidized cellulose (trade names, Oxycel and Surgicel) is available impregnated in treated gauze or cotton. Applied directly to a bleeding surface, it promotes clotting of capillaries and small vessels that cannot be controlled by other means. The gauze can be cut into strips or to the size desired and placed on the bleeding site dry, with a dry sponge to hold it in place. The oxidized cellulose is absorbed in two to seven days. It must not be packed tightly because it swells; also, it must never be left in the patient if used near the spinal cord, optic nerve, or any area where swelling can seriously damage surrounding tissues or nerves. Oxidized cellulose is not used as permanent packing in bone fractures because it interferes with bone regeneration. It should never be used with thrombin because it interferes with thrombin action.

Fibrin Gel.

Fibrin gel (also referred to as glue or sealant) is useful for controlling generalized oozing of blood, but it will not control vigorous bleeding. It is a biological adhesive that recreates natural physiological coagulation. In the presence of other ingredients, fibrinogen, which has been cryoprecipitated from human plasma, and thrombin, most often of bovine origin, are applied directly to tissue; the thrombin then converts fibrinogen to fibrin, forming a clot.[13] The gel can be prepared with either banked plasma or the patient's own (autologous) plasma, which is in one syringe, and thrombin (10,000 units per ampule) mixed with 10% calcium chloride in a separate syringe. Each solution is drawn into a separate syringe because combining them would rapidly form a fibrin clot. The two solutions are then sprayed (or injected) simultaneously on the bleeding site. The fibrin clot begins to form in a few seconds.

Albumin.   Albumin is frequently used to coat vascular prosthetic grafts to prevent bleeding through the porous graft surface. This not only contributes to hemostasis, but also makes the luminal surface of the graft smoother, decreasing postoperative thrombosis formation inside the graft. Vascular grafts precoated with albumin are available. If not on hand in the operating room, a non-precoated graft may be prepared by soaking it in albumin, wiping off any excess, and then steam sterilizing it for three minutes at 270 °F.

Epinephrine.   Epinephrine is used frequently with local anesthetic agents because it causes vasoconstriction, prolonging the effect of the local anesthetic and decreasing bleeding. Topically, gelatin sponges may be soaked in epinephrine and applied to a bleeding surface. Epinephrine should never be used for finger or toe surgery; sloughing may occur. It should not be used in patients with peripheral vascular disease for the same reason. Because epinephrine can cause increased blood pressure, tachycardia, and vasoconstriction, it is not usually recommended for patients with cardiac conditions.

SUMMARY

Perioperative nurses have long recognized the many potential risks facing patients during the intraoperative period. The RNFA, acting in the expanded perioperative nurse role, continues to monitor and ensure patient safety. The potential for patient injury exists even when nursing interventions are directed toward achieving a positive outcome, such as assisting with hemostasis and using hemostatic adjuncts. A review of the critical elements of providing hemostasis elucidates the following potential nursing diagnoses and consequent safety considerations:

1. Fluid Volume Deficit (intraoperative) related to inadequate control of bleeding
2. High Risk for Injury related to the use of electrical equipment (the ESU)
3. Altered Tissue Perfusion related to surgical interruption of blood vessels, the use of hypothermia, the tourniquet, controlled hypotension, and vasoconstrictive drugs
4. High Risk for Infection related to the use of vasoconstrictive drugs, electrosurgery, and tissue-reactive suture materials
5. Fluid Volume Deficit (postoperative) related to inadequate volume replacement or slippage of knot or suture

The RNFA, through the application of knowledge and skill, directs efforts toward providing patients with injury-free postoperative outcomes. When wounds are dry and hemostasis is achieved, attention has been paid to meticulous detail and the correct decisions have been made. Using a sound knowledge base, the RNFA has implemented techniques that prevent potential patient injury and wound complications.

Review Questions

1. The RNFA initially seeks to prevent blood loss by
   a. Appropriate use of the ESU and argon beam coagulator.
   b. Anticipatory control of blood vessels.
   c. Learning how to use the square knot.
   d. Using digital compression before other methods.

2. The body's natural defense of blood clotting will produce adhesion, aggregation, and initial plug formation within
   a. 1 to 2 seconds.
   b. 1 to 3 minutes.
   c. 5 to 10 minutes.
   d. 1 to 2 hours.

3. During assessment, the RNFA notes that the patient is undergoing cancer chemotherapy. This places the patient at risk for
   a. Deficiency in factor X concentration.
   b. Hemolytic transfusion reaction.
   c. Thrombocytopenia.
   d. Disseminated intravascular coagulation.

4. Which of the following would be the most appropriate question to ask a patient regarding any bleeding problems?
   a. "Can you tell me your normal clotting time?"
   b. "Have you had any problems with bleeding following dental extraction?"
   c. "Have you ever had a problem with a blood transfusion?"
   d. "Do you have problems with GI bleeding or hematuria?"

5. Prothrombin time measures
   a. The coagulant activity of the extrinsic system, including fibrinogen, prothrombin, and factors V, VII, and X.
   b. The presence of immune globulin on the surface of erythrocytes or in the plasma.
   c. Disorders of platelet function.
   d. Deficiencies of all plasma coagulation factors except VII and XIII.

6. Albumin aids in the maintenance of colloid osmotic pressure. An albumin level below _____ g/dL is of concern in assessing risk for fluid imbalance.
   a. 3
   b. 4
   c. 5
   d. 6

7. Initial attempts at reversing hemorrhagic shock are made by transfusing
   a. Plasma.
   b. Red blood cells.
   c. Crystalloid albumin.
   d. Intravenous fluids.

8. An example of the application of indirect pressure is applying it
   a. With a sponge on a stick.
   b. Between two fingers (bidigitally).
   c. To an area proximal to the bleeding vessel.
   d. With the tip of an instrument, such as the suction tip.

9. If a moist pack is used in an area of diffuse bleeding, it should be moistened with _____ saline.
   a. Cool
   b. Warm

10. When curved hemostats are used to clamp a vessel before transection, the hemostat tips should point _____ each other to facilitate cutting between the clamps.
    a. Toward
    b. Away from

11. When the RNFA must deal with multiple clamps as tying is about to proceed, he or she should
    a. Take two or three in the hand at a time to speed the process.
    b. Suggest using the ESU rather than tying.
    c. Pick them up for tying in the order that they were placed.
    d. Take the most accessible one first and proceed in a logical order.

12. Once the ligature is slid down the heel of a clamp, the clamp is lowered to a horizontal position and the tips are _____ without pulling.
    a. Directed downward
    b. Elevated

13. In general, during knot tying, the strand that is actively passed through the loop is held in which hand?
    a. Dominant
    b. Nondominant

14. Despite the type of knot to be used, a basic principle of knot tying is that
    a. The free end of a suture strand should be short.

    b. The free end of a suture strand should be long.

    c. Suture strands should not be sawed against each other.

    d. Knots are secured with three throws.

15. Keeping the suture strands loose and equal, forming a round loop as the knot is snugged down, prevents formation of an unwanted half hitch and
    a. The need to turn the body to properly orient the hands.
    b. The need to alternate throws.
    c. Sawing and fraying of the suture.
    d. Tying away from the body.

16. To prevent pulling up on the structure being tied (and to prevent reversing the throw into a half hitch), the RNFA should learn to complete the throw by putting the _____ finger of the hand holding the suture strand closest to the body down on the strand.
    a. Middle
    b. His or her strongest
    c. Thumb and middle
    d. Index

17. The first step of every throw is the formation of a loop over a finger or instrument. Keeping the finger _____ the structure being tied prevents twisting of the loop and crossing.
    a. Parallel to
    b. Perpendicular to
    c. Away from
    d. Pointing toward

18. A pneumatic tourniquet applied to a patient's arm is usually inflated to _____ mm Hg above the patient's systolic blood pressure.
    a. 25–50
    b. 50–75
    c. 75–100
    d. 100–150

19. When using an ESU, the RNFA should deactivate the current immediately on noting _____ of tissue about the vessel.
    a. Reddening
    b. Charring
    c. Darkening
    d. Erythema

20. Vascular prosthetic grafts may be coated with _____ to prevent bleeding through porous graft surfaces.
    a. Albumin
    b. Thrombin
    c. Fibrin glue
    d. Oxidized cellulose

■ Answer Key

1. b	8. c	15. c
2. b	9. a	16. d
3. c	10. a	17. a
4. b	11. c	18. b
5. a	12. b	19. c
6. b	13. a	20. a
7. d	14. c	

REFERENCES

1. Holcroft JW: Shock: Early recognition and emergency management. In: American College of Surgeons: Care of the Surgical Patient. Vol I. Critical Care. New York, Scientific American Medicine, 1997
2. American Society of Anesthesiologists: Practice guidelines for blood component therapy. Chicago, American Society of Anesthesiologists, 1995
3. Craig V, Bower JO: Blood administration in perioperative settings. AORN J 66(1):133–141, 1997
4. Vernon S, Pfeifer GM: Are you ready for bloodless surgery? AM J Nurs 97(9):40–47, 1997
5. Russell S: Bloodless surgery: Meeting patient needs. Point of View 35(2):8–14, 1997
7. Gruendemann BJ, Fernsebner B: Comprehensive Perioperative Nursing. Boston, Jones and Bartlett, 1995
8. Vancaille TG: Electrosurgery Principles and Risks. San Antonio, Center for Gynecologic Endoscopy, 1994
9. Emergency Care Research Institute: Controlling the risks of electrosurgery. Health Devices 18(12):430–432, 1989
10. Emergency Care Research Institute: The risks of laparoscopic electrosurgery. Health Devices 24(1):5, 1995
11. Recommended practices for electrosurgery. In: AORN Standards, Recommended Practices and Guidelines. Denver, Colo, Association of Operating Room Nurses, 1997, pp 163–168
12. Emergency Care Research Institute. The danger of laser plume. Health Devices 19(1):4, 1990
13. Pace RM: Intraoperative preparation of autologous fibrin gel. AORN J 62(4): 604–607, 1995

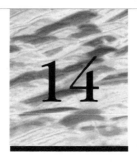

THE RN FIRST ASSISTANT
AND COLLABORATIVE PRACTICE

PATRICIA C. SEIFERT

■

New strategies, policy initiatives, delivery models, and payment methods are altering the way in which health care is delivered, and the successful transformation of the health care system will depend on effective collaboration between nurses and physicians as well as an expanding array of caregivers. The current patient care environment offers an ever-broadening range of treatment options and care strategies, and the interactions of caregivers can either create or divide alliances. Too often care is fragmented, and there is evidence of overreliance on physicians to direct care, lack of patient/family participation in setting health care goals, wasted resources, diminished effectiveness, and dissatisfaction among providers and patients.[1,2] Moreover, research on patient outcomes has demonstrated that physician behavior alone cannot account for the quality of patient care in hospitals: quality outcomes are more closely linked to teamwork, and specifically to nurse–physician interactions.[3-5]

In a managed care environment that values efficiency and effectiveness, fragmentation can produce costly conflict. Well-coordinated, integrated care not only promotes staff satisfaction and enhances patient outcomes, it also results in cost savings.[6] It is in this context that collaboration as a practice model is becoming more prominent in the health care community. As a result, collaborative models are being advocated by professional organizations, accrediting bodies, regulatory reformers, and governmental agencies.[7]

◼ DEFINITION OF COLLABORATIVE PRACTICE

According to Adler and colleagues, collaboration refers to the "process of different individuals working together toward a mutual goal."[8] This definition is broader than earlier ones that focused primarily on the nurse–doctor relationship. Although collaborative practice for nurses continues to reflect in large part nurse–physician interactions related to shared planning and decision making, joint problem solving, and cooperative and coordinated interventions, the nurse–physician prototype has been expanded to reflect the fact that many groups contribute to the delivery of quality care.

For the RNFA this expanded network may include not only surgeons, anesthesia care providers and physician assistants, but also social workers, pharmacists, physical and respiratory therapists, and nutritionists (Figure 14–1). It also includes the patient, whose well-being is the goal of health care professionals. In a capitated system, where there is a fixed reimbursment for each patient, education, preventive care, and counseling become especially important and highlight the value of nurses, whose education and training make them espe-

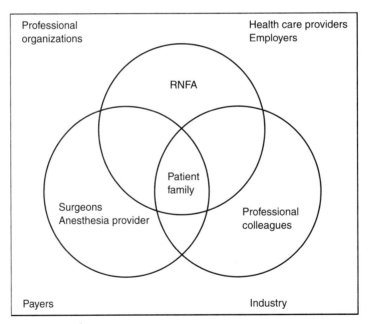

FIGURE 14–1

Collaborative model. The patient and family are the focus of the multidisciplinary health care delivery team. The RN first assistant also collaborates with health care providers, employers, industry representatives, payers, and members of professional organizations to improve patient care.

cially suitable to fulfill the goals of patients and payers.[9] These changing relationships and partnerships require new behaviors and ways of thinking.

■ BACKGROUND

Historically, the nurse–physician relationship was vertical, with most of the authority and decision making assumed by the physician. Nurses were not actively involved in planning patient care, nor were they privy to physicians' decision-making rationales. They were expected not to question orders and not to communicate to patients the reasons for those orders. This was described by Stein in 1967 as the "doctor–nurse game."[10] The "game" reflected hierarchical relationships that made communication difficult, and the education and training of both physicians and nurses, which fostered roles of leadership and subservience, respectively. Stein and colleagues returned to the subject when a number of social changes altered the health care environment.[11] Among these were deteriorating public esteem for physicians, the commercialization of health care, increasing recognition of the value of nursing care, and the growth of specialty trained and certified advance nurse practitioners who had independent duties and responsibilities to their patients. Perhaps most significant was the increasing dependence of physicians on nurses with special knowledge, skill, and experience.

In the past there were exceptions to the traditional hierarchical model that would influence the development of the RNFA role. In 1894, an operating team consisting of surgeons, nurses, and assistants was recommended and introduced at the Johns Hopkins Hospital in Baltimore.[12] At about the same time, in Rochester, Minnesota, the Mayo brothers were among the first to provide an opportunity to expand the role of nurses in the operating room and to include them in patient care by training them to provide anesthesia to their patients. Although the operating room nurse's duties at that time centered mainly on maintaining instruments, supplies, and equipment, managing the sterilizing room, preparing dressings, and passing instruments, the team concept did foster shared responsibilities and a growing mutual respect.[13]

By World War I, operating room nursing had evolved into a distinct specialty with formal education programs and specialized training. The nurse's focus shifted from technical concerns to more patient-centered activities. Responsibility for maintaining an aseptic environment, supervising nonnursing personnel, and preparing the surgical patient were added. First assisting was occasionally performed, and became increasingly more common as World War I progressed. The shortage of qualified medical first assistants influenced the decision to train nurses for this role.

First assisting was further promoted during World War II, when the demand for assistants became so great that even nonnursing technicians were trained to assist. After the war, the shortage of nurses forced hospitals to hire technicians trained in the armed forces. This increased use of technicians for scrubbing and first assisting, along with the concurrent reduction in the requirement for operating room rotations in student nursing programs, had the effect of producing a somewhat technical and isolated image of the operating room nurse. It also limited communication between nurses inside and outside the operating room. Of special significance for nurses outside the operating room was that deletion of an operating room rotation denied them contact with patients in surgery. It also reduced the interaction with nurses who could share the special knowledge and skills necessary for aseptic technique. That knowledge is still crucial to many nursing functions in all practice areas. In addition, first assisting by registered nurses, with its potential for increasing firsthand the nurse's knowledge of anatomy, physiology, and the impact of surgical interventions on patients, was largely delegated to technicians.

The formation of the Association of Operating Room Nurses (AORN) in 1954 signaled operating room nurses' concern for defining and promoting a high level of professional practice during surgery. AORN's formulation of the perioperative role in 1978, and its revision in 1985 describing perioperative nursing practice, addressed the nurse's responsibility for providing care in the preoperative, intraoperative, and postoperative phases of the patient's surgical experience. According to the AORN, the perioperative nurse "works in collaboration with other health care professionals to determine and meet patient needs and has primary responsibility and accountability for nursing care of patients having surgical intervention."[14] By 1992, the AORN had recognized that with changing practice patterns and care delivery settings, the focus of care could no longer be easily delimited by geographic boundaries (i.e., perioperative care was being delivered in settings other than traditional operating rooms) or time boundaries (i.e., the traditional preoperative, intraoperative, and postoperative phases of care had become blurred).[15] By redefining the concept of surgery to incorporate both "operative" and "other invasive procedures," the AORN anticipated the shift to ambulatory care centers and nontraditional settings such as cardiac catheterization laboratories, interventional radiology suites, mobile units, and physician offices.[16] The AORN has also addressed the growing demand for patient satisfaction and self-care skills by promoting greater community interaction. Not only does this increase the community's knowledge about surgical interventions and postoperative care, it also enhances recognition of the perioperative nurse's role in patient health maintenance and community well-being. RNFAs are well positioned, through their expanded knowledge and skill, to engage in these community partnerships.

The AORN has also fostered the RNFA role by creating the RNFA Specialty Assembly to serve as a forum for the discussion of issues, to provide educational opportunities, and to act as a representative in regulatory and legislative arenas. Professional recognition has been enhanced by a rigorous certification process for RNFAs, and by the development of a core curriculum and educational standards for the preparation of RNFAs.[17–19]

◼ DEVELOPMENT OF COLLABORATIVE PRACTICE

Because collaborative practice by most definitions involves a collegial relationship between and among professionals, it is crucial that the RN first assistant fulfill the professional perioperative role, because first assisting in and of itself is not nursing but rather a medically supervised supportive service.[20] This distinction has serious ramifications for the development of collaborative relationships. Joint or collaborative practice can be achieved only among persons or groups with accountability and authority for their own profession and practice. Collaborative practice, as H. Robert Cathcart, Chairman of the National Commission on Nursing, noted in 1981, is a "complementary relationship between nurses and physicians, not an unequal supervisor–subordinate type of relationship."[21] The practice of first assisting is an expansion of the perioperative role not only for assisting the surgeon intraoperatively, but also for preoperative patient assessment and postoperative evaluation. It is in this context that a complementary relationship can be established between nurses and physicians, rather than an unequal supervisor–subordinate type of relationship.

Recently the importance of collaboration was reaffirmed in two documents published by the Pew Health Professions Commission.[22,23] In the first document, which addressed the educational preparation of health care providers, the Pew Commission encouraged a more integrated professional training program for nurses and physicians, particularly in preclinical and clinical areas of study. In the second document, which reported on the regulation of the health care workforce, the commission stressed the importance of collaborative behaviors for fostering consumer well-being in the clinical setting. The need for effective teamwork becomes increasingly evident as the complexity and acuity of care expand.

National Joint Practice Committee

Formal attempts to establish nurse–physician collaborative practice models started in 1971, when the American Nurses Association (ANA) and the American Medical Association (AMA) established the National Joint Practice Commission (NJPC).[24] The creation of this national commission, consisting of equal numbers of nurses and physicians, had been recommended in "An Abstract for Action," a 1970 report by the National Commission for the Study of Nursing and Nursing Education.[25] Known as the Lysaught Report (after the commission's director, Dr. Jerome P. Lysaught), the study proposed, among other recommendations, institutional joint practice committees representing nursing and medicine. It also proposed the recognition and reward of increased competence in nursing practice.

The NJPC focused on the need for more collaboration and used the terms "joint practice" and "collaborative practice" interchangeably. Joint practice was defined as "nurses and physicians collaborating together as colleagues to provide patient care."[26] Reference to a collegial relationship represented a departure from the traditional notion that nurses had little to contribute to decision making in patient care management. The NJPC stressed that if nurses are to be accepted as colleagues, they must achieve clinical credibility and have it recognized by physicians, administrators, peers, and patients. In the past, reward systems in nursing encouraged competent nurses to move away from direct patient care and into administration or education. Emphasis on clinical performance fostered the development of performance standards and clinical ladders, which in turn rewarded clinical competence. Recognition of clinical competence also increased nurses' self-esteem and enabled them to become more confident in their contribution to patient management, and more willing to accept greater responsibility and accountability for nursing actions. The growing realization by nurses and physicians that each profession makes a unique contribution to the welfare of patients has been a major step toward achieving collaborative working relationships. And although the NJPC focused on hospital care—where most patient care was performed in that era—the findings did indicate overwhelmingly that communication was better, job satisfaction for both nurses and physicians was greater, and patients received better nursing care.[27]

Although the AMA withdrew support from the commission in 1981, positive benefits were achieved and the recommendations that were made are still valid today. Moreover, the commission's work encouraged other individuals and groups to develop collaborative practice models.[28] These interactions also helped to establish a climate of open communication, trust, and mutual respect, and paved the way for integrating informal as well as formal collaborative behaviors into clinical practice.

NJPC Recommendations

The NJPC's 1981 "Guidelines for Establishing Joint or Collaborative Practice in Hospitals" recommended five elements for the formal implementation of a collaborative practice model; most remain viable goals even with the profound changes that have occurred since the publication of that document. The recommendations were:

1. primary nursing
2. a joint practice committee of equal numbers of doctors and nurses who practice on the unit
3. unit doctors and nurses jointly evaluating their patient care
4. integrated patient records
5. encouragement of nurses' individual clinical decision making[29]

Primary Nursing

As defined by the NJPC, primary nursing is the performance of clinical nursing functions by RNs, with minimal or no delegation of nursing tasks to others.[30] Of all the NJPC recommendations, this one has been most affected by current cost considerations, which have mandated the performance of many task-oriented functions by assistive personnel. However, the impact of primary nursing on the development of collaborative practice was substantial, and it is worthwhile reviewing its introduction and transformation.

In the 1960s, primary nursing was established as a nursing care model that delegated decision making to bedside nurses. Prior to the institution of this model, head nurses were the primary decision makers and physician contacts. The aim of primary nursing was to encourage nurses to be individually responsible for a patient's comprehensive nursing care, thus enabling nurses to enter into a collegial relationship with physicians who provided the patient's medical care.[31]

Although primary nursing attempted to align nursing practice with professional nursing values, existing centralized and hierarchical decision-making structures conflicted with the primary nursing model. A shift to decentralization in the 1970s attempted to change the system that placed authority at the top. It was also an attempt to respond to growing financial pressures that necessitated a reduction of overhead expenses, in particular, personnel costs. Layers of middle management were reduced or eliminated, with the result that the remaining nurse managers assumed more responsibility for fiscal, human resource, and operational management and less direct supervision of caregivers. Consequently, greater staff involvement and participation in patient care decisions was promoted.[32]

The introduction of shared governance in the 1980s also increased nurses' involvement by promoting staff nurse accountability for professional standards and practice. This initiative anticipated the current trend toward integrated organizational frameworks by establishing committees or councils composed of staff, managers, and professional colleagues.[33]

In the early 1990s, patient-centered care expanded the scope of decentralization by recognizing the interdependence of every department in achieving quality care. Patient care came to be seen as a multifaceted, multidisciplinary activity. Consequently, decision making was delegated to those involved in patient care processes. At the same time, there was a shift in decision making and authority to patients, who are now increasingly portrayed as self-determined, able to influence their environment, empowered, and in charge.[34] These changes have important consequences for caregivers in general and RNFAs in particular. Collaborative practice now includes complementary as well as collegial relationships not only with physicians but also with other providers of care, as well as with the recipients of that care.

The effects of these changes on perioperative practice can be seen in the current environment, which values the processes of care mainly as they relate to the outcomes achieved. For example, preoperatively, RNFAs can enhance patient outcomes and reduce costs by educating patients and families about what to expect before, during, and after surgery; one report cites a 75% decrease in cancellations, delays, and unplanned admissions.[35] Other opportunities for collaborative practice in the preoperative period exist. Swan describes a collaborative ambulatory care model consisting of nurses and anesthesia care providers who worked together to perform preoperative assessments, obtain laboratory data, identify "at risk" individuals, and initiate the discharge planning process.[36] Preoperative assessment data can be used by the RNFA for proper positioning to prevent or minimize muscle or nerve injury. Information obtained during the preoperative assessment pertaining to activities of daily living, learning needs, and psychosocial concerns can be shared by the first assistant and other nurses to improve discharge planning and anticipate home care needs.

Intraoperatively, the RNFA engages in a cooperative effort with the surgeon to achieve a successful surgical intervention. Although responsible for supervising the first assistant's performance, the surgeon is nevertheless dependent on the first assistant for help with the operation. The first assistant must assume responsibility for self-performance. It is during this period that the surgeon and the first assistant are most closely associated and need most to rely on one another interdependently. Some of the factors necessary to accomplish this include:

- possessing the requisite knowledge and experience related to anatomy, physiology, microbiology, pharmacology, and behavioral sciences
- knowing the procedure and the rationale for it
- acquiring the manual skill and dexterity to perform the required maneuvers
- being familiar with the individual surgeon's preferences
- anticipating the needs of the surgeon and the patient
- communicating information relevant to the procedure
- concentrating on the operative field throughout the procedure
- protecting the patient from injury
- maintaining flexibility and adaptability when emergencies or unanticipated events occur
- possessing creativity in solving problems or dealing with difficulties during the procedure
- knowing one's limits as required by experience, conscience, professional ethics and responsibility, and legal and jurisdictional constraints
- becoming a lifelong learner

The RNFA's contributions extend beyond the immediate sterile field. One of the major benefits to be derived from assisting is the knowledge gained from directly observing and participating in the surgery itself. Sharing this knowledge with nonassisting nurses enhances these nurses' levels of practice and leads to a greater appreciation of the possible dangers and complications inherent in the procedure. Moreover, knowledgeably communicating with surgeons and other members of the health care team encourages active participation by staff and can also improve staff morale and self-esteem.

Postoperative evaluation provides an opportunity for the RNFA to investigate areas for improvement and to confirm the adequacy of aseptic technique, preoperative teaching, and prevention of thermal, chemical, or mechanical injury, and to participate in discharge planning. It also enables RNFAs and other perioperative nurses to contribute to the development and continual improvement of clinical paths and other time-related, standardized treatment plans.

Joint Practice Committees

The NJPC recommended "a joint practice committee equally representing practicing nurses and physicians, and supported by the administration, [that] will continuously monitor nurse–physician relationships and recommend appropriate actions supporting joint practice."[37] Joint practice committees enable the participants to communicate, to clarify roles, to discuss questions of competence and accountability, and to foster trust and mutual respect. Nursing must be represented, because it is ultimately in the practice setting itself that true collaborative practice can succeed. The Joint Commission on Accreditation of Healthcare Organizations supports policies and procedures designed to ensure effective collaboration among departments and services that provide nursing, surgical, and anesthesia services.[38]

In the operating room, committees consisting of nurses, surgeons, anesthesia care providers, and other key players (e.g., materials managers, case managers) have been successful in encouraging joint practice. Specific patient care issues may include the development of critical pathways, patient care protocols, recommended practices, and problem solving at the level of occurrence. Other agenda items specific to the operating room may include cost containment, value analysis/product selection, scheduling of cases, medical student orientation, and assignment of specialty personnel.[39–41]

RNFAs can provide pertinent insights into practice problems encountered in the operating room. Their familiarity with the surgeons' perceived needs and requirements specific to operative procedures can be invaluable in bridging the knowledge gap and promoting understanding between the professions. The interactive roles of nurses and physicians on joint practice committees underscore the value of discussion, negotiation, and compromise.

Nurse–physician committees consisting of perioperative nurses and surgeons have flourished on the national level for years. The AORN and the American College of Surgeons (ACS) hold conferences that provide an opportunity to discuss and resolve operating room issues.[42] Joint boards of medicine and nursing at the state level have addressed practice questions and jointly recommended guidelines for the role of the first assistant.

Even with the best intentions, joint practice committees cannot succeed without administrative support. The workplace culture should support an environment conducive to positive relationships between clinicians and support staff to improve the quality of service. In addition, committee discussions pertaining to practice issues that focus on licensure laws and hospital policies may require professional advice from risk managers and attorneys. For example, the question of what a nurse does, and more specifically what an RNFA does, may not be easily defined, especially with multistate health care systems. It is essential that committees addressing the scope of practice of the first assistant familiarize themselves with state nurse practice acts, governmental guidelines, and institutional policies.

Committee sessions need not always be harmonious. Complex subjects require careful exploration, frank appraisal, and sometimes reappraisal of roles and duties. This can lead to arguments. As long as disagreements focus on issues rather than on personalities, conflicts can form the basis for better understanding and teamwork. The important point is that communication be ongoing. Committee members approaching difficult issues in an open-minded manner foster trust and respect.

Joint Evaluation of Patient Care

The purpose of the joint review as described by the NJPC was to examine the nursing and medical care given to patients and to ascertain whether documentation reflected the care described.[43] This can create a teaching opportunity for physicians to discuss pathophysiology and the treatment provided; it can also offer nurses an occasion to describe nursing interventions based on patient responses to the disease and the medical therapy instituted. One research study has described collaborative research that focused on such patient practices as admission and discharge from a critical care unit, decubitus ulcers, incidental blood loss due to arterial lines, the occurrence and prevention of self-extubation, indwelling catheter infection rates, and prolonged ventilator times.[44] As part of the evaluation process, the joint review enables RNFAs and other surgical team members to assess the results of their own work within the overall team effort. For example, attention might be focused on the patient's skin healing in collaboration with wound care specialists; the development of surgical wound infections in collaboration with infection control staff; or nerve injury secondary to manipulation of arthritic extremities in collaboration with neurologists or physical therapists. Problems jointly discussed provide an avenue for mutually supportive actions and can form the basis for multidisciplinary research studies. The salient point of such collaboration in research is the ability to function together to change practice and effect positive patient outcomes. Group success, rather than individual reward, is the focus of a well-functioning team.

The value of joint reviews as teaching sessions can be appreciated not only by practicing clinicians, but also by medical, nursing, and other professional students. Students are exposed to role models after whom they can pattern their own professional behavior. Fagin and others have encouraged shared interdisciplinary learning experiences for nursing and medical students as one method of enhancing increased understanding between the two groups.[45,46]

Shared learning experiences are also appropriate for nurses and others, such as physiotherapists, occupational therapists, social workers, and others whose focus may be devoted to a specific population such as patients with orthopedic injuries.[47] And in the current environment, joint learning and joint evaluation of care with other members of the expanded health care team is consistent with efforts to integrate care. With shortened lengths of stay, for example, patients are likely to benefit from the professional assistance of social workers, home health nurses, and rehabilitation therapists, whose contributions to patient outcomes can be vital in an integrated care delivery system. RNFA interactions with these professionals can be beneficial not only for patients, but also for the professional growth of the individual caregivers involved.

Joint patient care conferences, morbidity and mortality conferences, trauma reprises, and specialty meetings are all useful forums for fostering increased understanding among professionals and promoting integrated patient care. Informal meetings between the RNFA and the physician also facilitate comprehensive care. Postoperative discussions focusing on surgery just performed are useful for future planning. The insights gained from each operation contribute to the first assistant's store of knowledge and experience.

Integrated Patient Records

According to the NJPC, "a patient record system integrating the observations, judgments, and actions of both nurses and physicians will reflect collaborative practice and contribute to it, and will provide a formal means of doctor–nurse communication in the care of patients."[48]

Initially, this element of the joint practice guidelines aroused the greatest concern in physicians and nurses on pilot units. The former feared increased legal liability risk; the latter expressed anxiety about the quality of their charting. Once nurses developed the necessary skill in writing notes and physicians came to appreciate the information documented, integrated progress notes and flow sheets fostered coordination of patient care.[49] One obvious benefit of this recommendation is the reduction of duplicate information; another is a better mutual understanding of the care and concerns of nurses and physicians. This leads to improved continuity of care and has the potential for reducing errors.

Complete integration of the patient record may not be feasible or advisable. However, documentation of a patient's preoperative mental status or ability to participate in activities of daily living is of importance to the surgeon and could justifiably be noted in the progress notes or assessment forms. Surgeons also want to be aware of intraoperative activities, such as correct sponge, needle, and instrument counts, and they ought to know what actions are taken for the preparation and protection of patients during surgery. The RNFA should be aware of the admitting diagnosis and indication for surgery, as well as pertinent laboratory data and the results of the history and physical examination. Knowing that the patient has been taking aspirin, for example, allows the RNFA to anticipate the potential for prolonged bleeding and the possible need for platelets. The patient with a history of arthritis may have special positioning needs. By documenting individualized nursing care, RNFAs educate others and accept responsibility for their own actions. The surgeon's operative reports also provide the same learning opportunities for RNFAs. And RNFAs can serve as "translators" of operative reports for others, such as rehabilitation therapists, whose clearer understanding of the surgical procedure can facilitate rehabilitative protocols and prescriptions.

Postoperative evaluations should be documented as well. RNFAs will want to assess and note the effects of their interventions, the adequacy of preoperative preparation and teaching, and the need for additional support and education.

In hospitals where integrated nurse–physician records are not yet a reality, integrated records are certainly appropriate for nurses themselves. Where charting commonly includes "Patient to OR via stretcher," followed immediately by "Patient returned from OR via stretcher," continuity of care would be facilitated by the inclusion of a perioperative note. This would benefit both unit nurses and perioperative nurses by increasing awareness of their individual roles. Collaboration between nurses can prepare the nurse for interdisciplinary joint practice. Given the increasing complexity and specialization that exists in health care provision, cooperation and mutual understanding are important for achieving consistent outcomes.

Encouragement of Nurses' Individual Clinical Decision Making

Individual decision making is essential for the collegial practice of nurses and physicians according to the NJPC.[50] To exercise their professional skills to the fullest, nurses must be encouraged to make individual clinical nursing decisions using both medical and nursing consultations and have this decision making capability reflected in the institution's defined "scope of nursing practice."

Probably no other element of the NJPC guidelines tests the level of trust and respect as greatly as does the encouragement of nurses' individual clinical decision making. Physicians must trust and respect their nursing colleagues, but so too must supervisors, administrators, patients, and peers. These attitudes are derived from the recognition of clinical competence, and this fact is the basis for any form of collaborative practice. Because the focus of all our efforts is ultimately the patient, nurses and patients cannot afford to accept anything less than the highest level of practice. Although the NJPC no longer exists formally, discussions between the ANA and the AMA concerning qualifications, competence, and supervision have been ongoing and have focused on the role of advanced practice nurses.[51]

For the RNFA, clinical competence incorporates experience, an educational/intellectual component, and demonstrated manual skill and dexterity. Not all perioperative nurses have such skill, nor will all choose to assist during surgery. While first assisting is considered to be an acceptable expanded role, it is not necessarily integral to perioperative practice. Rather, it is an option, and a nurse's choice not to assist must be respected. Surely no surgeon or supervisor can expect the highest level of performance from a nurse who is forced to engage in this activity.

For those nurses who desire to assist competently, the importance of highly developed technical surgical skills cannot be overstressed. Many areas of clinical nursing, whether critical care units or perioperative care units, require technical skills. The RNFA's clinical competence demands such skill in conjunction with knowledge. Although there is a trend to delegate the "technical" aspects of care to ancillary, nonprofessional personnel, not all technical skills are simple or benign. Many of the technical skills demonstrated by RNFAs, such as suturing or exposing tissue, require additional knowledge and experience if they are to be performed safely. The potential for injury to major organs, blood vessels, or nerves during retraction, for example, necessitates a level of critical thinking and decision making that can be developed only with professional education and training. Even when one allows a distinction between simple and complex cases, the determination of what constitutes simple versus complex requires professional judgment. There is little merit to the notion that the execution of technical skill is somehow demeaning to the image of professional nursing. The high public esteem for surgeons is due in no small part to surgeons' technical skill, and physicians are no less admired because they work with their hands as well as their minds.

A surgeon's competence is judged mainly on her or his ability to produce a successful operative repair. This entails mental as well as manual skills in preparing for and executing the procedure. The RNFA accepts the same dual demands. The reward is the satisfaction of participating in what can be an aesthetically pleasing creation as well as a meticulously scientific intervention. Appreciating an assistant's work from different aspects yields greater satisfaction and pride. This in turn inspires continued efforts for improvement.

Conscientious practitioners should be aware of their limitations and use extra caution in situations where experience is lacking. Basic principles of anatomy and surgical technique form a foundation for safe practice while the RNFA develops expertise. Knowing what one doesn't know, and practicing accordingly, is a sign of wisdom, maturity, and professional responsibility. Asking questions or requesting assistance should not be rebuked; it should be encouraged and respected for the courage it entails. The RNFA with a secure self-concept accepts such risk taking as necessary for the coordination of joint practice. Professionals who realize their limitations and seek to fill knowledge gaps better understand the learning needs of others. Taking the opportunity to share expertise with students and visitors often benefits the teacher as well. The selection and synthesis of information required to teach tests the educator's grasp of the subject. The RNFA can provide learning experiences and foster collegiality in interactions with students by offering formal and informal educational sessions.

Developing closer collegial relationships with other specialty nurses can also enhance patient outcomes and strengthen performance. The RNFA cannot fulfill all patient needs or solve all patient problems. Physicians accept this fact and have referral systems and consultation mechanisms for problem solving. Nurses also need to develop such systems to tap the rich diversity of resources available to them. For example, medical nurses caring for preoperative patients might call on perioperative and surgical nurses for insights and information relating to their patient's problems, concerns, and knowledge deficits about surgery.

The RNFA's wealth of knowledge about anatomy, surgical technique, and indications for a particular procedure is more than just intellectually interesting to critical care or trauma nurses facing emergency thoracotomies. The RNFA's background in aseptic technique is helpful for nurses instituting standard precautions or investigating the increase in urinary tract or surgical site infections.

RNFAs have much to gain by consulting pediatric or psychiatric clinicians about reducing preoperative fear or anxiety in children or adults. Surgical intensive care nurses can provide a greater appreciation for a well-delivered postoperative report by explaining the rationale for including baseline pulmonary or cardiac ventricular function studies or preoperative mental status assessments.

The need for consultation may not always exist, but when it does, consultation should be available. This not only encourages better patient care, it also creates a feeling of mutual respect for the knowledge and skills that nurses have to offer one another. This in turn fosters self-esteem and pride in one's accomplishments and promotes professional growth. Turning to a nurse or physician colleague for professional advice reflects strength and a desire to use all the resources available to provide the best care possible.

■ CONSIDERATIONS AND IMPLICATIONS OF COLLABORATIVE PRACTICE

The previous discussion offers suggestions for the implementation of collaborative practice in the perioperative setting by members of the health care team, specifically physicians, perioperative nurses, and RNFAs. The knowledge and experience gained by RNFAs from observing and participating in the surgery itself offer additional advantages as well.

As a key facilitator, the RNFA can contribute special knowledge and understanding to non-first assisting nurses. Consequently, confidence in the ability to anticipate needs is greatly improved and overall performance enhanced. The clinical knowledge of and familiarity with the devices and implants used in surgery enables RNFAs to foster patient safety by complying with the provisions of the Safe Medical Devices Act. Intraoperative care paths can be developed and refined with the clinical expertise of RNFAs who are well positioned to participate in case management roles. Procedures that are frequently performed and resource intensive (e.g., orthopedic implants, coronary artery bypass grafts), can be streamlined and made more efficient by RNFAs with in-depth knowledge and experience.

Managers and administrators are more apt to encourage and reward this expanded role when job satisfaction, cost savings, and better productivity can be achieved. Job satisfaction reduces costs because it reduces staff turnover and the subsequent expense of hiring and orienting new personnel. Greater efficiency in the delivery of care and increased flexibility in job performance are facilitated by the presence of nurses who are cross-trained to scrub, circulate, and assist. Moreover, the RNFA's insights into surgeons' preferences can minimize unnecessary and wasted supplies; familiarity with the proper use of complex equipment can prolong the life of these expensive items and reduce repair costs. Opportunities to develop partnerships between nurses and hospitals have expanded with the growth of managed care. Cost-cutting measures commonly include labor and supply reduction strategies, especially in the operating room, which consumes 60% of a hospital's supply expenses.[52] RNFAs can demonstrate their cost-effectiveness by working to streamline operating systems and negotiating with in-house departments and outside suppliers to reduce costs.

Reimbursement issues may pose challenges. In situations where the RNFA is an employee of an institution, the performance description may include scrubbing or circulating when the nurse is not functioning as an assistant; interpersonal relations can be jeopardized if there is inequitable distribution of assigned procedures to assistants or inadequate compensation for the increased responsibilities associated with the role. Supervisors must be alert to prevent resentment against first assistants during staffing shortages. Ideally, adequate staff should be available to supply all needs. Effective leadership can also prevent negative interactions between nurses and residents, physician assistants, or other first assisting staff. Collaborative practice between RNFAs and other caregivers is based on trust in one another's abilities, respect for each other's capabilities, and mutual concern for the patient undergoing surgery.

Self-employed RNFA's continue to pursue equitable payment for services from Medicare, Medicaid, and third-party payers; involvement in the political process is one way to influence change.[53] Development of business skills and an understanding of global and local economic factors are also necessary, as is the ability to communicate the economic and social value of the RNFA's contributions to health care.

SUMMARY

Although the concept of collaborative practice has broadened to include not only physicians and nurses but also other members of the health care team, the traditional nurse–physician partnership remains the cornerstone of collaborative practice. Collaborative practice between the RNFA and the surgeon is based on trust. It forms the foundation for a patient care partnership wherein the people in it perceive one another as equally important peers who mutually contribute to the same desired outcome—excellence in perioperative patient care. The NJPC and others have noted that, first and foremost, patients received better nursing care and were more satisfied with their care.[54] Communication between doctors and nurses improved, respect and trust increased, and job satisfaction was greater for both nurses and physicians. Additional studies are needed to confirm the correlation between collaborative practice and improved patient outcomes.

The establishment of joint practice committees and integrated patient records can promote collaborative practice models, but committees and documentation forms in and of themselves are neither necessary nor sufficient for true teamwork. Working together in a collaborative framework brings forth a joint intellectual effort, a sharing in planning, making decisions, solving problems, setting goals, and assuming responsibility, as well as cooperation, coordination, and communication. One physician has listed three reasons why a collegial, unified relationship between nurses and physicians can improve patient care.[55] First, collegiality is a moral imperative requiring respectful interactions that encourage sharing of information. Second, physicians and nurses should advocate for patients jointly in order to further the patient's best interest, especially when threatened by external pressures to maximize efficiency. Finally, collaboration allows nurses and physicians to educate one another and thereby improve their ability to achieve patient well-being. These reasons underscore the value of teamwork for patients and caregivers. Teamwork can be achieved only when physicians, nurses, and other health care providers each decide that working together in the interest of consistent, quality patient and family care will bring them to their fullest professional potential.

Review Questions

1. List four reasons why RNFAs are cost-effective.
   1. _____
   2. _____

3. _____

4. _____

2. The RNFA role should be integrated into the perioperative nursing role because:
   a. Perioperative nursing provides the collegial foundation for collaborative practice.
   b. It is necessary for the performance of the perioperative nursing role.
   c. It provides a rationale for reimbursement.
   d. The surgeon will not have to assume responsibility for the RNFA.

3. Benefits of the RNFA role include (1) achieving new dimensions of clinical competence, (2) having greater responsibility and accountability, (3) allowing participation in collaborative practice, and (4) maintaining positive nurse–physician relationships.
   Which of these statements are true?
   a. 1, 2, and 4
   b. 1, 2, and 3
   c. 1 and 3
   d. 1, 2, 3, and 4

4. Factors necessary for successfully fulfilling the RNFA role include (1) knowing the reason for the operation, (2) being familiar with a surgeon's preference, (3) anticipating the patient's needs, (4) communicating relevant information to the postoperative care unit, and (5) possessing manual skills.
   Which of these statements are true?
   a. 1, 3, and 5
   b. 1, 2, 3, and 4
   c. 2, 4, and 5
   d. 1, 2, 3, 4, and 5

5. One of the independent nursing functions that an RNFA performs is
   a. Determining the need for surgery.
   b. Performing patient assessments.
   c. Positioning the patient for optimal exposure.
   d. Suturing and dressing the surgical incision site.

6. One of the initiating factors for the development of the National Joint Practice Commission (NJPC) and its subsequent work was to improve
   a. Role ambiguity for professional nurses.
   b. Incongruent expectations between nursing education and service.
   c. Nurse–physician relationships.
   d. The positional status of hospital-employed nurses.

7. The NJPC definition of collaborative practice is
   a. To work together in a mutual undertaking.

    b. To work together, side-by-side, in a cooperative effort.

    c. A process whereby a nurse works with a physician to deliver health care services within the scope of the practitioner's professional expertise.

    d. Nurses and physicians collaborating together as colleagues to provide patient care.

8. The interpersonal milieu for collaboration must be founded on
    a. Self-esteem and professional confidence.
    b. Truth, active listening, and sincerity.
    c. Open communication, trust, and mutual respect.
    d. Negotiation, compromise, and working within one's sphere of influence.

9. An essential element in establishing nurse–physician collegiality is
    a. Clinical credibility.
    b. Advanced educational preparation.
    c. Advanced, specialty certification.
    d. Joint attendance at professional meetings (like the AORN/ACS meeting).

10. The NJPC recommended that five elements be present for the formal implementation of joint practice models. Which of the following is least likely to be part of a managed care system?
    a. Joint practice committees
    b. Primary nursing
    c. Joint care reviews
    d. Integrated patient records

11. The RNFA who is appointed to a joint practice committee should expect that the committee's primary focus will be on
    a. Clinical outcomes.
    b. Critical pathways.
    c. Practice guidelines.
    d. Nurse–physician relationships.

12. In preparing for a Joint Commission accreditation team visit, the RNFA should know that the Joint Commission expects to see
    a. Confirmation that the state board of nursing has determined that first assisting is within the scope of nursing practice.
    b. Medical bylaws that define the institutional role of the RNFA.
    c. Policies and procedures ensuring effective collaboration among departments .providing surgical services.
    d. Peer review by RNFAs and surgeons.

13. When involved in committee discussions, the RNFA should be careful to avoid
    a. Having to compromise.
    b. Discussing personalities.

c. Negotiating on patient care issues.

d. Conflict and disagreements.

14. In joint care reviews, one way of examining care provided is to review
    a. Documentation on the patient care record.
    b. Survivor rates.
    c. Nurse job satisfaction.
    d. The success of PPOs.

15. If collaborative practice aims to truly promote joint efforts and communication about patients, then:
    a. Clinical ladders should include advancement opportunities for RNFAs.
    b. Nurses should use the medical model, not nursing diagnoses.
    c. RNFAs should learn to do histories and physical examinations.
    d. RNFAs and surgeons should write on the same progress notes.

16. For the RNFA, clinical competence incorporates (1) experience, (2) an intellectual component, (3) the ability to assist in any surgical procedure, (4) demonstrated manual skills, and (5) cross-training in critical care. Which of these statements are true?
    a. 1, 2, and 5
    b. 1, 3, and 4
    c. 1, 2, and 4
    d. 1, 2, and 3

17. In the preoperative admitting area, the RNFA is reviewing the history of a 20-year-old woman who is the mother of an 8-month-old child. While discussing postsurgery discharge plans and whether the patient will be able to manage decreased activity for the next 24 hours, the patient expresses her frustration over her baby's crying behaviors, revealing her fears of harming the baby. Which of the following would be the most appropriate action of the RNFA?
    a. Instill confidence in the patient that she is experiencing normal frustrations with a teething infant.
    b. Determine whether the mother, as a child, was physically abused by her parents.
    c. Provide empathy, support, and therapeutic touch.
    d. Request a consultation with the psychiatric nurse clinical specialist.

Indicate whether each of the following statements is true (T) or false (F).

18. _____The RNFA has an obligation to share knowledge derived from assisting with perioperative nursing colleagues.

19. _____If quality improvement is really the goal of joint care reviews, then the committee should focus on correcting problems; quality improvement efforts don't need to focus on what is already working well.

20. _____Probably no other element of the NJPC guidelines tests the level of trust and respect as much as the encouragement of nurses' individual clinical decision making.

■ Answer Key

1. Some of the reasons include: decreased staff turnover from increased nurse satisfaction; improved operating room efficiency from using a flexible RN staff (RNs can scrub, circulate, first assist); more effective and efficient use of costly supplies; improved time management; less potential for damage to instruments and supplies; improving care paths and protocols; negotiating with vendors on supply costs; informed selection of surgical products.

2. a	9. a	15. d
3. b	10. b	16. c
4. d	11. a	17. d
5. b	12. c	18. T
6. c	13. b	19. F
7. d	14. a	20. T
8. c		

REFERENCES

1. Marcus LJ, Dorn, BC, Kritek PB, Miller VG, Wyatt JB: Renegotiating Health Care: Resolving Conflict to Build Collaboration. San Francisco, Jossey-Bass Publishers, 1995
2. McEwen M: Promoting interdisciplinary collaboration. Nurs Health Care 15(6): 304–307, 1994
3. Prescott PP: Nursing: An important component of hospital survival under a reformed health care system. Nurs Economic$ 11(4 July–August):192–193, 1993
4. Knaus WA, Draper EA, Wagner DP, Zimmerman JE: An evaluation of outcome from intensive care in major medical centers. Ann Intern Med 104:410–418, 1986
5. Alpert HB, Goldman LD, Kilroy CM, Pike AW: Gryzmish: Toward an understanding of collaboration. Nurs Clin North Am 27(1):47–59, 1992
6. Fagin CM: Collaboration between nurses and physicians: No longer a choice. Acad Med 67:295–303, 1992
7. Henneman EA, Lee JL, Cohen JI: Collaboration: A concept analysis. J Adv Nurs 21:103–109, 1995
8. Adler SL, Bryk E, Cesta TG, McEachen I: Collaboration: The solution to multidisciplinary care planning. Orthop Nurs 14(2):21–29, 1995
9. Mundinger MO: New alliances: Nursing's bright future. Nurs Admin Q 20(3): 50–53, 1996
10. Stein LI: The doctor–nurse game. Arch Gen Psychiatry 16:699–703, 1967
11. Stein LI, Watts DT, Howell T: The doctor–nurse game revisited. N Engl J Med 322(8):546–547, 1990
12. Kneedler JA, Dodge GH: Perioperative Patient Care: The Nursing Perspective. Boston, Jones & Bartlett Publishers, 1994, p 20

13. Clapesattle H: The Doctors Mayo. Garden City, NJ, Garden City Publishing, 1941, p 429
14. A model for perioperative nursing practice. AORN J 41:188–194, 1985
15. Members discuss important issues. AORN J 55:1401, 1992
16. A model for perioperative nursing practice. In: AORN Standards and Recommended Practices. Denver, Colo, Association of Operating Room Nurses, 1997, pp 77–79.
17. Vaiden RE, Fox VJ, Rothrock JC: Core Curriculum for the RN First Assistant, rev ed. Denver, Colo, Assocation of Operating Room Nurses, 1994
18. Revised AORN Recommended Education Standards for RN First Assistant Programs (position statement). AORN J 65(2):404–406, 1997
19. RN First Assistant certification; clinical internship; job descriptions; insurance coverage; specialty assembly. AORN J 64(1):115–118, 1996
20. Davis NB: Charting a course for the first assistant. AORN J 32:1032–1038, 1980
21. Nursing Commission issues preliminary report. Hospitals 55(18):20, 1981
22. Pew Health Professions Commission, Third Annual Report. Critical Challenges: Revitalizing the Health Professions for the Twenty-First Century. San Francisco, Center for Health Professions, University of California, 1995
23. Pew Health Professions Commission: Reforming Health Care Workforce Regulation: Policy Considerations for the 21st Century. San Francisco, Center for Health Professions, University of California, 1995
24. National Joint Practice Commission: Guidelines for Establishing Joint or Collaborative Practice in Hospitals. Chicago, National Joint Practice Commission, 1981, p 2
25. Lysaught JP: An Abstract for Action. New York: McGraw-Hill Book Co, 1970
26. National Joint Practice Commission, p 2
27. Fagin, 1992
28. King KB, Parrinello, Baggs JG: Collaboration and advanced practice nursing. In: Hickey JV, Ouimette RM, Venegoni SL, eds: Advanced Practice Nursing: Changing Roles and Clinical Applications. Philadelphia, JB Lippincott, 1996
29. National Joint Practice Commission, p 7
30. National Joint Practice Commission, p 11
31. Ellis JR, Hartley CL: Nursing in Today's World: Challenges, Issues and Trends. Philadelphia, JB Lippincott, 1995
32. Klakovich MD: Connective leadership for the 21st century: A historical perspective and future directions. Adv Nurs Sci 16(4):42–54, 1994
33. Adams R, Baker M, Briones E, et al: The "energized" nursing department: Design for change. In: Flarey DL, ed: Redesigning Nursing Care Delivery: Transforming Our Future. Philadelphia, JB Lippincott, 1995
34. Donley R: Advanced practice nursing after health care reform. Nurs Economic$ 13 (2):84–88, 1995
35. Collaborative practice patterns cut cancellations. RN (May) 16C–17C, 1997
36. Swan BA: A collaborative ambulatory preoperative evaluation model. AORN J 59(2):430–437, 1994
37. National Joint Practice Commission, p 11
38. Joint Commission on Accreditation of Healthcare Organizations: Accreditation Manual for Hospitals. Chicago, Joint Commission on Accreditation of Healthcare Organizations, 1997
39. Moss MT: Collaborative care design: A global tool for managed care. Surgical Services Management 1(6):25–29, 1995
40. Lassen AA, Fosbinder DM, Minton S, Robins MM: Nurse/physician collaborative practice: Improving health care quality while decreasing cost. Nurs Economic$ 15(2):87–91, 1997

41. Black ER, Weiss KD, Erban S, Shulkin D: Innovations in patient care: Changing clinical practice and improving quality. J Qual Improve 21(8):376–386, 1995
42. American College of Surgeons, Nursing Management, American Academy of Nursing, Nursing Organization Liaison Forum, nurse attorneys conference reports. AORN J 61(1):222–227, 1995
43. National Joint Practice Commission, p 12
44. Denholm B, Lehr P: Physician–nurse cooperative efforts. AORN J 55:262, 1992
45. Fagin, 1992
46. Laschinger HKS, Weston W: Role perceptions of freshman and senior nursing and medical students and attitudes toward collaborative decision making. J Profess Nurs 11(2):119–128, 1995
47. Prentice A: Multidisciplinary teaching: The wave of the future. Can Nurse (January)53–54, 1995
48. National Joint Practice Commission, pp 11–12
49. Ibid, p 18
50. Ibid, p 11
51. Nurses and physicians attempt to define collaboration and practice roles. AORN J 62(1):107–110, 1995
52. Moss MT: Perioperative nursing in the managed care era: Collaborative relationships in the operating room. Part II. Hospital and nurses: Strategies for partnerships. Nurs Economic$ 13(5):310, 1995
53. Romig CL: Legislation for RN first assistant third party reimbursement. AORN J 65(3):643–646, 1997
54. Alpert et al, 1992
55. Gianakos D: Physicians, nurses, and collegiality. Nurs Outlook 45(2):57–58, 1997

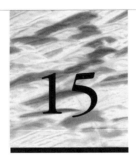

CLINICAL APPLICATIONS

DALE A. SMITH
CHRISTINE C. ESPERSEN
BARBARA M. WILSON
CHRISTOPHER C. HLOZEK

■

■ THE RN FIRST ASSISTANT IN ORTHOPEDIC SURGERY

Orthopedics may be the most physically demanding for the RNFA, who must balance the finesse of handling tissue and instrumentation with the strength needed for manipulation of an extremity or joint during some procedures. The spectrum of orthopedic surgery varies widely, from arthroscopic procedures in healthy young adults to emergency fixation of unstable pelvic and long bone fractures in patients with multiple traumatic injuries. It is important for the RN first assistant to have an overall understanding of coexisting medical problems and their implications, commonly used anesthetic and surgical techniques, postoperative complications, and various prophylactic measures used to minimize postoperative morbidity.[1]

The RNFA faces the challenge of combining technical advances with personalized, humanistic care. In the specialty of orthopedics, the RNFA must maintain skills in the tried-and-true techniques (e.g., internal and external fixation, total joint replacement) while also acquiring knowledge of and assisting expertise with new interventions and techniques (e.g., minimally invasive approaches, laser surgery, advanced manufacturing techniques for implants). Recent research findings need to be incorporated into clinical practice. The Total Knee Replacement Patient Outcomes Research Team (PORT), supported by the Agency for Health Care Policy Research, is only one example of ongoing investigations on topics of importance to RNFAs. RNFAs should also be involved with interdisciplinary quality improvement efforts and the development of clinical paths. These specify the interdisciplinary clinical interventions that move the orthopedic patient through a sequence of clinical steps to a final outcome (Box 15–1).[2] Such efforts also examine the cost of services provided as well as the efficiency and effectiveness of outcomes, demanding a high level of communication and coordination across disciplines involved in the orthopedic patient's care.[3] Because the development of clinical paths is often begun with high-volume diagnoses and procedures, the RNFA in orthopedic surgery is ideally positioned to participate in these, and other initiatives that seek to contain costs while maintaining or improving quality of care.[4] The RNFA must also participate in the evaluation of patient outcomes and assist patients in meeting home care recovery requirements, contributing to databases that measure effectiveness and provide cost-benefit analyses of the delivery of required patient care services.

Preoperative Patient Management

Preoperative management of the orthopedic patient requires the RN first assistant to first consider the type of procedure planned for the patient and then identify any special needs or patient care requirements. Communication with the other members of the perioperative staff about specific patients needs will help decrease morbidity and increase quality patient care. Orthopedic procedures may include arthroplasty (construction of a new movable joint), arthrodesis (joint fusion), osteotomy (cutting of the bone or creation of a surgical fracture), synovectomy (removal of the inflamed lining of a joint), bone grafting (for stabilization and encouragement of bone regeneration), tendon grafting or transplantation, arthroscopy (exploration of a joint with fiber-optic light and a camera, for both diagnosis and treatment), or multiple procedures for the polytraumatized patient. The planned procedure may guide the RNFA's review of the history and physical examination findings, or the RNFA may initiate the history and physical examination to assist in determining the planned treatment.

Review of History and Physical Examination Findings.   The RNFA uses the preoperative evaluation findings to determine the appropriate plan of care. Whether the RNFA actually takes the history and performs physical examination or uses the information obtained by another practitioner, an evaluation of all body systems is necessary.

The history should begin with a review of subjective complaints and the patient's description of specific ailments (e.g., pain, edema, weakness in affected part, activity or movement limitations, gait disturbance), past medical

BOX 15–1

Critical Pathway Total Knee Arthroplasty

Outcome Criteria

1. Discharge to rehab on postop. day 4
   - Demonstrated rehab potential per PT
   - Afeb. VSS | Hg > 8

2. Discharge to home on postop. day 5
   - Independent with ambulation on level surfaces, stairs, and functional distances per individual needs
   - [I] With active knee exercises and use of immobilizer as needed
   - Active knee flexion 80 degrees or more

	PAT Date:	Day of Operation Date:	Postop. Day 1 Date:	Postop. Day 5 Date:
Assessments/ Consults	History and physical (include dental status and BOO symptoms) PT, SS (V#1) + NSG assessment Risk assessment	Postop. assessment*	ROSA* Skin assessment*	ROSA
Laboratory Tests and Diagnostics	CBC PT/PTT CHEM 7 CXR ECG	T&C	HG/HCT PT	PT
Interventions		Knee immobilizer,* elevation (pillow under heel),* TEDS/Kendalls,* incentive spirometry q 1 hr W/A,* hemovac, orthoevac,* straight cath/Foley prn,* don't gatch bed,* postop. routine VS,* NV checks q 2 hr	Knee immobilizer,* elevation (pillow under heel),* no pillow under knee,* TEDS/Kendalls,* incentive spirometry q 1 hr W/A,* D/C hemovac/Foley prn,* don't gatch bed,* VS, q 4 hr,* NV checks q 4 hr	Knee immobilizer,* prn, TEDS/Kendalls,* incentive spirometry q 1 hr W/A,* DSG change/Ace, don't gatch bed,* VS q shift,* NV checks q shift*
Diet/GI	Nothing by mouth after MN	Clears → house as tolerated	House or per order	
IVs		IVFs*	IVFs → HL or KVO if using PCA*	
Meds	NSAIDs discontinued	ABX × 48 hr,* PCA or IM analgesic,* heparin or coumadin*	PCA or IM analgesic,* heparin or coumadin,* antibiotics,* Revw meds; home meds, vitamins DVT prophylaxis, analgesics	PO analgesic,* heparin or coumadin,* home meds/vitamins*

(continued)

BOX 15-1 *(continued)*

Critical Pathway Total Knee Arthroplasty

	PAT Date:	Day of Operation Date:	Postop. Day 1 Date:	Postop. Day 5 Date:
Activity		Bed rest* Bed exercises q 1 hr W/A*	OOB → chair 2–3 hr bid am and pm,* bed exercises,* to PT WBAT/PWB, gait training with walker, AROM 0–40°, initiate knee-strengthening exercises	OOB → chair/ambulate with walker bid,* bed exercises q 1 hr W/A,* review of home exercise program by PT, review all previous gains, CPM as days 4 and 5*
Teaching	Review critical path,* review bed exercises,* review knee booklet,* review incentive spirometry*	Review bed exercises q shift,* review incentive spirometry, C + DB exercises q shift*	Review previous teaching prn*	Family teaching by PT if needed, review discharge instructions,* wound care/reportable signs and symptoms, and F/U visit*
Discharge Planning and Follow-Up	Initial discharge planning with patient and family		SS visit #2	Review discharge plans* discharge to home, give written instructions,* give card w/phone number*

KEY: *NSG care activities

V=Variance	V V V	V V V	V V V	V V V
N=No variance	N N N	N N N	N N N	N N N
Nursing care performed	☐ ☐ ☐	☐ ☐ ☐	☐ ☐ ☐	☐ ☐ ☐
→	1. _____	1. _____	1. _____	1. _____
Signatures: →	2. _____	2. _____	2. _____	2. _____
→	3. _____	3. _____	3. _____	3. _____

Abbreviations: ABX, antibiotics; BOO, bladder outlet obstruction; C+DB, cough and deep breathing; D/C, discharge or continue; HL, heparin lock; IVF, intravenous fluids; KVO, keep vein open; OOB, out of bed; PCA, patient controlled analgesia; PT, physical therapy; PT (in lab tests and diagnostics), prothrobin time; ROSA, review of systems assessment; SS, social service, V#1, visit number one; W/A, while awake.

(Source: Smeltzer SC, Bare BG: Brunner and Suddarth's Textbook of Medical-Surgical Nursing, 8th ed. Philadelphia, Lippincott–Raven Publishers, 1995, p 1876.)

history, concurrent diseases or conditions, past illnesses and surgical procedures, family and social history, current medication use, and allergies. During assessment, the RNFA needs to ascertain to what degree, if any, the patient's condition has disrupted activities of daily living. This information will aid in determining the patient's motivation to participate in the discharge plan, which specifies necessary postoperative activities.

The RNFA then focuses on the nature of the existing condition, injury, fracture, or disability. A description of the onset, the progression of symptoms, and any limitations of mobility must be included. The physical examination includes a thorough inspection of the functions of all body systems, with a particular focus on the affected extremity or joint. An inspection of posture, gait, body movements, and the degree of mobility/immobility (both active and passive range of motion [ROM] testing) is performed. The skin of the affected body part is assessed for color, temperature, and sensation; any edema, bruises, length and location of lacerations, rashes, or lesions are noted. Pain or tenderness is also assessed and documented, including its extent, nature, onset, and any exacerbating or relieving factors. (See Box 15–2) for an overview of examination techniques for the musculoskeletal system.)

With advanced physical examination skills, the RNFA brings considerable knowledge to patient assessment. For example, for a suspected injury as simple as a meniscal tear, the RNFA will understand common mechanisms of injury, the relative prevalence of different tears (e.g., the medial meniscus is torn much more often than the lateral meniscus and is frequently associated with anterior cruciate ligament tears), and the classification of tears according to shape (longitudinal, transverse, flap, horizontal, complex), location (peripheral versus central), and extent (complete versus incomplete). Evaluating the patient's history will help the RNFA determine whether the tear is traumatic (following a twisting injury) or degenerative (often following a minor twist or squat) and confirm symptoms such as pain, swelling, a sensation of "giving way," and mechanical symptoms (e.g., locking, catching, clicking). On physical examination, the RNFA assesses for joint line tenderness, effusion (using ballottement or the bulge sign to determine the presence of excess fluid or an effusion in the knee), quadriceps atrophy, and certain signs such as McMurray's sign (manipulation of the tibia with the leg flexed produces a subtle click and sometimes actual locking of the joint if the meniscus has been injured) or Apley's sign (clicks, locking, and pain in the knee on prone examination, with the knee flexed 90 degrees and rotated externally and internally) (Figure 15–1).[5]

Patient Education. The RNFA is well prepared to augment perioperative patient teaching. In the immediate postoperative period, the importance of coughing and deep breathing and safe movement must be stressed. Coughing and deep breathing techniques, ROM exercises of unaffected extremities, and postoperative restrictions and limitations should be discussed and taught to the patient and family or significant others. For a patient undergoing total hip arthroplasty, additional teaching requirements include gluteal and abdominal contractions, quadriceps setting, dorsiflexion and plantar foot flexion, hip spiking, isometric exercises, the use of assistive devices such as a trapeze, and continuous passive motion, as well as the importance of leg abduction or adduction postoperatively. The correct use and rationale for use of antiem-

BOX 15–2

General Techniques for Examination of the Musculoskeletal System

TECHNIQUES OF EXAMINATION

General Approach

While examining the musculoskeletal system, direct your attention to function as well as to structure. During the interview, you should have evaluated the patient's abilities to carry out normal activities of daily living. Also keep these abilities in mind during your physical examination.

In your initial survey of the patient you have assessed general appearance, bodily proportions, and ease of movements. Now, using inspection and palpation, you will examine individual joints or groups of joints, their range of motion, and the tissues surrounding them.

Note Particularly:

Examples of Abnormalities

■ Any *limitation* in the *normal range of motion* or any unusual *increase* in the *mobility* of a joint (instability). Range of motion varies among individuals and decreases with aging.

Decreased range of motion in arthritis, inflammation of tissues around the joint, fibrosis in or around a joint, or bony fixation (*ankylosis*).

■ Any *signs of inflammation*, such as:

■ *Swelling* in or around the joint. Swelling may involve the synovial membrane, which then feels boggy, or doughy, to your fingers, or may be produced by excessive synovial fluid within the joint space. Swelling sometimes originates not in the joint itself but in tissues around it, such as bones, tendons, tendon sheaths, bursae, and fat. Trauma to any of these structures may also cause swelling.

Palpable bogginess, or doughiness, of the synovial membrane indicates synovitis. Palpable joint fluid indicates an effusion in the joint. Synovitis and joint fluid often coexist.

■ *Tenderness* in or around the joint. Try to define the specific anatomical structure that is tender. Trauma may also cause tenderness.

Arthritis, tendinitis, bursitis, osteomyelitis.

■ Increased *heat*. Use the backs of your fingers to compare the joint with the symmetrical joint on the opposite side or, if both joints are involved, with the tissues near them.

Tenderness and warmth over a thickened synovium suggest rheumatoid arthritis.

■ *Redness* of the overlying skin. This is the least common sign of inflammation near the joints.

Redness of the skin over a tender joint suggests septic or gouty arthritis, or possibly rheumatic fever.

■ *Crepitus (crepitation),* a palpable or even audible crunching or grating produced by movement of a joint or tendon. Crepitus is more significant when it is associated with other symptoms or signs than when it exists by itself. Cracking or snapping sounds, which result from movement of tendons or ligaments over bone, may occur in normal joints such as the knees.

Fine, soft crepitus may be felt over inflamed joints. Coarser crepitus suggests roughened articular cartilages, as in an inflamed joint or osteoarthritis. A creaking, leathery crepitus may arise in inflamed tendon sheaths.

(continued)

BOX 15–2 (continued)

General Techniques for Examination of the Musculoskeletal System

- *Deformities,* such as:

  Those produced by restricted range of motion.

  Dupuytren's contracture, flexion deformity of the hip.

  Malalignment of bones.

  Bowlegs, knock-knees.

- The *condition of the surrounding tissues,* including muscle atrophy, subcutaneous nodules, and skin changes.

  Subcutaneous nodules in rheumatoid arthritis or rheumatic fever.

- *Muscular strength.*

  Muscular weakness and atrophy in rheumatoid arthritis.

- *Symmetry* of involvement. Note whether arthritic changes involve several joints symmetrically on both sides of the body or affect only one or perhaps two joints.

  Involvement of only one joint increases the likelihood of bacterial arthritis. Rheumatoid arthritis typically involves several joints, symmetrically distributed.

When handling a person with painful joints, be gentle and move slowly. Often patients can move more comfortably by themselves. Let them show you how they manage.

(Source: Bates B: A Guide to Physical Examination and History Taking, 6th ed. Philadelphia, JB Lippincott, 1995, pp 464–465.)

bolism stockings and sequential compression devices should be included on the perioperative teaching checklist. Specific teaching plans can assist the patient in structuring a self-care program. Preoperative physical therapy instruction on safe and effective methods of postoperative movement is important in preparation for discharge planning.

Pain management strategies, including the use of patient-controlled analgesia, continuous epidural analgesia, and intramuscular and oral agents, should be reviewed.

The patient's anxiety about and fear of pain and functional ability postoperatively may confound postoperative participation in rehabilitation. In a recent study of preoperative nursing diagnoses encountered in patients undergoing total hip replacement, knowledge deficit, anxiety, and fear occurred most frequently.[6] Accurate education for pain management and pain assessment are vital to effective pain management and preventing postoperative complications. The physical effects of untreated pain are well documented and include diminished respiratory effort, which can lead to retained pulmonary secretions and pnuemonia, and decreased mobility and early ambulation, which can lead to deep vein thrombosis. The patient must be assessed thoroughly to determine proper treatment as well as to evaluate the effective-

The Bulge Sign. With the ball of your hand, milk the medial aspect of the knee firmly upward two or three times to displace any fluid. Then press or tap the knee just behind the lateral margin of the patella.

A bulge of returning fluid indicates an effusion within the knee joint.

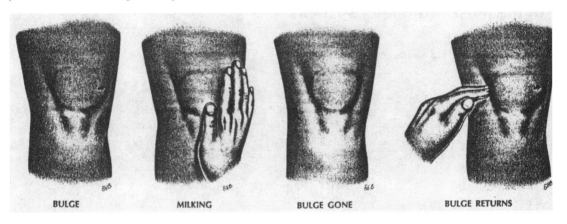

FIGURE 15–1

Using the bulge sign to detect suspected fluid in the knee joint (Source: Bates B: A Guide to Physical Examination and History Taking, 6th ed. Philadelphia, JB Lippincott, 1995).

ness of interventions. Accurate assessment allows the clinician to assist the patient in making judgments about what is and what is not working.[7]

Diagnostic Studies. The most common diagnostic study for orthopedic patients is radiography. Minimally, x-rays will be obtained of the affected extremity or joint. Magnetic resonance imaging (MRI) has become a valuable orthopedic diagnostic tool, especially for knee, shoulder, and back complaints. MRI facilitates the examination of both osseous and soft tissue structures, which was not possible with older imaging methods such as plain radiography and computed tomography (CT). The RNFA can learn to interpret both x-rays and MRI films with the assistance of the operating surgeon or a staff radiologist.

If the patient is scheduled to receive a general anesthetic, the facility may require a chest radiograph if the patient is over age 60 or in American Society of Anesthesiologists (ASA) category III, IV, or V, which includes most patients undergoing total joint replacement or revision.

Preoperative laboratory work also is required. The specific tests vary but should include as a minimum a complete blood cell count, urinalysis, electrolyte determination (sodium, potassium, carbon dioxide, and chloride), and, for total joint procedures, blood type and cross-match. Renal function is assessed by determining blood urea nitrogen and serum creatinine levels. For the orthopedic patient undergoing extensive surgery, such as a total joint revision, coagulation studies (bleeding time and platelet count, prothrombin time, and partial thromboplastin time) are usually performed. Most institutions require an electrocardiogram for patients over age 45 or with a history of cardiac problems.

The diagnosis of prosthesis infection is occasionally obvious (as when an abscess appears around the prosthesis) but is more often accompanied by nonspecific signs and symptoms. Pain is a principal sign of infected total hip prostheses. Sinus tracts that communicate with the prosthesis may be present in either late or chronic infection. Contrast arthrography can demonstrate loosening of the prosthesis and the presence of abscesses and sinus tracts; plain radiographs and bone scans are helpful in demonstrating osteomyelitis associated with an infected joint prosthesis. CT and conventional ultrasonography (US) are of limited usefulness owing to the artifacts generated on the image by the implant components. Combined technetium and gallium scanning may help distinguish joint prosthesis infection from aseptic loosening. An erythrocyte sedimentation rate will be requested. Normally, the erythrocyte sedimentation rate returns to normal preoperative levels within three to six months after arthroplasty; if infection occurs, it remains elevated. C-reactive protein levels are also likely to be elevated with prosthetic infection.[8] The best method of detecting infection and identifying the organism is biopsy, either open capsular biopsy or aspiration of the joint fluid.[9] Because infection of a total joint prosthesis nearly always necessitates removal of the prosthesis, preventing infection is a primary nursing consideration.

Preoperative Measures to Prevent Infection. Beginning one to two days preoperatively, the patient should bathe or shower with an antimicrobial soap containing hexachlorophene or an iodophor. A patient undergoing a major orthopedic procedure will receive prophylactic antiobiotic therapy preoperatively. An initial dose of a cephalosporin is administered within two hours before surgery, to ensure that adequate tissue levels are present at the start of the operation. If a tourniquet is used, its inflation should be delayed for at least five minutes after intravenous administration of an antibiotic, to allow achievement of adequate tissue levels. Antibiotic prophylaxis may be continued. It is important for the RNFA to note any patient allergies before the administration of any perioperative medication.

Intraoperative Patient Care

The choice of anesthesia is determined not only by the nature of the procedure, (e.g., the length, extent, position of the patient, and location of the incision), but also by the age, physical condition, and history of the patient. Pediatric, trauma, arthritic, and elderly orthopedic patients each have special anesthesia needs. For procedures involving an extremity and the use of a tourniquet, the choice between a regional anesthetic technique (specific nerve blockades, intravenous regional anesthesia, plexus anesthesia, spinal or epidural blockade) and a general anesthetic is usually determined by the interplay of patient and surgical parameters just listed. For orthopedic procedures involving soft tissue, a local infiltration technique may be selected. For orthopedic procedures involving the bone, a regional or general anesthetic is desirable. During administration of a local anesthetic agent, the patient must be closely monitored for signs and symptoms of an overdose or allergic reaction. Epinephrine should be avoided in digital blocks or blocks in other areas where circulatory compromise to the tissues is a concern.

Probably no other specialty uses as many varied surgical positions as orthopedics. Positions for orthopedic surgery are usually variations on the supine, lateral, and prone positions. For procedures involving the extremities, such as knee arthroscopy or carpal tunnel release, the patient is placed in the supine position. For procedures involving the shoulder or elbow, a sitting or semi-sitting position is preferred. Surgery involving the hip joint requires that the patient be in a lateral position to allow efficient access.

Each position presents a challenge for the perioperative team. Complications from improper positioning can result in nerve compression, interference with venous return and cardiac output, compression of the eye or possibly corneal abrasions, accidental removal of the endotracheal tube, joint strain, and other position-specific sequelae. In a position where the operative site is higher than the right atrium (such as the sitting position for cervical laminectomy), the patient may be at risk for venous air embolism; an esophageal stethoscope, transthoracic Doppler device, and end-tidal carbon dioxide monitor will be required. A right atrial catheter may be inserted in high-risk patients to permit removal of air.

The RNFA in orthopedics must maintain a practical knowledge of the use of positioning aids and operative beds, including increasingly complex fracture tables with special attachments. These present special patient care considerations as well; ensuring safety for the unconscious and paralyzed patient during positioning maneuvers must be a joint effort of the anesthesia provider, surgeon, and perioperative nursing team.

Skin preparation and draping techniques also vary according to the surgical intervention and patient characteristics. Many different products can be used for the skin prep, including film-forming iodophor complexes, povidone-iodine in solutions or gels, and iodine soap suspensions. Agents containing iodine are bactericidal against gram-negative and gram-positive organisms. Alcohol in combination promotes the rapid action of the agent's bactericidal properties. However, the flammability and volatility of storing alcohol-based solutions may preclude their use in some operating rooms. The area to be prepared is always inspected for integrity. If the skin is broken, even slightly, an alcohol-based agent is not recommended for use.

Applying surgical drapes, initiating aseptic technique, and providing adequate surgical site exposure are important RNFA activities. Many orthopedic operations involve manipulation of an extremity or a joint at some point in the procedure. The drapes must be placed to allow this activity. Many facilities use disposable drapes, many of which are designed to meet manipulation requirements as well as surgical site exposure and barrier requirements. In general, whichever type of draping system is chosen, the drapes should be nonlinting, provide an effective fluid and bacterial barrier, provide maximum patient coverage, permit freedom for manipulation, transmit heat and water vapor, and be nonflammable or flame retardant. The basic principles for aseptic technique and the handling of sterile drapes are observed. When plastic incise drapes are used, those with an antiseptic incorporated into the adhesive may be selected.

To begin the surgical procedure, the surgeon makes the skin incision with a scalpel blade and may dissect the fascia with the electrosurgical pen tip or scalpel. As the incision progresses, the surgeon uses electrosurgical current to cauterize and ligate blood vessels and transect muscle. The RNFA assists by applying slight pressure with a lap sponge to the area already exposed. The lap sponge can also be used to provide retraction of the skin edges, depending on the procedure.

Self-retaining retractors may be used during the procedure, placed in the shallow area of the incision. The position of the self-retaining retractor may need to be changed frequently to provide exposure. Whenever a retractor is placed, care must be taken to observe all structures it is to retract. The nerves and blood vessels must be identified before retractor placement. As the procedure progresses, the type of retractor needed changes from one designed for tissue retraction to one designed to elevate or secure bone. Caution is needed when manipulating any type of retractor. Too much upward force can result in a fracture; too little will not provide the correct exposure. Also, the downward pressure exerted while using a retractor may place unwanted stress on the underlying structures, causing interruption in the blood flow and possible damage to the muscle and nerves.

A hand-held retractor such as a rake retractor is often used superficially, to retract the skin or superficial fascia. It may also be used at the beginning of the procedure, after the skin incision has been made, to assist in the discovery of blood vessels severed during the incision. Used to retract the skin, this instrument permits exposure so that hemostasis can occur. A rake can also be used to retract the fibrous tissue covering a bone or joint capsule and ensure that the tissue is not twisted onto the drill bit, preventing visual inspection during the drilling procedure and possibly obscuring the hole after drilling.

A power saw, drill, or reamer (nitrogen, electrical, or battery-driven) is frequently used to resect, perforate, or cannulate a bone. Care must be taken to protect the surrounding tissue from injury related to mechanical (pressure from the angle of use or wound entry) or physical (thermal effects from the friction between the metal and the bone) events. The Midas Rex equipment is frequently used in total hip revisions. This particular instrumentation is very effective in removing old cement. Pulsating irrigation systems are used with antibiotic irrigating solutions throughout many orthopedic procedures to remove bone or cement fragments.

Tourniquets are often useful in minimizing blood loss. The RNFA may either apply the tourniquet or assist with application. In general, the width of the tourniquet cuff should be more than half the limb diameter, and the cuff should be applied over smooth padding that is kept wrinkle-free and dry. During prepping, it may be necessary to protect the cuff with an impermeable plastic drape placed just distal to the cuff. A properly applied and monitored pneumatic tourniquet is reasonably safe. The RNFA should carefully implement the AORN's recommended practice for the use of the pneumatic tourniquet.[10]

Hemostasis is maintained during surgery by means of pressure, suctioning, irrigation, and the electrosurgical unit (ESU). When the electrosurgical pencil is used, care must be taken to touch only the hemostat holding the bleeding end of the blood vessel or the area of uncontrolled bleeding. The ESU should be activated only after contact is made between the blade of the ESU pencil tip and the hemostat. Touching any other tissue can cause thermal damage and increase the risk of postoperative wound infection. Because blood loss can be significant in certain procedures, RNFAs must participate in measures to calculate blood loss by observing the amount of blood on sponges and in suction canisters, estimating the amount of blood on the drapes, and tracking the amount of irrigation fluid. If chemical or topical hemostatic adjuncts are required, oxidized regenerated cellulose is less likely to promote infection than are gelatin sponges or microfibrillar collagen.[8] This may be especially important when other foreign bodies, such as a prosthesis, are also left in the wound.

Wound closure techniques and materials will vary depending on the location of the surgical incision. Generally, an interrupted technique is used for closure. Each stitch is placed separately so that if one stitch breaks or loosens, the remaining sutures will still maintain the integrity of the closure. Stress on the primary suture line is of particular concern in procedures involving a joint. For procedures involving a capsule (hip or shoulder), a nonabsorbable synthetic multifilament braided suture is used to secure the internal tissue approximations. Next to surgical steel, this type of suture is the strongest available, and it retains its tensile strength for a long time. The nonabsorbable suture remains embedded in the body tissues (unless it is surgically removed), becoming encapsulated in fibrous tissue during wound healing. A retention suture—interrupted nonabsorbable suture material placed through tissue on each side of the primary suture line—may be used to relieve tension.

For smaller incisions, incisions in areas of less stress (e.g., the arm), or incisions in areas where sutures will not be removed, an absorbable synthetic multifilament braided suture is used. The suturing technique will be either continuous or interrupted, depending on the site and surgeon's preference. This suture is usually absorbed within 60 to 90 days by a process of slow hydrolysis.

Skin closure commonly is achieved using skin staples. Drains are used to reduce the chance of hematoma and decrease the risk of infection. The drain is placed by means of a secondary stab wound made distal to the surgical wound. Depending on the location, this drain may be secured with a heavy silk suture or taped securely in place as part of a bulky dressing.

Postoperatively, the orthopedic extremity must be stabilized. This is achieved by means of a cast, a splint, a sling, or a restricting device (such as an abduction pillow for the postoperative total hip replacement patient). The patient may remain under anesthesia while the orthopedic appliance is secured. Postoperatively, the extremity is elevated to minimize swelling and discomfort; an ice pack may be applied to reduce swelling and decrease pain, and antiembolic stockings may be indicated if the patient's mobility is limited by the surgery performed. Before transfer from the operating room, the patient's neurovascular status is checked. This includes assessment of the pulses in the operate extremity, tissue perfusion, and sensorimotor function. A grave complication in patients with a cast or other orthopedic conditions is compartment syndrome (Table 15–1). For patients at risk, the five "Ps" of the signs and symptoms of compartment syndrome are carefully evaluated: pain, pallor, paresthesia, paresis, and pulselessness.

Summary

Advances in orthopedic surgery have changed and will continue to change the types of patients and patient procedures with which RNFAs are involved. As the population continues to age, there will be more age-related orthopedic problems presenting for surgical treatment. New materials from space-age technology will invite new applications in orthopedics. Lasers are being considered in future orthopedic procedures; for arthroscopic procedures, the carbon dioxide laser has proved effective. Fortunately, for all patients who need orthopedic surgery, the surgeon and RN first assistant, along with biomechanical engineers, will continue to contribute innovation and the knowledge of experience to alleviate pain and improve patients' functional abilities.

■ THE RN FIRST ASSISTANT IN CARDIAC SURGERY

The advent of minimally invasive cardiac surgery and "off pump" coronary artery bypass procedures is already changing the face of what was considered to be a well-established, commonly performed surgical procedure. The RNFA is challenged to prepare for the changes occurring in the practice setting of assisting at cardiac surgery and to concurrently provide quality care for cardiac surgery patients. The explosion of minimally invasive procedures is driven by economic as well as patient preference factors.[11] Those who might have been denied surgery because of multiple risk factors or advanced age are sometimes being offered less invasive procedures or procedures done without the use of cardiopulmonary bypass.[12] The RNFA on a cardiac service has the opportunity—and, indeed, the responsibility—to contribute to im-

T A B L E   1 5 – 1 .   COMPARTMENT SYNDROME

Description: An abnormal increase in pressure within a confined anatomical space, resulting in impaired circulation, nerve injury, and loss of muscle function

Etiology and Incidence:

1. Compartment syndrome can result from a decrease in compartment size or an increase in compartment volume.
2. A decrease in compartment size can result from constrictive dressings or casts.
3. An increase in compartment volume can result from swelling or bleeding.
4. Patients at risk for compartment syndrome include those with fractures or crushing injuries of the limbs; the legs and forearms are the most common sites.

Pathophysiological Processes and Manifestations

1. Normal intracompartment pressure is about 6mm Hg; pressures above 30mm Hg are considered high enough to impair capillary perfusion.
2. If pressure increase is sufficiently high and remains unrelieved for several hours, permanent damage to nerve and muscle cells, with resulting loss of function and limb contractures, may occur.
3. Severe pain caused by the stretching of skin and soft tissue occurs. Patients may describe it as deep, throbbing, and nonstop.
4. Paresthesia occurs as nerves are compressed. Patients often describe it as a burning or tingling sensation, or as a loss of feeling.
5. Limited muscle movement or diminished reflexes occur, with muscle ischemia.
6. Distal pulses may be present and normal; this occurs because the major arteries palpated in pulse-taking lie outside the muscle compartment.
7. Muscle trauma releases myoglobin, an intracellular muscle protein, into the urine, causing a dark, red-brown pigmentation.

Overview of Nursing Interventions

1. Assess at-risk patients frequently.
2. Instruct the patients in the use of a pain-rating scale; interpret the degree and type of pain according to the patient's evaluation.
3. Assist the physician with invasive pressure measurement using a wick catheter or needle placed directly into the muscle compartment.
4. Remove any constricting material to reduce pressure
5. Avoid elevating the extremity because it decreases arterial pressure, thus reducing the amount of tissue pressure needed to stop circulation.
6. Prepare the patient for fasciotomy, if indicated, to allow blood flow.

(Source: Paradiso C: Lippincott's Review Series—Pathophysiology. Philadelphia, JB Lippincott, 1995, pp 151–152.)

proving the quality of patient care and the achievement of optimal patient outcomes. Collaboration with nursing colleagues, physicians, and other members of the surgical team in the operating room and within the health care facility contributes to an efficient and coordinated cardiac surgery service, adding to the potential for improvements in patient care.

Today, owing to a multiplicity of economic factors, many patients undergoing elective cardiac surgery are admitted the day of surgery and have already been evaluated for their cardiac disease and any concurrent medical or surgical conditions. Assumptions should not be made, however, that such patients are completely prepared, either physically or emotionally, for their surgery or recovery from it. Careful attention should be given to medical records from previous admissions and to any physical or emotional changes that the patient might have experienced in the interim. RNFAs need to be innovative in their approach to preoperative assessment because the patient undergoing elective surgery is in the hospital for such a short time preoperatively.

Preoperative Patient Preparation

Preoperative assessment and preparation of the cardiac surgery patient is extremely important. Common routine diagnostic studies (usually performed on an outpatient basis for elective surgery) might include chest radiography, electrocardiography, stress testing, angiography, carotid Doppler study, and a gated equilibrium heart scan. The RNFA might provide valuable information intraoperatively if she or he has reviewed the patient's angiogram preoperatively. Pulmonary function tests and room air arterial blood gas analysis should be considered in patients scheduled for elective surgery who have an extensive smoking history or other significant lung disease that might result in chronic hypercarbia. In managing these patients postoperatively, it is important to know if they are dependent on hypoxic drive for respiration. Among other diagnostic studies performed on a selected basis are echocardiography, venous Doppler studies, venography, electrophysiological studies, and any other patient-specific studies deemed necessary (e.g., gastroscopy examination for the patient with a history of gastric ulcer disease).

In addition to these diagnostic studies, routine laboratory data are also vitally important. Traditional preoperative laboratory studies include a complete blood cell count, electrolyte determination, coagulation studies, blood urea nitrogen, creatinine, and urinalysis. (See Appendix III for information on these and other laboratory studies.) Other important laboratory studies for the patient undergoing cardiac surgery might include evaluation of medication levels (e.g., digoxin), cardiac enzymes, blood chemistries, and lipid levels. Unfortunately, these laboratory data are sometimes given lower priority than the cardiac diagnostic studies. For the cardiac surgery patient whose routine laboratory data are not within normal limits, overlooking the data can have disastrous consequences.

Issues related to quality of life and psychosocial patient characteristics should not be overlooked.[14,15] Research has indicated that patients over the age of 55 years who did not find comfort and strength from religion and who lacked group participation accounted for 20% of those who died after cardiac surgery.[16] The RNFA could provide valuable input, after assessing the patient, in helping the surgeon determine these and other risk factors that are present.

Review of History and Physical Examination. The admission history and physical examination are very important elements in the preoperative assessment of cardiac surgery candidates. Identifying previous surgical procedures is essential, with special attention paid to whether the patient has undergone vein stripping and ligation, commonly performed 20 years ago. Although vein stripping does not necessarily destroy incompetent perforators or remove varicosities of the branches, it is currently recognized that preservation of the long saphenous vein for coronary artery or peripheral vascular conduits is advisable. However, because vein stripping was once common, some of today's cardiac surgery patients underwent the procedure. In these patients, consideration may need to be given to using the lesser saphenous vein, if veins are considered to be the conduit of choice for a particular patient. Either internal mammary artery, the gastroepiploic artery or the radial artery can also be used as a conduit. If the radial artery is being considered for grafting, Allen's test must be done to evaluate the arterial supply to the hand (Figure 15–2). A positive test indicates inadequate flow to the hand from the ulnar artery or its distal branches; that artery should not be used, even for arterial pressure monitoring. The test results should be documented and conveyed to the surgeon. Usually the radial artery is harvested from the nondominant hand.[17] Arm veins and homologous veins have fallen into disfavor because of their low patency rates.[18] Other important information when taking the patient's history includes medication use (including cardiac medications, anticoagulant/antiplatelet agents, antiarrhythmics, birth control pills), allergies, smoking history, height and weight, activity intolerance, and any concurrent medical problems. The use of vitamins and nutritional supplements should also be queried. Although vitamin C is essential for normal wound healing and bromelain (found in pineapple) decreases the time required for hematoma resorption, garlic, vitamin E, and fish oil have the potential to increase surgical bleeding, especially when taken in conjunction with other antiplatelet agents.[19]

During the physical examination, particular attention should be paid to the respiratory and cardiovascular systems. The patient's general appearance, breathing pattern, respiratory rate, skin color, nail bed and nail configuration, chest wall configuration, and tracheal position should be inspected. Chest percussion should note areas of resonance, hyperresonance, tympany, dullness, or flatness. Chest auscultation should be performed to detect normal breath sounds (vesicular, over most of the lung fields; bronchovesicular, over the main bronchus and upper right posterior lung; and bronchial, over the trachea) and abnormal breath sounds (decreased breath sounds, crackles, wheezes, rales). The presence of murmurs, rubs, or gallops should also be documented. If the internal mammary artery is being considered as a graft, the subclavian artery should be checked for bruits; bruits could indicate stenosis of the subclavian artery, adversely affecting blood flow in the internal mammary.[20] Patients undergoing cardiopulmonary bypass are subjected to hemodynamic changes that are not generally seen in other major operative procedures. For these patients and for those undergoing minimally invasive

Ask the patient to make a tight fist with one hand; then compress both radial and ulnar arteries firmly between your thumbs and fingers. Next, ask the patient to open the hand into a relaxed, slightly flexed position. The palm is pale.

Extending the hand fully may cause pallor and a falsely positive test.

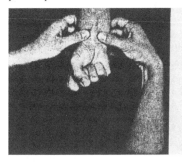 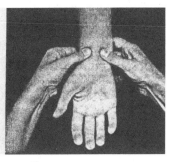 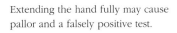

Release your pressure over the ulnar artery. If the ulnar artery is patent, the palm flushes within about 3 to 5 seconds.

Persisting pallor indicates occlusion of the ulnar artery or its distal branches.

Patency of the radial artery may be tested by releasing the radial artery while still compressing the ulnar.

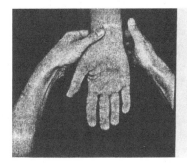 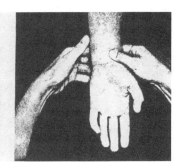

FIGURE 15–2

Evaluating the arterial supply to the hand. (Source: Bates B: A Guide to Physical Examination and History Taking, 6th ed. Philadelphia, JB Lippincott, 1995, p 441.)

as well as "off pump" procedures, careful respiratory and cardiac assessment is essential.

Patient Education. A large research base supports the importance of effective psychological and educational interventions in postsurgical outcomes.[21] In today's managed care environment, with decreased lengths of stay, research on psychoeducational interventions continues to be of critical importance in nursing's research agenda. Which interventions, their timing, for which patient populations, in what form, and leading to what quantifiable outcomes are research questions that RNFAs should seek answers to. Modern medicine and the sophisticated technology that allows complex surgical intervention do not completely "cure" a patient's illness. These major advances may allow a longer life and enhance the quality of that life; however, they are not fully adequate in dealing with the psychosocial and lifestyle modification issues that underlie the disease process. The RNFA is well positioned and educated to assist patients and their families in meeting these psychosocial needs and assisting them to a fuller, more meaningful surgical recovery.

Research on the timing of preoperative education of cardiac surgery patients indicates that patient knowledge, postoperative mood states, and physiological recovery improve when such education is initiated 5 to 14 days before surgery.[22] If it is not possible for the RNFA to participate this early in the preoperative phase, a collaborative patient education program should be designed. Educational interventions might be begun by nursing staff in the angiology laboratory. After angiography, patient education should continue if the patient is referred for surgery. A questionnaire might be developed to determine the learning needs of the patient, thus enabling beneficial use of time.[23] As the RNFA becomes involved in educating the patient and family, a positive relationship is established and lines of communication are opened.

Although much media attention has been given to cardiac surgery, the patient still may have misconceptions about the actual surgery and the recovery period. Before patient teaching can begin, it must be determined what the patient knows and how much the patient wants to know. Information included in preoperative teaching has often been determined by health care professionals and assumed to be important for all patients. Although there is certain general information that all patients should have access to, the patient and the RNFA may not have the same perceptions of what is stressful.[24] Identifying the perioperative events and conditions that the patient considers stressful and anxiety producing allows the RNFA to determine which are amenable to nursing intervention, and to design a plan of care accordingly.

Cardiac surgery and recovery from it may elicit mental distress, such as anxiety and fear about outcomes; the physical and physiological demands of the diagnostic workup may magnify psychological stress. Preliminary research on the rank order of perceived stressors by coronary artery bypass surgery patients indicates that having the surgery is most stressful, followed by such concerns as resuming lifestyle, pain and discomfort, dying due to illness or surgery, absence from home or business, progress in recovery, activity level, and the interval before the surgery.[25] Elucidation of individual stress-generating events can guide psychoeducational preparation.

Patient education should involve the family and significant others, as appropriate, and begin from a baseline of their understanding. Explanations regarding the procedure itself, the location of the incision, and the anticipated length of recovery need to be reinforced. Usually, when a patient understands the reason for a request, compliance is improved. Perioperative events may be described in the order of their occurrence. The importance of showering with an antimicrobial soap should be explained. The scheduled start time of the operation should be reviewed, along with the possibility of postponement and cancellation. The routine for transporting the patient to the operating room should then be explained. Presurgery procedures, such as the insertion of monitoring lines in a holding area or in the operating room, possibly under local anesthesia, need to be reviewed. Relaxation techniques, such as guided imagery and deep breathing, can be reinforced at this time. The patient needs to know that perioperative staff will be in constant attendance, providing ongoing explanations, support, and comfort during this period.

Postoperative care regimens should be reviewed and explained preoperatively. The patient should understand that he will wake up in a special care unit, and special monitoring equipment should be described in terms that the patient can understand. A tour of the intensive care unit might have a perceived benefit for some patients but does not appear to significantly reduce the anxiety of the patient or family members.[26] Explaining methods for the patient to communicate while intubated is very important, as is reassuring the patient that the "tube in his throat" will be removed as soon as he is awake enough to breathe on his own. If the patient is scheduled for a type of minimally invasive surgery, he may be extubated in the operating room.[27] Simple but factual information regarding intravenous or blood replacement therapy, oxygen therapy, monitors, drainage tubes, and devices will help prepare both the patient and family for what they will see and hear. The patient and family also should be reassured that the nurses in the special care units are very proficient in taking care of postoperative heart patients and able to discern their needs. Patients often have fears of mistakes by health care providers; preoperative preparation can alleviate such fears by increasing patients' confidence in nursing expertise.

The patient should be taught that the early postoperative period is the time when he can really "help himself" by performing deep breathing and coughing, incentive spirometry, foot and leg exercises, and frequent positional changes. These maneuvers should be demonstrated and time allowed for the patient to practice them. Because anxiety regarding postoperative pain is common, and some degree of pain or discomfort is inevitable after cardiac surgery, the patient should be reassured that medication is available for any discomfort related to the surgery and should be taken if needed. If patient-controlled analgesia is going to be used, this should also be explained. In the past, the stay in the special care unit was one to two days. However, with the implementation of rapid recovery approaches, which intend to reduce lengths of stay and costs for cardiac surgery patients, extubation often takes place on the day of surgery and the intensive care unit stay might be only hours. The urinary catheter and invasive monitoring lines are usually removed before transfer from the special care unit to a postsurgical unit.

After moving to the postsurgical cardiac unit, the patient should be instructed to gradually increase activities as tolerated. Depending on the institution, the patient may be enrolled in a cardiac rehabilitation program that could extend postdischarge. Such programs assist cardiac patients to regain physical abilities and resume functional and productive lives.

Home care requirements and needs should be reviewed. With decreased lengths of stay, many patients may not be able to master self-care requisites during hospitalization. In a study eliciting descriptions of recovery experiences from coronary artery bypass surgery patients, concerns centered on pain management and return to independence in activities of daily living; patients reported depression, anxiety, fatigue, difficulty sleeping, and physical sensations related to their chest incisions and shoulder and neck muscles.[28] Telephone teaching programs for at-home follow-up can reinforce previous teaching, clarify information, and provide additional information to enhance home health maintenance after hospitalization. Other available resources such as at-home patient visits might be an option to explore. An important point for the cardiac surgery patient to understand is that although he might have days when he does not feel quite as good as he did the day before, in general he should experience an upward trend during recovery. Postoperative recovery is a dynamic time during which changes in physical activity and emotions may provoke some patient anxiety. The RNFA can develop a follow-up program with the patient to provide information and interpretation of both physiological and psychological reactions to enhance performance of recovery behaviors.

Intraoperative Patient Care

The overall quality of patient care has increased dramatically due to the development of invasive monitoring techniques and the increased knowledge and skill of those professionals involved in their use. Routine invasive monitoring lines include the arterial pressure line (peripheral or central), central venous pressure line, and pulmonary artery catheter. The pulmonary artery catheter may be omitted if the patient is hemodynamically stable and has a good (greater than 50%) left ventricular function, and if the benefits of catheter insertion do not outweigh the risks. During placement of these lines, the electrocardiogram should be monitored closely for any dysrhythmias. In addition to the electrocardiogram, other monitoring devices include a urinary catheter (with temperature probe attached) and a blood pressure cuff. Transesophageal echocardiography (TEE), which provides clearer images than traditional transthoracic Doppler electrocardiography, is increasingly used to evaluate functional repair of the mitral valve; it allows evaluation of regurgitation and stenosis at the time of repair. Residual mitral regurgitation, as assessed by transesophageal color flow mapping in the operating room, correlates highly with the ultimate mitral regurgitation by cineangiography. TEE is also useful for assessing function of the tricuspid and aortic valves and for measuring the aortic root size and valve annulus to aid in determining the size of the prosthesis required. Perioperative TEE is a primary tool for assessing the chambers for air after valve replacement.

The supine position is the position of choice for most cardiac procedures. However, the left lateral position might be used for a redo coronary artery bypass graft (CABG), depending on the vessels to be grafted and the patency of existing grafts. The right lateral position might be selected for a redo mitral valve repair or replacement. The rationale for these deviations is primarily the presence of fewer adhesions as well as the preservation of existing grafts. A 30-degree lateral position might be the position of choice for a minimally invasive procedure.

During routine patient positioning (see Chapter 7, Anesthesia and Patient Positioning, for a full discussion of patient positioning), special attention is given to the hand. If a radial line is used, care must be taken to position the hand so that the arterial pressure trace is not dampened. The elbows must be in a forward position to prevent stretching of the nerve trunks and padded to protect the ulnar nerve and the radial artery as it crosses the inner aspect of the humerus. In addition, the occiput must be protected from dependent pressure. The patient's head may be positioned on a piece of foam and turned from side to side every half hour to prevent alopecia or necrosis, which might arise from a low-perfusion state and a certain degree of hypothermia. Care must also be taken when positioning the legs to ensure that the heels are well padded and that the "frog leg" position is not so acute as to cause peroneal nerve injury, resulting in footdrop. Injury to the lateral femoral cutaneous nerve might cause numbness and paresthesia on the anterolateral aspect of the thigh.

First Assisting Skills

An analogy can be drawn between first assisting and a choreographed dance. Each member of the operative team performs in a manner that enhances the performance of the others. To do this, all members must have perfected their skills. The RNFA must know the sequence of steps in the operative procedure as well as the special preferences of the individual surgeon. Procedures that are inherently difficult become easier when the individuals involved are familiar with each other's routines.

The importance of exposure during cardiac surgery cannot be overemphasized. Good visibility and illumination of the field are essential. The proper method of exposure needs to be selected at the right time. As with any type of surgery, instrumentation and techniques used for exposure during cardiac surgery vary depending on the procedure. Adjustable fixed instrumentation for sternal retraction has evolved from the Burford rib retractor, normally used for thoracotomy approaches, to the Kuyper or Pilling retractor. The sternotomy incision should not be too widely retracted with these retractors, especially in elderly patients or in female patients with osteoporosis; either the sternum or the ribs and costal margins could be fractured. Unnecessarily wide retraction may lead to bleeding in the costovertebral articulation and consequent intercostal nerve injury. The retractor blades also need to be placed carefully; cephalad placement may fracture the first rib. Retractors for dissecting the internal mammary artery have progressed from hand-held army-navy and rake retractors to such self-retaining devices as the Favalaro, Rultract, and Pilling. Proper exposure for mitral valve surgery, previously gained by using two green retractors (or hand-held atrial retractors) to retract the left atrium, can now be achieved using modified Carpentier-type sternal/atrial retractors. Although fixed retractors have obvious benefits, the RNFA needs to use clinical judgment in helping to determine when a self-retaining retractor might be better replaced by hand-held retractors, such as atrial retractors. Disposable retractors are available for minimally invasive procedures, and their use will have to be evaluated in relation to cost-effectiveness and patient outcomes.

Providing exposure during CABG surgery is a critical RNFA nursing behavior. During this procedure, the RNFA assumes very important responsibilities. The assistant retracts the heart with his or her hand. By applying gentle pressure with fingers on either side of the coronary artery, an experienced assistant exposes the wall of the incised coronary artery for the surgeon. Utmost care must be taken when doing this so as not to lacerate the epicardium or injure the myocardium. The hand of the assistant should be positioned as flat as possible. Maintaining a clear and dry field requires thoughtful and deliberate suctioning. If suction is used it should be placed as far as possible from the artery to avoid damage to the vessel and provide the surgeon with an unobstructed view. The use of medical air (passed through a sterile filter and tubing) and irrigation fluid can also be useful in providing exposure in certain cases.

Hemostasis is achieved in cardiac surgery using the same techniques described for all surgeries. (See Chapter 13, Providing Hemostasis, for a thorough discussion of achieving hemostasis during surgery.) The traditional cardiac surgery patient, however, is heparinized and hemodiluted. If an incision is closed (e.g., vein harvest site in the leg) before cardiopulmonary bypass, even though the heparin has been given, then the amount of drainage from that site is less at the conclusion of the procedure. The fact that the wound is closed and not open to air decreases the risk of wound infection.

Gentleness is the key word when discussing tissue handling. During any procedure, all of the operating surgeon's skill cannot make up for rough handling of tissues by an assistant. This is particularly true when harvesting a saphenous vein or radial artery. The RNFA must be constantly aware of the ramifications of his or her actions. The technique for harvesting conduits varies somewhat from institution to institution and from surgeon to surgeon. Vein branches left long and untied are much easier to deal with than are those torn by rough dissection. Branches tied too far away from the vein are more easily dealt with than those tied too close to the vein, compromising the vein lumen. Whether the vein is harvested from a single incision, multiple incisions, by using a bridge at the knee, or endoscopically, sound surgical principles still apply.

Although harvesting veins for use as bypass grafts is a relatively simple procedure, the RNFA needs to use meticulous technique to ensure an adequate, unimpaired conduit. Scott-Conner and Dawson recommend the following steps when harvesting the saphenous vein:

1. Make a short longitudinal incision over the distal vein near the medial malleolus.
2. Ligate the vein distally and secure it proximally with either a vascular clamp or ligature.
3. Dissect the vein free from the subcutaneous tissue, avoiding undermining the incisional edges, and ligate all branches near the wall of the vein, taking care not to narrow the lumen or injure the vein (Figure 15–3).
4. Carefully dissect the vein free from the adjacent sensory nerves to avoid injuring them.
5. The vein can be removed via a continuous longitudinal incision or short incisions (Figure 15–4). The latter technique is less likely to result in necrosis of the adjacent skin (which may occur secondary to devascularization associated with continuous skin incisions).
6. After removal of the vein from its bed, the vein is irrigated and then a small vascular clamp is placed on the proximal portion.
7. The closed venous segment is gently injected to test for any leaks. Excessive pressure is avoided, as this may injure endothelial cells and increase graft thrombogenicity. Small tributaries are ligated; small holes may be closed with fine prolene suture.[29]

In endoscopic harvesting, illuminated dissectors and retractors are used to follow the course of the saphenous vein and separate it from surrounding subcutaneous tissue. Endoscopic clip appliers are used to ligate side

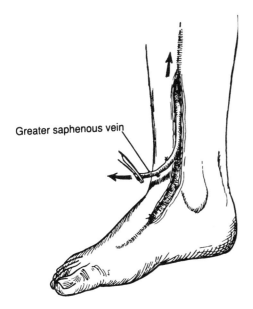

Greater saphenous vein

FIGURE 15–3

When harvesting, the RNFA needs to keep in mind the course of the saphenous vein. At the ankle, it is anterior to the medial malleolus. As it ascends, it passes posteromedially; at the level of the knee, it is 8 to 10 centimeters posterior to the patella. As it ascends through the thigh, it passes anteromedially to pass through the saphenous hiatus, on the anterior side of the upper thigh lateral to the pubic tubercle, subsequently draining into the (common) femoral vein. (Source: Scott-Conner C, Dawson DL: Operative Anatomy. Philadelphia, JB Lippincott, 1993, p 633.)

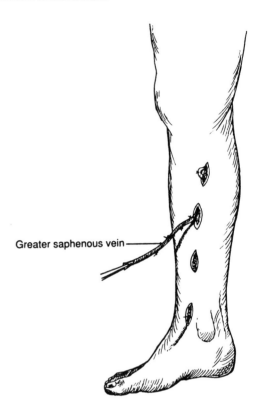

Greater saphenous vein

FIGURE 15–4

Even with short incisions, which are less likely to cause necrosis of the adjacent skin, the RNFA should avoid undermining the incisional edges during dissection. (Source: Scott-Conner C, Dawson DL: Operative Anatomy. Philadelphia, JB Lippincott, 1993, p 633.)

branches, which are then divided with endoscopic scissors. One to three small incisions suffice for vein removal. While research is ongoing regarding the integrity and quality of the endoscopically harvested vein compared to open harvesting, it is likely that RNFAs will increasingly need to learn this minimally invasive approach.[30]

The RNFA needs skill in suturing and assistive behaviors during suturing to ensure smooth teamwork and prevent problems. For example, if the first assistant follows the suture too closely, the second assistant and scrub nurse will not be able to see the operative field. All members of the team need to be able to see to anticipate the next step in the procedure. The first assistant must follow the suture in a manner that respects the needs of other team members. The same principle applies to suctioning, suturing, retracting (with or without the use of instrumentation), and dissection. Practice, practice, and more practice is essential to attain the skills necessary for quality first assisting. The RNFA must be diligent about maintaining proper technique in the operating room and must constantly assess her efforts as part of quality improvement efforts and professional performance standards for nursing.

Summary

Postoperatively, RNFAs can also contribute to quality care for the cardiac surgical patient. Removal of sutures, epicardial pacing wires, and chest tubes is within the scope of practice of RNFAs in some institutions.[31,32] The RNFA is well positioned to be involved in this aspect of postoperative care through knowledge of intraoperative placement and the potential for injury on removal. An opportunity also exists at this time to answer a patient's questions and to encourage the patient to write down questions as they might arise. Signs and symptoms of infection should be reviewed with the patient and family. Superficial infections are usually marked by elevated temperature, erythema, poorly approximated wound edges, and serous drainage; deeper infections are often marked by persistent chest pain that is unrelieved by analgesics at a point when the sternal incisional pain should be waning. Sternal instability, detected by sternal clicking on palpation along the entire sternal length, and bone motion, detected by asking the patient to cough while hand pressure is applied, require immediate attention; these indicators may be the prelude to sternal dehiscence with deep sternal infections. Signs and symptoms of wound infection usually appear as late as the sixth or seventh day, so discharge planning and patient teaching must incorporate what to look for in the risk for wound infection.

The future promises many changes and challenges for the RNFA involved in the care of cardiac surgery patients. Minimally invasive procedures, "off pump" techniques, endoscopic vein harvesting, and the use of arterial conduits (other than the internal mammary artery) are all evolving. The long-term outcomes of some of these innovative changes are not known. RNFAs involved with these procedures should become part of the research effort in their own institutions and throughout the country. Case management, the delivery innovation of the 1990s, focuses on interdisciplinary collaboration; RNFAs need to be involved in the design of models that improve patient care while decreasing lengths of stay and the total cost of care. Evaluation of patient progress toward specific outcomes and modifications of care regimens based on those observations are part of the opportunities for RNFAs to participate in improving quality while keeping resource use at an appropriate level.

RNFAs need to share their experiences, not only with their colleagues in the operating room but also with colleagues throughout the institution in which they practice and in their professional organizations. Much research needs to be undertaken and many studies need replication. Physiological and psychological factors often affect the cardiac surgery patient's anxiety about surgery and confidence in the capacity for postoperative recovery. The RNFA can be a critical intervener during the entire perioperative experience and recovery process, providing the help and assistance the patient requires from a nurse caregiver.

▨ THE RN FIRST ASSISTANT IN ENDOSCOPIC AND MINIMALLY INVASIVE SURGERY

In the past two decades, remarkable advances in endoscopic and minimally invasive procedures have been made that allow new approaches to surgical interventions in many specialties. With the exception of gynecological procedures, most endoscopic and minimally invasive techniques have been developed and utilized only within the past 10 to 15 years.[33] As video technology advances, new surgical applications are being developed. The endoscopic surgeon is at the end of a long chain of technology and all of the knowledge necessary to run it, and therefore relies heavily on the operating team. A skilled assistant is essential to the success of all but the simplest of endoscopic and minimally invasive procedures. An in-depth knowledge of the procedure, instrumentation, and technical equipment is mandatory for the RNFA to deliver safe and effective perioperative care.

Laparoscopic surgery had its beginnings in gynecology. Procedures frequently performed pelviscopically include lysis of adhesions, coagulation or laser ablation of endometrial implants, salpingectomy for ectopic pregnancy, fimbrioplasty, myomectomy, oophorectomy, and ovarian cystectomy. More recent advances include laparoscopically assisted vaginal hysterectomy and laparoscopic bladder suspension procedures. In general surgery, the most commonly performed procedure is laparoscopic cholecystectomy, with or without routine intraoperative cholangiography. Introduced in 1989, by 1992 close to 80% of cholecystectomies were being performed via laparoscopy.[34] Laparoscopic appendectomy has become an accepted method of removing both the normal and the acutely diseased appendix, but the laparoscopic approach should not be used in the presence of an appendiceal abscess or gangrene at the base of the appendix when secure stump closure cannot be ensured with a stapling device. Procedures such as laparoscopic lymphadenectomy and Nissen fundoplication are quickly gaining popularity as surgeons and RNFAs master these more advanced techniques. Other applications, such as laparoscopic inguinal hernia repair, continue to be somewhat controversial; questions remain as to whether a laparoscopic procedure, requiring general anesthesia and a longer operating time, should be used instead of an ambulatory procedure performed under local anesthesia, given the lack of data proving a reduction in recurrence rates in laparoscopic repairs.[35] Thoracic surgeons are routinely performing such procedures as thoracoscopic pulmonary wedge resection for biopsy or bullous disease, pleurodesis, lymphadenectomy, drainage and debridement of empyema, and pericardial window.[36] In some trauma settings, endoscopy is being performed to evaluate penetrating abdominal trauma and small-volume hemothorax.[37] Video technology has the benefit not only of minimizing the body wall invasion of a large incision, but also affords excellent illumination and magnification of the surgical site. This improves visualization in many cases, theoretically lowering the risk of inadvertent injury to surrounding structures. Many procedures such as laparoscopic bowel resections (Figure 15–5), thoracoscopic lung resections, and even anterior lumbosacral fusions are employing these technological advances, and are more accurately termed "laparoscopic-assisted" or "video-assisted."

For perioperative patients, endoscopic and minimally invasive surgery has some significant advantages over open laparotomy or thoracotomy. Patients experience less incisional pain, a shortened hospital stay, and earlier return to normal activity. Increasing numbers of these procedures are being performed on an ambulatory surgery basis, reducing hospitalization costs. For many patients, the cosmetic result is also an important benefit. Potential postoperative complications from large abdominal incisions, such as wound dehiscence, as well as the possible indirect cardiovascular and respiratory complications resulting from delayed early exercise or decreased respiratory excursion are significantly reduced. As a result, elderly or debilitated patients may have a more positive outcome from a less invasive approach to their surgical needs.

Preoperative Preparation

Patient Assessment and Workup.   Preoperative patient assessment and workup vary with the disease being treated. A complete history and physical examination, along with the diagnostic studies normally required for the patient's age, diagnosis, and proposed surgical procedure, remain part of the preoperative workup. During a focused history and physical examination, the RNFA notes any significant information, such as the presence of an abdominal or pelvic mass or hepatosplenomegaly. Previous abdominal operations, especially those in close proximity to the proposed surgical site, alert the surgeon and RNFA to the likely presence of adhesions that may alter the surgical technique. The RNFA should carefully note any relative contraindications to laparoscopic surgery, such as severe intestinal distention, third trimester of pregnancy, abdominal carcinoma, massive obesity, or generalized peritonitis. Any medical history, such as severe cardiopulmonary disease, hypovolemic shock, cardiac or respiratory failure, all of which may indicate a potential intolerance to pneumoperitoneum, should be recognized as a contraindication.[38]

For laparoscopic surgery on the biliary tract, patients with cholangitis, preoperative jaundice, or common bile duct stones found on ultrasound are very likely to have stones; identifying these indicators during the history and diagnostic workup enables the RNFA to predict the possibility of common duct exploration and stone extraction.[39] Liver function studies are usually ordered; an elevated amylase or alkaline phosphatase level would also increase the likelihood of common duct exploration.[40] For video-assisted colectomy, colonoscopic placement of metallic markers proximal and distal to the lesion may be done the day before or the day of surgery to facilitate laparoscopic

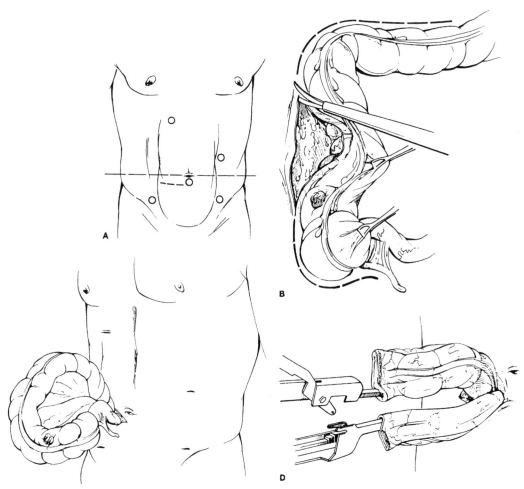

FIGURE 15–5

(A) Trocar sites for a laparoscopic-assisted right colectomy. A supraumbilical site may be chosen for the camera and for the subsequent incision. **(B)** Mobilization of the right colon using laparoscopic Babcock clamps and cautery scissors. Planes of dissection are identical to those for conventional surgery. The ileocolic and right colic arteries can be divided using laparoscopic instruments or in an extracorporeal fashion. **(C)** Prolapse of the mobilized right colon through a small "minilap" incision. **(D)** After resection of the specimen, an extracorporeal anastomosis is performed using a side-to-side stapled technique (shown here) or a handsewn technique. **(A, B,** and **C** redrawn from Bleday R, Babineau TJ, Forse RA. Laparoscopic surgery for colorectal cancer. Semin Surg Oncol 9:59, 1993. Reprinted by permission of Wiley-Liss, Inc., a subsidiary of John Wiley & Sons, Inc. **D** redrawn from Bleday R, Wong WD. Recent advances in surgery for colorectal cancer. Curr Probl Cancer 17:1, 1993. Mosby, Inc., St. Louis, MO.

location of the lesion.[41] Similarly, wires may be placed in a small pulmonary nodule under CT guidance prior to thoracoscopic resection.

Patient and Staff Education. The importance of educating the patient and family has gained respect among health care professionals. With shortened stays and ambulatory procedures, it is imperative that the patient understand what to expect throughout the surgical experience. However, the RNFA is confronted with conducting patient and family education efficiently, owing to these shortened stays. In assessing patient and family education needs and responding to those needs, RNFAs should keep in mind the questions in Box 15–3, which represent the vital information needed for patient and family education and discharge planning. The RNFA possesses the nursing knowledge as well as the perioperative clinical expertise to serve as the ideal patient educator (Box 15–4). Because many patients have misconceptions about endoscopic and minimally invasive surgery, as part of patient and family education the RNFA should explain where the incisions will be and how many to expect. The patient should also be told that although postoperative pain is significantly reduced with endoscopic surgery, some discomfort is to be expected. The possibility of referred shoulder pain following laparoscopy should be discussed. This is the result of peritoneal and phrenic nerve irritation, caused by the combination of carbon dioxide and water making carbonic acid. When this occurs under the right hemidiaphragm, the patient experiences shoulder pain because the phrenic nerve innervates both that portion of the diaphragm and the shoulder.[42]

Length of stay depends on the procedure and overall health status of the patient. For example, patients undergoing laparoscopic hernia repair may be

---

BOX 15–3

Basic Information to Determine in Educating the Patient

Because of shortened stays, and the ambulatory nature of many minimally invasive and endoscopic procedures, RNFAs need to focus patient and family education and discharge planning on vital information.

- What information does the patient need?
- What attitudes should be explored?
- What skills does the patient need to perform health care behaviors?
- What factors in the patient's environment may pose barriers to the performance of desired behavior

(Source: Rankin SH, Stallings KD: Patient Education: Issues, Prinicples, Practices. 3rd ed. Philadelphia, Lippincott-Raven Publishers, 1996, p 126.)

BOX 15-4

The Four Characteristics of the Excellent Nurse-Teacher

RNFAs possess the characteristics of excellent nurse-teachers.

Confidence

- Selects what to teach
- Alleviates the patient's anxiety
- Provides appropriate learning environment
- Prepares appropriate teaching plan and material

Competence

- Decides what is important to teach
- Ensures the patient's safety
- Provides individualized written instructions
- Teaches home management of special problems

Communication

- Gives clear directions
- Uses simple pictures or models
- Speaks the patient's language

Caring

- Has empathy
- Recognizes patient concerns
- Provides encouragement
- Ensures adequate time
- Sensitive to patient's mood

(Source: Rankin SH, Stallings KD: Patient Education: Issues, Prinicples, Practices. 3rd ed. Philadelphia, Lippincott-Raven Publishers, 1996, p 149.)

ready for discharge within a few hours, while those admitted for thoracoscopic surgery may need to stay several days to allow for management of their chest tubes. For many laparoscopic procedures, the patient may anticipate going home within 24 hours, provided that a regular diet can be tolerated and bowel and bladder function have resumed.

Because endoscopic and minimally invasive surgical approaches and techniques are constantly evolving, the RNFA can play a vital role in educating perioperative staff members as well as other health care providers. A preoperative appraisal of room setup, instrumentation, and equipment will facilitate a smooth and efficient surgical course. The RNFA can also serve as a valuable resource to perianesthesia or other facility personnel who are providing care to the patient undergoing minimally invasive or endoscopic surgery.

Intraoperative Patient Care

Anesthesia. Although some limited diagnostic laparoscopies and thoracoscopies are performed with local or regional anesthetics, the most common anesthesia technique is general with endotracheal intubation. This permits maximum abdominal wall relaxation, which is necessary to keep intra-abdominal pressures as low as possible upon insufflation. During thoracoscopic procedures, a dual-lumen endotracheal tube and one-lung ventilation allow for the complete collapse of the lung on the affected side, excellent exposure of the pleural space, and safe control of the patient's airway and hemodynamic status.[43]

Patient Positioning. Patient positioning varies with the operative procedure. For most gynecological procedures, the patient is put in a low lithotomy position, with her arms padded and secured on arm boards or at her sides. The addition of the Trendelenburg position helps displace bowel out of the pelvis. The RNFA stands across from the surgeon, with the viewing monitor positioned toward the patient's feet. For laparoscopic cholecystectomy, the patient will be supine, in the reverse Trendelenburg position, with the right side elevated. This permits optimal visualization by causing the bowel to fall away from the gallbladder. The patient's arms can be abducted on arm boards, or the left arm may be padded, protected, and tucked at the patient's side. The RNFA stands to the patient's right, across from the surgeon. Two monitors are placed toward the head of the bed so that the surgeon and RNFA each view a separate screen across the patient. Laparoscopic gastric procedures may be performed with the patient supine or in a low lithotomy position with the surgeon standing between the patient's legs. When visualization of the surgical site requires that the patient be placed in the reverse Trendelenburg position, as in upper abdominal procedures, sequential compression stockings are usually applied to inhibit venous stasis in the lower extremities and thus lower the risk of deep vein thrombosis.

Patients undergoing elective thoracoscopy are most often placed in the lateral decubitus position, as for thoracotomy. A bean bag mattress can be used to stabilize the patient. The legs are padded and supported with pillows, the upper arm is extended anteriorly, and an axillary roll is used to prevent brachial plexus injury. Flexing the operating room bed at the level of the patient's waist facilitates a wider range of camera and instrument manipulation by dropping the iliac crest out of the way.

Peritoneal Entry and Insufflation. Achieving pneumoperitoneum has long been regarded as the most important, and many times the most difficult, step in any laparoscopic procedure. There are four basic techniques for peritoneal entry. The *blind*, or *direct* trocar entry is very risky and the least used. The *percutaneous* method involves the blind insertion of a Veress needle, which has a sharp beveled outer sheath and a spring-loaded blunt inner sheath. Once the Veress needle has been introduced through the abdominal wall, its tip placement should be verified by means of several saline tests before insufflation is begun. Once an adequate pneumoperitoneum is established, creating a theoretical buffer space between the abdominal wall and the underlying viscera, the Veress needle is replaced with an operative trocar.[44] The *Hasson* or *open* technique is a microlaparotomy in which a small skin incision is made, dissection is carried down to the fascial layer, and the fascia and peritoneum are divided between clamps. Stay sutures are placed on either side of the fascia and used to secure the cone-shaped trocar shaft in place. These sutures can then be used for closing the port site at the end of the procedure. Although many surgeons choose to utilize this technique routinely, others may reserve it for extremely obese patients and those with suspected adhesions along the anterior abdominal wall. The newest technique involves the use of a *visual* or *optical clear trocar,* which has a sharp conical tip. The laparoscope is inserted into the trocar in order to visualize the penetration of each tissue layer.

Once the peritoneum has been entered, carbon dioxide gas is used to displace the anterior abdominal wall, creating a suitable working space. Upon initial insufflation through a large-diameter trocar, the flow rate should remain at 1 to 3 L/min until an intra-abdominal pressure of 5 to 6 mm Hg has been achieved. This reduces the risk of hemodynamic instability associated with rapid pressure changes. Once an adequate pneumoperitoneum has been achieved, the intra-abdominal pressure should be monitored closely, as high pressures may interfere with ventilation, impede venous return, or induce air embolism. The RNFA must be keenly aware that intra-abdominal pressure settings should be individualized to each patient. Although the standard pressure setting for the average healthy adult is between 12 and 16 mm Hg, the patient's age, size, or underlying disease processes will influence his or her ability to tolerate abdominal distention.[45]

The choice of trocar placement will depend on the procedure to be done and on the individual patient's anatomy. Optimal trocar placement should facilitate tissue manipulation during the procedure. Consideration should be given to distance, angle, and relationship to the camera, as well as to anatomical structures to avoid. Once the initial trocar and scope are in place, subsequent trocars should be introduced slowly, deliberately, and under direct visualization. If visualization of the trocar tip is lost for any reason, downward pressure on the trocar should be halted until it is regained. Trocar sizes are determined by the types of instruments to be used.

Equipment and Instrumentation.

Endoscopy is a highly technical specialty that requires the use of an optical system, an electronic insufflator, a suction/irrigation system, operative cannulas or ports, and various surgical instruments designed and developed as techniques advance. The RNFA should be familiar with the function, normal operation, and troubleshooting of the equipment. Troubleshooting in an orderly fashion, from the patient back to the power source, facilitates expedient correction of the problem. Common equipment-related problems include loss of pneumoperitoneum, inadequate picture quality, and lens fogging. The inability to maintain pneumoperitoneum may be the result of excessive suctioning, an open stopcock at one of the ports, leakage around a port, a break in the integrity of the tubing, low flow rate or pressure settings, or an empty carbon dioxide tank.

Problems with the video system may be as simple as the inadvertent disconnection of a cable or complex enough to require the attention of biomedical experts. Before each procedure, the camera and telescope lens should be checked for clarity, focus, and the absence of cracks or moisture at the coupling. "White-balancing" is necessary to ensure the accuracy of color. When the laparoscope enters the body cavity, the rapid temperature and humidity change can fog the laparoscope's lens. Rinsing the scope in warm water or applying a sterile antifog solution before inserting it through the cannula helps to reduce fogging. If the lens becomes fogged or soiled, it may be withdrawn and cleaned with a wet sponge, or rinsed with the irrigator probe inside the body cavity.

Endoscopic instruments are now available in a wide variety of styles. Basic instruments include traumatic and atraumatic tissue graspers, dissecting forceps with finer jaws, and various types of scissors. Electrosurgery probes are available in various forms such as hooks, spatulas, and suction/coagulator combinations. Some of these probes have the ability to irrigate and aspirate as well as to coagulate and cut. A suction/irrigation system is utilized to clear the surgical site of blood and debris, as well as for smoke evacuation. For procedures that require intracorporeal suturing, various endoscopic needle holders should be available according to surgeon preference. Needle holders differ from tissue graspers in that the jaws are generally smaller, single action, and smooth in order to prevent the suture from catching on the hinges. The RNFA must know and understand each instrument's intended use, its capabilities and limitations, and its availability within the institution.

Use of an electrosurgery unit (ESU) is common during laparoscopic surgery. The RNFA must know the special precautions needed when using these devices. With monopolar energy, breaks in the instrument's insulation may result in current leakage, arcing, or jumping, and subsequent burns. Direct coupling, when the active electrode tip comes in direct contact with another conductive instrument such as a metal cannula or the laparoscope itself, diverts electrical current to unintended target tissue, resulting in stray energy burns. The RNFA must bear in mind that both of these situations will most likely occur outside the camera's field of vision, and may therefore go unnoticed. The use of metal cannulas anchored by plastic stability threads should be avoided, as this promotes capacitive coupling, a phenomenon characterized by the disruption of a safe electrical pathway back to ground.[46] Stray current from capacitative coupling results in thermal tissue damage. In 1994, 31 insurers reported a total of 614 claims arising from laparoscopy; bowel perforations were the most commonly reported injury for laparoscopic pelvic procedures.[47] Thus, RNFAs should use risk-reduction strategies to prevent patient injury with the use of electrosurgery during endoscopic and minimally invasive procedures. Chapter 13 reviews these precautions in detail. In summary, an ESU with return electrode monitoring or active electrode monitoring should always be used. High-power settings should be avoided, as should high-voltage waveforms (spray coagulation). Instead, the RNFA should opt for low-power, low-voltage settings, using a cutting waveform; this produces adequate tissue dessication at lower voltages than the coagulation waveform. The operator should avoid touching the ESU active electrode (pencil tip) with other metal instruments; this leads to direct coupling and stray energy burns. The ESU is activated only when the assistant is ready to cut or coagulate the target tissue, and short activations are used to allow surrounding tissue to cool down. Extreme care should be used if cutting long, thin adhesions with the ESU; these can carry current to unseen locations, such as the bowel.[48]

When using a free-beam laser, careful control and visualization of the beam must be maintained at all times. The RNFA must make sure that retracted tissue does not fall into the path of the beam during laser operation. As with any laser or electrosurgical device, meticulous technique and adherence to safety precautions are of paramount importance in preventing thermal injury.

Surgical Skills.   The adaptation of surgical skills to endoscopic and minimally invasive techniques may not proceed as smoothly or as rapidly as the surgeon or the RNFA desires. A learning curve is to be expected when making the transition to endoscopy and minimally invasive techniques, as well as with each new procedure attempted. The RNFA must first develop a conscious awareness of the loss of depth perception and three-dimensional view, and compensate accordingly. The handling of elongated instruments and the loss of tactile sensation brings a new "feel," vastly different from that of traditional open surgery. Accurately judging the degree of tension being applied to tissue requires considerable endoscopic experience. Care must be taken to avoid overly aggressive retraction or tissue manipulation, to reduce the incidence of laceration.

The camera operator is a surgical team member unique to endoscopy. This role is crucial to the success of the procedure, as the surgeon and RNFA rely on the camera to visualize the surgical field. After inspecting the tip of the instrument for type (i.e., traumatic versus atraumatic) and integrity, the RNFA should carefully introduce instruments under direct visualization. It may be necessary to request and wait for the camera operator to locate the instrument before advancing. Skillful manipulation of endoscopic instruments requires slow and deliberate movements in order to avoid undue injury. As a general rule, tissue should be grasped, cut, coagulated, or otherwise manipulated only if clearly visualized. During a procedure, as the camera is focused on the action of the surgeon's instruments, those providing exposure or retraction held by the RNFA may be outside the camera's field of view. The assistant should remain keenly aware of the position of these instruments at all times. The RNFA should not hesitate to ask the camera operator to verify the location of an instrument; taking a few extra seconds is preferable to risking the possibility of organ or tissue damage.

Hemostasis and tissue approximation can be accomplished through various endoscopic techniques. Endoclips and endoscopic stapling/cutting devices are frequently used when dividing structures. Endoligatures are pretied loops of suture used to ligate vessels or other structures with a pedicle. After the loop is introduced through a sleeve, a grasper is placed through the loop and onto the structure, the knot pusher advanced, and the knot tightened around the pedicle. The suture is then cut, leaving a one-quarter-inch tail.[49]

As endosurgical techniques advance, so will the need to develop the skills of endoscopic suturing. Suturing endoscopically allows the surgeon and RNFA to more closely duplicate open procedures (such as Nissen fundoplication), and to approximate delicate tissues with precision (such as the common bile duct), and it affords a means of addressing intraoperative occurrences without necessarily converting to an open procedure. Endoscopic suturing is often the most time-consuming, tedious, and frustrating part of the entire procedure. The design of endoscopic needle holders used depends on surgeon preference, as does the type of needle—straight, curved, or ski needle. Knots are tied using either the intracorporeal or extracorporeal technique. Intracorporeal knot tying is accomplished inside the body cavity, in much the same fashion as an instrument tie. This technique, the superior choice for delicate tissue, is quite challenging to the surgeon and RNFA. Extracorporeal knots are either slip knots or individual throws that are tied on the outside and then advanced down the trocar to the tissue with the aid of a knot pusher.

Complications. Despite the general public's view of endoscopic and minimally invasive procedures as "quick and easy minor surgeries," minor and major complications, including death, have been reported. The carbon dioxide gas itself may contribute to dysrhythmias, hypotension and acid–base disturbances. Venous air embolism may manifest as a sudden decrease in systolic blood pressure, desaturation, increased end-tidal carbon dioxide, dysrhythmias, frothy sputum, cyanosis, and the classic "millwheel" murmur. Any disruption in the integrity of the diaphragm will result in pneumothorax, quickly leading to tension pneumothorax.[50] The majority of complications are procedure related, as in biliary leaks or obstruction associated with laparoscopic cholecystectomy or common bile duct exploration. Gastrointestinal injuries, associated with significant morbidity and mortality, may be the result of thermal damage or laceration. A Veress needle or trocar inserted blindly can easily puncture or lacerate even nondistended bowel. Serosal tears often result from overly-aggressive manipulation or the use of an inappropriate grasping instrument. Bowel or other tissue burns may be related to an energy source such as monopolar current, or contact with the telescope itself. Urinary tract injuries may occur when the bladder is full, or when a free beam laser is fired along the pelvic side wall. Large vessel injury is uncommon, but has been reported with the initial insertion of the umbilical trocar.[51] As most intraoperative injuries may be related to poor exposure or visualization, the skill of the camera operator and the quality of the video image are of paramount importance. Maintaining surgical standards and meticulous technique helps prevent complications.

In the past, visceral herniation and incarceration through a trocar insertion site were rare. However, with the use of more numerous trocar sites and larger trocars, this complication is being reported with more frequency. The depth and small size of trocar sites make fascial closure difficult. For trocar sites more than 5 millimeters in diameter, a double-ended polydioxanone suture swaged to a J-shaped, taper needle with a 180-degree curve has been recommended, using the following technique: (1) After desufflation, grasp and elevate the fascial edges with allis clamps. (2) Insert the J needle parallel to the fascial edge—the curve of the needle permits an adequate bite of fascia. (3) After the needle has been brought through the fascia, the second needle is similarly inserted on the opposite side. The suture is then tied in the usual fashion.[52]

There is always the possibility of the need for conversion to an open procedure. The perioperative team should have a preestablished plan of action should the need for laparotomy develop emergently. The nature of the endoscopic procedure and the patient's medical history also influence the degree of preparedness for conversion to an open procedure. Because of the critical nature of bleeding events involving thoracic anatomy, thoracotomy instruments should be a standard component of any thoracoscopy setup.

Postoperative Assessment

Because patients typically recuperate at home, postoperative follow-up is limited. The surgeon and RNFA must rely on the effectiveness of their preoperative teaching and the patient's or caregiver's level of understanding. Routine postoperative monitoring and precautions are usually similar to those appropriate for the corresponding open procedure. As a general rule, endoscopic surgical patients should improve each postoperative day, even after advanced operative procedures. The surgeon and RNFA should heed any patient complaints of increasing postoperative pain or general signs of regression, bearing in mind the potential for undetected thermal bowel injury and subsequent peritonitis.

BOX 15–5

Impact and Value of LAVH in a Community Hospital

A study by an RNFA and surgeon assessed the impact and value of laparascopically assisted vaginal hysterectomy (LAVH) in a community hospital. Clinical parameters examined included the type of hysterectomy, level of difficulty, additional procedures performed, length of stay, patient's weight, procedure time, size of uterus, estimated blood loss, complications, instrumentation, and technique. Initiation of the LAVH procedure, after the RNFA and surgeon had undertaken the necessary training, inverted the ratio of abdominal to vaginal hysterectomies from 80%/20% before LAVH was available in the institution to 20%/80%. The RNFA and surgeon found the procedure to be safe and effective, and quantified patient outcomes in terms of high levels of acceptance, shorter hospital stay, and earlier return to work and daily activities, which was approximately two weeks sooner than with abdominal or traditional vaginal hysterectomy. RNFAs who participate in research such as this add value to perioperative patient care by collaborating in the important work of quantifying patient outcomes as new endoscopic and minimally invasive procedures are undertaken in their practice setting.

(Source: Reisner JG, Miollis M: Laparoscopically assisted vaginal hysterectomy in a community hospital. Reprod Med 42(9):542–546, 1997.)

Summary

The application of laparoscopic surgery has expanded dramatically from the early, simple gynecological procedures performed on young, healthy women. Today, minimally invasive techniques can lend their benefits to a broader population, from young children to the very aged, the healthy to the severely debilitated. As improved patient outcomes, a reduction in overall health care costs, and technology continue to advance, so will the quest for alternative procedures for diagnosing and managing surgical patients. Within this framework, the role of the RNFA will become increasingly valuable (Box 15–5). Many surgeons consider the skill of the first assistant to be of greater importance during endoscopic and minimally invasive procedures than during open surgery. To achieve this level of excellence in perioperative nursing, RNFAs must value education and lifelong learning, acquiring new skills and expertise to underscore their professionalism and accountability to the patients for whom they care.

▨ THE RN FIRST ASSISTANT IN VASCULAR SURGERY

Vascular surgery, while considered its own specialty, is also encountered in other areas of specialty practice, such as plastic and reconstructive, cardiothoracic, and neurosurgical procedures. The term *vascular* is a derivative of the

Latin term *vasculum*, meaning "small vessel." Early reports of vascular surgery date back to the late 1800s: as early as 1877, Eck anastomosed the portal vein to the inferior vena cava, and in 1888 Matas developed techniques in aneurysm repair.[53] The era of modern vascular surgery was founded on basic principles and techniques implemented in 1902 by Alexis Carrel, a French surgeon.[54] Progress in related medical fields such as hematology, pharmacology, and radiology helped move this specialty into its current golden era.

In the United States, Canada, and the United Kingdom, RNFAs are performing complex surgical maneuvers (e.g., harvesting inferior epigastric and radial arteries) and assisting with them (e.g., minimally invasive open heart or partial left ventriculectomy surgery).[55,56] In order for the RNFA in vascular surgery to achieve optimal patient outcomes and excellence in clinical practice, an understanding of preoperative patient considerations, vascular anatomy, intraoperative patient care, and postoperative patient care and discharge planning is necessary.

Preoperative Patient Considerations

As part of preoperative assessment, the RNFA examines the medical record, reviewing the history and physical examination results. Results of the diagnostic workup, invasive and noninvasive studies (such as Doppler ultrasound flow studies, oscillometry, angiography, digital subtraction angiography, exercise tests, CT, and MRI), and laboratory values should be noted. Particular attention should be paid to clotting values as well as to current medications (including over-the-counter preparations) the patient is taking. The RNFA also needs to determine whether the patient is diabetic. Many patients presenting for vascular surgery have diabetes, and if they are taking NPH insulin, the dosage of protamine given intraoperatively will need to be adjusted.

The RNFA's assessment of the peripheral vascular system to corroborate findings and begin plans for intraoperative care relies primarily on the patient's history (presenting complaint) and inspection of the symptomatic area and system (arterial or venous) involved, along with palpation of the pulses. Arms are inspected for symmetry, size, and skin and nail bed color and texture. The radial pulse should be palpated in both arms and described as normal, increased, diminished, or absent. If there is arterial insufficiency, the brachial pulse may be palpated in the antecubital space or higher in the arm in the groove between the triceps and biceps. A similar examination may be performed for the patient with lower extremity disease, additionally looking for any pigmentation, rashes, or ulcers. Arterial circulation is assessed by palpating the femoral, popliteal, dorsalis pedis, and posterior tibial pulses. Indications of chronic arterial and venous insufficiency are listed in Table 15–2.

It is not unusual for an RNFA to be involved in caring for a patient with a traumatic injury to an extremity. These injuries are often categorized as blunt

T A B L E 1 5 – 2 . FINDINGS OF CHRONIC ARTERIAL INSUFFICIENCY VERSUS CHRONIC VENOUS INSUFFICIENCY

	Chronic Arterial Insufficiency (Advanced)	Chronic Venous Insufficiency (Advanced)
Pain	Intermittent claudication, progressing to pain at rest	None to an aching pain on dependency
Pulses	Decreased or absent	Normal, though may be difficult to feel through edema
Color	Pale, especially on elevation; dusky red on dependency	Normal, or cyanotic on dependency. Petechiae and then brown pigmentation appear with chronicity.
Temperature	Cool	Normal
Edema	Absent or mild; may develop as the patient tries to relieve rest pain by lowering the leg	Present, often marked
Skin Changes	Trophic changes: thin, shiny, atrophic skin; loss of hair over the foot and toes; nails thickened and ridged	Often brown pigmentation around the ankle, stasis dermatitis, and possible thickening of the skin and narrowing of the leg as scarring develops
Ulceration	If present, involves toes or points of trauma on feet	If present, develops at sides of ankle, especially medially
Gangrene	May develop	Does not develop

(Source: Bates B: A Guide to Physical Examination and History Taking, 6th ed. Philadelphia, JB Lippincott, 1995, p 443.)

or penetrating. It is with penetrating injury that vascular (and neurological) injury is a primary problem, although such injuries may also occur with blunt trauma. Blunt trauma usually results in thrombosis of a blood vessel (as opposed to transection); the vessel stretches, and the tunica intima and media disrupt first, leaving the tunica externa to maintain vessel integrity.[57] Unless there is massive hemorrhage, an initial assessment of the injured extremity starts with a history; this may be taken at the same time the examination is being conducted. The mechanism of injury, circulatory status (blood pressure, temperature, and pulses in injured and contralateral extremity), discomfort, pain, or paralysis are priorities in assessment and management decisions. If there is a pulseless extremity and a fracture-dislocation is present, reducing the fracture often results in reestablishment of circulation and pulses. If pulses do not return, the RNFA and surgeon assume there is a vascular injury; arteriography or Doppler evaluation will likely be required. Continuous assessment of any injured extremity is required whenever the possibility of compartment syndrome exists; although it may have many causes, the most common in an injured extremity is the hemorrhage and edema in the damaged soft tissue accompanying a fracture (see the orthopedics section of this chapter for the classic signs of compartment syndrome). A diagnosis of acute compartment syndrome requires immediate surgery.

Lacerations in an injured extremity range in severity. Simple lacerations may be closed by the RNFA following irrigation and debridement if necessary. In a randomized prospective evaluation, patients with simple lacerations of the extremities (excluding those on hands, feet, or joints) were allocated to have skin closure with octylcanoacrylate adhesive or monofilament suture. Tissue adhesive was a faster method of wound repair and less painful, with no differences in either cosmetic results or wound evaluation scores.[58] Conducting research is critical to advancing the science of surgical patient care, but utilization of research findings is just as critical for RNFAs as they develop expert nursing practice.[59]

Throughout the period of preoperative assessment and evaluation of the elective or emergently scheduled vascular surgery patient, the RNFA collaborates with the entire perioperative team to ensure a safe and successful outcome (see Chapter 14 for a discussion of the elements of collaborative practice). Patient and family education is begun during this time. In addition to a description and explanation of anticipated perioperative events and their sequence, the RNFA should participate in psychoeducational interventions aimed at modification of risk factors and management of peripheral vascular problems. Because of the wide spectrum of vascular disease, patient and family education will vary in relation to specific postoperative care regimens and discharge planning needs. Nonetheless, broad educational interventions relate to strategies for managing and improving alterations in peripheral tissue perfusion, pain management, maintaining tissue integrity, wound care, medication regimens, and self-care activities. Written instructions should be provided and referrals made as appropriate (e.g., smoking cessation, diabetes management, weight loss, stress management, exercise programs).

Vascular Anatomy

Adequate perfusion for oxygenation and nutrition of body tissues relies in part on a well-functioning cardiovascular system—an efficient pumping action of the heart, patent and responsive blood vessels, and an adequate blood volume. Systemic circulation is subdivided into five anatomical and functional categories: arteries, arterioles, capillaries, venules, and veins. All systemic arteries arise from the aorta, which originates from the left ventricle of the heart. The aorta passes upward and deep to the pulmonary trunk (ascending aorta), giving off the right and left coronary arteries within the sinuses of Valsalva immediately above the aortic valve. The ascending aorta turns left to form an arch, then descends to the level of the fourth thoracic vertebra (descending aorta), passes through the diaphragm (abdominal aorta) at the level of the third and fourth lumbar vertebrae, then divides into the right and left common iliac arteries. These pass downward and divide into the internal and external iliac arteries. The internal iliac artery forms branches that supply the psoas major, quadratus lumborum, and medial side of each thigh, and the urinary bladder, rectum, prostate, ductus deferens, uterus, and vagina. The external iliac arteries pass through the pelvis, enter the thighs under the inguinal ligament, and become the right and left common femoral arteries; these branch into the deep femoral and superficial femoral arteries. The deep femoral artery continues down to become the popliteal; between the knee and ankle, the popliteal becomes the posterior tibial artery. Below the knee, the peroneal artery branches off the posterior tibial to supply structures on the medial side of the fibula, calcaneum, and heel. In the calf, the anterior tibial artery branches off the popliteal, running along the front of the leg, and becoming the dorsalis pedis at the ankle. Here the posterior tibial artery divides into medial and lateral plantar arteries, which anastomose with the dorsalis pedis to supply blood to the foot.

Blood from the lower extremities is returned by superficial (the saphenous system) and deep sets of veins, which are connected together by communicating, or perforating, veins. The deep veins of the leg carry approximately 90% of the venous return from the lower extremities and are well supported by surrounding tissue. In contrast, the superficial veins have relatively little support, owing to their subcutaneous location. Veins have one-way valves, allowing blood to flow against gravity; this is facilitated by muscular activity. As muscles contract, blood is forced up against gravity; the valves prevent it from flowing backward. The great saphenous vein begins at the medial end of the dorsal venous arch, passes in front of the medial malleolus, and then ascends upward along the medial aspect of the leg, emptying into the femoral vein in the groin below the inguinal ligament. The small saphenous vein begins at the lateral end of the dorsal venous arch, passes behind the lateral malleolus, and ascends along the back of the leg, receiving blood from the foot and posterior portion of the leg and emptying into the popliteal vein behind the knee. The posterior tibial vein is formed by the lateral and medial plantar veins, behind the medial malleolus. It descends deep in the muscle in the back of the leg, receiving blood from the peroneal vein and uniting with the anterior tibial vein just below the knee. The anterior tibial vein is an upward continuation of the dorsalis pedis vein, running between the tibia and fibula, uniting with the posterior tibial to form the popliteal vein, which continues upward as the femoral vein. Eventually, the veins merge with the inferior vena cava, which extends upward through the abdomen and thorax to the right atrium of the heart, where the deoxygenated blood is returned.

While veins are the capacitance system (their thin, less muscular walls allow greater distensibility and compliance, permitting large volumes of blood to be stored under low pressure), the arteries are the resistance system, having low volume and high pressure. Arteries have two main properties—elasticity and contractility. An artery is comprised of three layers (or tunics) known as the *tunica interna* (or intima), *tunica media,* and *tunica externa* (or adventitia). The innermost layer is in contact with the blood and is composed of a layer of endothelial cells on a thin layer of elastic fibers. The middle layer is composed of elastic tissue, collagen, and smooth muscle, giving the arterial wall its characteristic properties of elasticity and extensibility. The third or outer layer is composed of smooth muscle collagen fibers. Although

T A B L E 1 5 – 3 . PHYSIOLOGICAL RESPONSES TO VASCULAR DYSFUNCTION

Arterial Responses

1. *Ischemia*
   a. Ischemia refers to reduced oxygenation to a body part, which can occur when vessels are so diseased that they are unable to transport oxygen-rich blood.
   b. It results in pain to the affected part
2. *Paresthesia:* Decreased sensation in the extremities, described as tingling or numbing.
3. *Pain*
   a. Pain occurs in the feet and leg muscles and may be described as burning, throbbing or cramping.
   b. Usually it is brought on by exercise but may also occur with the elevation of lower extremities.
4. *Intermittent claudication*
   a. Pain in exercising muscles; most commonly occurs in the calf but may occur anywhere in the lower extremity.
   b. It is directly related to decreased blood supply during activity and recedes with rest.
5. *Temperature changes:* Extremities are cold due to decreased blood supply.
6. *Skin color changes:* Skin is pale, especially on elevation; dependent rubor, or redness, occurs as blood rushes downward in the extremity.
7. *Reactive hyperemia:* Reduced blood flow to an extremity results in arteriolar dilatation; when the blood supply is restored, the affected area becomes warm and red from the congestion.
8. *Pulse changes*
   a. Peripheral pulses may be diminished or absent.
   b. A notable difference in the strength or character of pulses from one side of the body to the other may exist.
9. *Prolonged capillary refill:* 3 seconds or more is required for filling.
10. *Ulcers:* Open lesions occurring on the feet resulting from diminished distal perfusion.

Venous Responses

1. *Pain*
   a. Pain occurs in the feet and leg muscles and is described as aching or throbbing.
   b. It results from venous stasis and usually increases as the day progresses, especially with prolonged dependent positioning (eg, sitting or standing)
2. *Temperature changes:* Skin will be warm to the touch because blood can enter but not leave the affected area.
3. *Skin color changes:* Skin may be reddened or cyanotic.
4. *Edema:* pooling of fluid resulting in swelling or enlargement of affected parts.
5. *Venous stasis ulcers:* Skin breakdown due to increased pressure resulting from chronic pooling of blood.
6. *Decreased mobility:* May result from edema.

(Source: Paradiso C: Lippincott Review Series: Pathophysiology. Philadelphia, JB Lippincott, 1995, pp 56–57.)

the thinnest of the three layers, its composition is what gives the arterial wall much of its strength and resistance to overexpansion.

In the capillary bed, blood circulates from arteries to veins, as hydrostatic pressure, especially close to the arteriolar end, forces fluid out into the tissue spaces. An equilibrium is maintained by interstitial colloid osmotic pressure within the tissue and hydrostatic pressure, attracting and opposing fluid movement. As blood moves through the capillary bed toward the venous end, the hydrostatic pressure begins to fall, and the colloid osmotic pressure of the plasma proteins pulls fluid back into the vascular bed. This microcirculation constitutes the site of exchange of nutrients and metabolic wastes between the circulatory system and tissues. Lymphatic capillaries, closely associated with the vascular tree, remove excessive fluid and protein from the interstitial space. A disturbance in any of these mechanisms results in increased interstitial fluid, clinically manifested as edema.

Arterial wall changes are precipitated by numerous factors. The aging process is accompanied by thickening of the medial and intimal wall, with a consequent loss in elasticity. Atherosclerosis, and the plaque associated with it, initially causes the intima and media to lose elasticity as lipids, fibrous tissue, and calcium deposits form and accumulate (Figure 15–6). Risk factors for atherosclerotic lesion formation include smoking, diabetes, hytertension, a family history of peripheral vascular disease, and lipid abnormalities. Eventually, blood flow in veins and arteries is obstructed, leading to symptoms such as intermittent claudication, ischemic pain at rest, ischemic ulceration, and vascular compromise (Table 15–3). Surgical treatment may involve bypassing lesions, such as carotid endarterectomy, femoro-popliteal, aortofemoral, or femoro-femoral bypasses. Less invasive procedures such as angioplasty and intravascular stenting, continue to evolve as alternatives to traditional bypass surgery.[60]

Intraoperative Patient Care

In the operating room, the RNFA reviews the patient's chart, records a preoperative note, and communicates vital assessment information to other members of the perioperative team. Any radiographic studies, such as arteriograms or CT, MRI, and Doppler scans, should be hung on a view box and reviewed with the surgeon. The RNFA may assist with the insertion of arterial, central venous pressure, or Swan Ganz lines; application of EEG or ECG electrodes, blood pressure cuff, pulse oximeter, and other standard monitoring devices; may clip operative hair (if necessary); may help the circulating nurse and anesthesia provider with patient positioning and application of a forced warm air device (or other means for thermoregulation); may place a nasogastric tube, indwelling urinary catheter, or additional intravenous line insertions; or may start an insulin drip (if necessary). After intubation, the RNFA prepares the patient's skin for the surgical procedure and applies surgical drapes. Positioning, preparing, and draping vary according to the type of vascular procedure and, in the absence of a standardized clinical path, surgeon preference.[61]

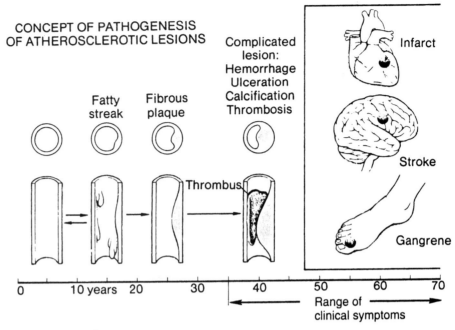

FIGURE 15–6

Schematic concept of the progression of atherosclerosis. Fatty streaks are one of the earliest lesions of atherosclerosis. Many fatty streaks regress, whereas others progress to fibrous plaques and eventually to atheroma. These may then become complicated by hemorrhage, ulceration, calcification, or thrombosis and may produce myocardial infarction. (Adapted from Hurst JW, Logue RB: The Heart. New York, McGraw-Hill.)

In vascular surgery, the RNFA needs to understand the goals and monitoring techniques of the anesthesia provider in order to collaborate in their effective achievement. These may vary according to the surgical procedure and patient co-morbidity. For example, in surgery for cerebrovascular insufficiency, anesthetic goals are to protect the heart and brain from ischemia. This may require injection of the carotid bifurcation with lidocaine and constant assessment of the EEG to guide afterload reduction; if the EEG becomes abnormal, the RNFA should anticipate the need to shunt carotid flow.[62] Light anesthesia may be employed, and patient movement should be communicated, signaling that the anesthesia is inadequate. The anesthesia provider will most likely want to have the patient awake at the end of the procedure; this requires communication between the RNFA and anesthesia team as to how rapidly closure is proceeding.

Suture materials for peripheral vascular surgery are selected according to the structure or layer being closed. In general, blood vessels tend to heal rapidly, allowing use of a synthetic nonabsorbable suture to achieve an anastomosis that has lasting strength and is leakproof. It is important that the suture material be nonreactive; tissue reaction at the anastomosis could lead to a narrowed lumen or thrombus formation. The more inert synthetics, such as nylon and polypropylene, are therefore good choices, although a polyester that allows clotting within the interstices may help prevent leakage at the suture line. The RNFA should also evaluate suture material for its drag; a "slippery" surface on suture allows it to be drawn through the vessel with less friction. With large vessels, a continuous technique is usually used to distribute tension evenly along the anastomotic line. In microvascular repair, an interrupted technique is more usual. When suturing a prosthetic graft, either interrupted or continuous technique may be selected, but the suture material must retain its durability and strength indefinitely; coated polyesters meet this requirement. Chapter 10 discusses suture materials, techniques, and vascular needles and needleholders.

Depending on the RNFA's level of expertise and institutional protocols, wound closure may be assumed by the RNFA while the surgeon sees the patient's family or significant others. The technique for groin closure is described here as an example of the need for clinical judgment and proficiency. Before groin closure, the RNFA assesses the vessel's suture lines and wound for hemostasis and any lymphatic drainage. The deep fascia and subcutaneous tissue layers are often closed with 0 and 2-0 polyglactic absorbable suture using a running technique. It is very important to avoid the femoral nerve, which lies lateral to the artery and could be injured with deep or careless suturing. The skin is closed either with 3-0 interrupted nylon sutures or with surgical staples. The RNFA's goal is to achieve a wound that heals without complication, regardless of the suturing technique or material used.

At the end of the procedure, the RNFA applies the wound dressing, then assists the scrub nurse in removing the sterile drapes. In some institutions, the RNFA writes an operative note in addition to the surgeon's operative note. The RNFA's note includes a description of the procedure performed, type of suture, methods used for vessel and wound closure, and condition of the patient, which might look like the following:

> Secondary procedure. R common femoral vessels exposure and groin closure for CABG: R CFA/R CFV exposed via transverse incision. Fem-Fem CPB. Vessels without plaque/clots. Inguinal ligament and profunda identified. Following decannulation, vessels free of trauma/injury. R CFA repair/closure with 5-0 interrupted silk. R CFV repair/closure with 5-0 running prolene. Vessels without deformities post closure/repair. Suture lines secure. Groin closed with running 2-0 Dexon and skin with prolene, interrupted mattress. Incision intact, without bleeding/lymphatic drainage. C. C. Hlozek, RN, BSN, RNFA

Postoperative Patient Considerations

The RNFA collaborates with the surgeon, anesthesia, perianesthesia, and critical care team in patient assessment and management. The primary goal of postoperative patient care is to maintain adequate circulation through the vascular repair. Two specific assessment considerations include checking the pulses, temperature, and color of the affected lower extremity, and checking the wound for signs of complications. Urine output, central venous pressure, mental status, and pulse rate and volume are monitored to assess fluid balance. Collaboration between the RNFA and the entire health care team continues throughout the patient's recovery in the intensive care unit, on the regular nursing unit, and upon discharge. Patient education is reiterated during this phase of the perioperative process and continues even when the patient returns for follow-up appointment.

Summary

Patients with peripheral vascular disease are frequently encountered in vascular surgical practice. Diet, smoking, sedentary lifestyles, abnormalities in coagulation, hereditary factors, and the increasing age of patients all contribute to this prevalence. RNFAs on a vascular team need to recognize clinical manifestations of vascular disorders, understand their physiological impact, interpret diagnostic test results that determine the location and extent of the physiological impairment, and participate collaboratively in the surgical or endovascular intervention. Over the past few years, RNFAs have published many articles on specific surgical procedures and techniques that are performed in a variety of practice settings. RNFAs are harvesting vascular conduits (e.g., greater and lesser saphenous vein, inferior epigastric arteries, radial arteries) for vascular and cardiac surgery and performing many types of complex wound closure. To do these procedures, and do them well, RNFAs are meticulous in their technique and follow all basic principles of surgery. Clinical talent combined with a deep sense of professional self and regard for the code of ethics of nursing are the hallmarks of RNFA practice. Thus, RNFAs in vascular surgery, as in other areas of surgical practice, concern themselves with safeguarding and promoting the health, safety, and well-being of their patients, and accept responsibility for assessing and ensuring their own competence, seeking opportunities for professional growth, being accountable for their own actions, and collaborating with other health professionals to improve the quality of care they provide to their patients and the community they serve.[63]

◼ Review Questions

1. The RN first assistant in orthopedics often is involved in trauma patient care. When a patient with a compound fracture of the shaft of the right femur is admitted, the RNFA is present with the trauma team. What is the first thing the nursing team should do?

    a. Cover the patient's open wound.

    b. Determine the patient's blood pressure.

    c. Clean the fracture site.

    d. Assess respiratory status.

2. To determine the presence of effusion in the knee, the RNFA will use

    a. McMurray's test.

    b. Apley's test.

    c. Ballottement.

    d. Passive and active range of motion assessment.

3. A common postoperative device that is patient guided and provides passive exercise is

    a. PCA.

    b. CPM.

    c. TENS.

    d. ROM.

Answer questions 4 through 7 regarding the following scenario: John Carry is admitted for arthroscopic knee surgery.

4. When Mr. Carry's tibiofemoral joint is palpated on each side of the patella, with his leg flexed to 90 degrees, what finding may indicate a damaged meniscus?

    a. Nodules

    b. Edema

    c. Tenderness

    d. Bogginess

5. During preoperative patient education, the RNFA should explain to Mr. Carry

    a. The importance of early weight-bearing.

    b. The type of general anesthesia he will receive.

    c. Methods of crutch walking.

    d. The type of immobilization device used postoperatively.

6. In the postanesthesia care area, the RNFA will be alert to the nursing diagnosis of Altered Peripheral Tissue Perfusion. Accordingly, the RNFA will:

    a. Monitor the neurovascular status of the operative leg.

    b. Encourage range-of-motion exercise of the affected knee to improve tissue perfusion.

    c. Check that perioperative antibiotics have been prescribed.

    d. Encourage Mr. Carry to increase ambulation as tolerated.

7. A potential complication for Mr. Carry is compartment syndrome. If left untreated, this could cause

    a. Gas gangrene.

    b. Necrosis with loss of the extremity.

    c. Liver failure.

    d. Metabolic alkalosis.

8. Following total hip arthroplasty, the RNFA would expect the patient's erythrocyte sedimentation rate to return to perioperative levels within
    a. 1 to 2 months.
    b. 2 to 3 months.
    c. 3 to 6 months.
    d. 6 to 9 months.

9. The antibiotic usually selected for prophylaxis for major orthopedic procedures is a
    a. Cephalosporin.
    b. Second-generation tetracycline.
    c. Penicillin or penicillin derivative.
    d. Aminoglycoside.

10. Which of the following are the physical examination techniques used for assessment of the musculoskeletal system?
    a. Inspection and palpation.
    b. Palpation and percussion.
    c. Inspection and percussion.
    d. Percussion and auscultation.

11. When examining the musculoskeletal system, the extent of the examination depends on the patient's condition and symptoms as guided by which of the following?
    a. Patient reports of tenderness and nonverbal signs of distress
    b. Degree of passive range of motion until RNFA is stopped by joint limitation
    c. Patient's ability to complete active range-of-motion exercises
    d. Patient's pain response elicited on range-of-motion exercises

12. After receiving his pain medication, a patient with a fracture of the humerus complains that his pain is greater than ever. The RNFA assesses the limb, finding palpable pulses, no impingement of the digits by the cast, and rapid capillary refill. The patient complains of pain when his fingers are extended. At this time, the most appropriate analysis by the RNFA is:
    a. The patient may be habituated to his usual pain medication.
    b. The patient may need pain medication more frequently, in smaller doses.
    c. Some increase in pain can be anticipated due to the normal inflammatory response to tissue injury.
    d. Progressive pain may be indicative of a serious complication.

13. On assessment of a 53-year-old male patient scheduled to have all arterial grafts (including radial artery), the RNFA performs Allen's test. The test is positive on the patient's nondominant arm. What action is appropriate?
    a. Do nothing; a positive Allen's test is good.
    b. Tell the patient that he will lose his hand if the radial artery is used.

    c. Document the results in the chart and inform the surgeon.

    d. Ask the anesthesia provider to inform the surgeon.

14. Patients taking vitamin and nutritional supplements are better candidates for surgery and have fewer risk factors.

    a. True

    b. False

15. Results of minimally invasive coronary artery bypass surgery have shown good long-term results.

    a. True

    b. False

16. A patient is scheduled to undergo a minimally invasive procedure on the left anterior descending artery after a failed angioplasty. The RNFA might expect the surgical position of choice to be

    a. Supine or a 30-degree lateral.

    b. Right lateral.

    c. Left lateral.

    d. Modified lawn chair.

17. During the induction of anesthesia in a patient scheduled for reoperation, the RNFA should:

    a. Review the angiogram.

    b. Make postoperative patient rounds.

    c. Assist in monitoring the patient.

    d. Prepare to perform the Sellick maneuver.

18. A primary tool for assessing the chambers for air after valve replacement is:

    a. ECG.

    b. Arterial waveform.

    c. TEE.

    d. MUGA scan.

19. When the greater saphenous vein is to be harvested, the RNFA should:

    a. Assess the quality of the vein in both legs.

    b. Assess the distal pulses.

    c. Question the patient about claudication in either leg.

    d. All of the above.

20. Mr. Smith is a 74-year-old patient whose past surgical history includes a vein stripping on the right leg and previous CABG surgery utilizing the greater saphenous vein on the left. Which conduits should not be considered?

    a. Lesser saphenous vein

    b. Internal mammary artery

    c. Homologous vein

    d. Arm vein

Answer questions 21 through 27 regarding the following scenario: Mrs. Darden is admitted to the hospital with nausea and right upper quadrant pain. After a thorough workup, she is diagnosed with cholecystitis and scheduled for laparoscopic cholecystectomy.

21. During the preoperative interview, Mrs. Darden asks the RNFA about the advantages of laparoscopic cholecystectomy. An appropriate explanation would include
    a. Smaller incisions.
    b. Less postoperative pain and discomfort.
    c. A shortened hospital stay and earlier return to usual activities.
    d. All of the above.

22. The most important question for the RNFA to ask Mrs. Darden during preoperative assessment would concern
    a. Any previous abdominal surgery.
    b. Her menstrual history and possibility of current pregnancy.
    c. Previous episodes of dyspepsia following carbohydrate ingestion.
    d. Frequency of eructation and sensation of fullness.

23. Which of the following would be a relative contraindication to the laparoscopic approach for Mrs. Darden?
    a. The presence of severe pain
    b. Massive obesity
    c. Clay-colored, fatty stools
    d. The need for common duct exploration

24. Most likely, Mrs. Darden will be placed in the supine position with which of the following modifications?
    a. Reverse Trendelenburg, left side elevated
    b. Slight Trendelenburg, right side elevated
    c. Reverse Trendelenburg, right side elevated
    d. Low lithotomy, Trendelenburg

25. Because Mrs. Darden has had previous abdominal surgery, the surgeon and RNFA anticipate abdominal wall adhesions. In this situation, they might decide to change their usual Veress needle entry to
    a. An infraumbilical site.
    b. An open Hasson technique.
    c. A right upper quadrant site.
    d. The cul de sac.

26. To prevent the risk of air embolism or adverse cardiovascular changes in a healthy adult patient like Mrs. Darden, the RNFA will ensure that the intra-abdominal pressure monitor is set for an upper limit of
    a. 4–6 mm Hg.
    b. 6–12 mm Hg.
    c. 12–16 mm Hg.
    d. 16–25 mm Hg.

27. During Mrs. Darden's surgery, the intra-abdominal pressure monitor sounds. The RNFA should first
    a. Discontinue insufflation.
    b. Reduce the flow rate.
    c. Close the trocar valve.
    d. Check for kinks in the insufflation tubing.

28. In which endoscopic knot-tying technique is the knot tied outside the abdomen and slid down the trocar to be secured with a knot pusher?
    a. Extracorporeal
    b. Pretied endoligature
    c. Ski needle technique
    d. Suture-introducing technique

29. To prevent inadvertent thermal injury during laparoscopic electrosurgical coagulation, the RNFA should use
    a. A blend-cut waveform, set on high power.
    b. A coagulation waveform, set on low power, low voltage.
    c. A cutting waveform, set on high power, high voltage, in short bursts.
    d. A cutting waveform set on low power, low voltage.

30. Endoscopy is best utilized in the trauma setting
    a. For small-volume hemothorax, especially in conjunction with another surgical intervention.
    b. For evaluation of a gunshot wound to the abdomen.
    c. For the hypotensive patient with blunt abdominal injury.
    d. For the chest trauma patient with ECG changes.

31. Preoperative laboratory tests for a laparoscopic cholecystectomy patient reveal an elevated amylase level and elevated alkaline phosphatase level. These would alert the RNFA to
    a. Change to an open Hasson technique.
    b. Abort the endoscopic approach.
    c. Have the laparoscopic choledochoscope and baskets available.
    d. Order a postoperative ICU bed.

32. To prevent visceral herniation through a trocar insertion site, the most important consideration is that the RNFA
    a. Use polydiaxanone suture material.
    b. Select a J needle.
    c. Use an upper abdominal port site for desufflation.
    d. Take adequate bites of fascia.

33. Which technique of peritoneal entry poses the least risk of injury to intra-abdominal contents?
    a. Direct trocar entry
    b. Veress needle insertion
    c. Open Hasson technique
    d. Optical trocar

34. Which of the following would the RNFA *not* consider as a risk factor for artherosclerosis?
    a. Diabetes mellitus
    b. Heredity
    c. Smoking
    d. Anemia

35. On postoperative rounds, the RNFA notes that the patient has pain, redness, and edema in the calf. These symptoms may indicate which of the following?
    a. Arterial embolism
    b. Varicose veins
    c. Thrombophlebitis
    d. Compartment syndrome

36. A diabetic patient on NPH insulin will likely need to have the intraoperative dosage of _____ adjusted.
    a. Heparin
    b. Lidocaine
    c. Protamine
    d. Papaverine

37. In clinically determining that the patient has an arterial (rather than venous) insufficiency, the RNFA relies on findings of
    a. Intermittent claudication, decreased pulses.
    b. Aching pain on dependency of extremity.
    c. Normal temperature in extremity but marked edema.
    d. Normal pulses, but ulceration at medial side of ankle.

38. The RNFA is called to the emergency room to suture a clean, simple laceration on an extremity. Based on the RNFA's knowledge of current research, he or she may opt to use
    a. Subcuticular nylon.
    b. Interrupted mattress suture with fine silk.
    c. Octylcyanoacrylate adhesive.
    d. Continuous suture of coated polyester.

39. In devising a patient and family educational intervention, the RNFA would likely use which of the following nursing diagnoses?
    a. Arterial Insufficiency, surgical
    b. Alteration in Tissue Perfusion
    c. High Risk for Pulmonary Embolism secondary to thrombophlebitis
    d. Potential for Compartment Syndrome

40. The two main properties of arteries are
    a. Elasticity and contractility.
    b. Capacitance and distensibility.
    c. Elastic tissue and smooth collagen fibers.
    d. Hydrostatic pressure and colloid osmotic pressure.

41. When taking the history of Mr. Smith, the RNFA notes that he has sought health care advice because he has been experiencing pain in exercising his muscles, particularly in his calf; the pain recedes when he rests. The RNFA would label this physiological response to vascular dysfunction
    a. Ischemia.
    b. Reactive exercise intolerance.
    c. Intermittent claudication.
    d. Decreased mobility.

42. During carotid endarterectomy, the anesthesia provider notes an abnormal EEG. The RNFA may therefore anticipate the need to
    a. Administer heparin, as the patient is likely having a CVA.
    b. Massage the carotid sinus.
    c. Lighten the anesthesia and proceed with a quick closure.
    d. Assist in inserting a carotid shunt.

43. Suture selection by the RNFA for vascular anastomoses should be guided by the need for material that is
    a. Nonreactive and nonabsorbable.
    b. Inert, synthetic and absorbable.
    c. Nonabsorbable, with interstices to promote clotting.
    d. Coated to decrease tissue drag, absorbable or nonabsorbable.

44. RNFAs on a vascular surgery team need to be able to interpret diagnostic test results. The "gold standard" for anatomical diagnosis is
    a. A directed physical examination.
    b. A noninvasive study, such as CT or MRI.
    c. A cost-effective, simple study that can be performed in the office.
    d. Angiography.

45. The *Code of Ethics for Nursing* suggests that RNFAs
    a. Obtain a BSN.
    b. Become certified (CRNFA).
    c. Assess and ensure their competency.
    d. Expand their roles to include preoperative patient education.

◻ Answer Key

1. d	6. a	10. a
2. c	7. b	11. a
3. b	8. c	12. d
4. c	9. a	13. c
5. c		

14. False. Some vitamins and nutritional supplements have the potential to increase the risk for bleeding, especially when taken with other antiplatelet agents.

15. False. While some of these procedures have had "good" results, the long-term effects (such as a possible increase in the need for postoperative stenting or angioplasty, the necessity of earlier repeat surgery for obstructed grafts, or the need to

bypass additional vessels because of incomplete revascularization) have not been fully researched.

16. a	26. c	36. c
17. c	27. d	37. a
18. c	28. a	38. c
19. d	29. d	39. b
20. both c and d	30. a	40. a
21. d	31. c	41. c
22. a	32. d	42. d
23. b	33. c	43. a
24. c	34. d	44. d
25. b	35. c	45. c

REFERENCES

1. Goldman D, Brown F, Guarnieri D: Perioperative Medicine, 2nd ed. New York, McGraw-Hill, 1994, p 139
2. Horne M: Involving physicians in clinical pathways: An example for perioperative knee arthroplasty. Qual Improve 22(2):115–124, 1996
3. Murphy J: Critical pathways and standardization: Useful tools for improving patient care. Proceedings of the 1997 World Conference of Operating Room Nurses—X, September 1997
4. Lagoe RJ, Aspling DL: Benchmarking and clinical pathway implementation on a multihospital basis. Nurs Ecomomic$ 15(3):131–137, 1997
5. Seidel HM, Ball JW, Dains JE, Benedict GW: Mosby's Guide to Physical Examination. St Louis, CV Mosby, 1996, pp 686–689
6. Grindel CG: Building nursing's minimum data set: The results of a pilot study. Medsurg Nurs 5(6):449–456, 1996
7. Salerno E, Willen J: Pain Management Handbook. St Louis, CV Mosby, 1996, pp 25–26, 233–241
8. Dougherty SH: Prosthetic devices. In: American College of Surgeons: Care of the Surgical Patient. New York, Scientific American Medicine, 1991, pp 2.1–2.22
9. Cuckler JM, et al: Diagnosis and management of infected total joint arthroplasty. Orthop Clin North Am 22:523–530, 1991
10. Association of Operating Room Nurses: Recommended Practices for Use of Pneumatic Tourniquet. In: AORN Standards, Recommended Practices and Guidelines. Denver, Colo, Association of Operating Room Nurses, 1997, pp 231–236
11. Mailhot C: Mini-coronary artery bypass grafting. Nurs Management 27(6):56–57, 1996
12. Mizell J: Minimally invasive direct coronary bypass surgery. Crit Care Nurse 17(3):22–27, 1997
13. Mathias JM: MIS techniques could transform heart surgery. OR Manager 12(7):1, 1996
14. Kinney MR, Burfitt SN, Stullenbarger E, Rees B, Debolt MR: Quality of life in cardiac patient research: A meta-analysis. Nurs Res 45(3):173–176, 1996
15. Frye RL (for the Writing Group for the Bypass Angioplasty Revascularization [BARI] Investigators): Five-year clinical and functional outcome comparing bypass surgery and angioplasty in patients with multivessel coronary disease. JAMA 277(9):715–721, 1997
16. Oxman TE: Lack of social participation or religious strength and comfort as risk factors for death after cardiac surgery in the elderly. Psychosom Med 57:5–15, 1995

17. Reyes AT: Technique for harvesting the radial artery as a coronary artery bypass graft. Ann Thorac Surg 59:118–126, 1995

18. Reardon MJ: Coronary artery bypass conduits: Review of current status. J Cardiovasc Surg 38:201–209, 1997

19. Petry J: Nutritional supplements and the surgical patient. AORN J 65(6):1117–1121, 1997

20. Coulson AS, Backshaw S, Quarnstrom J, Mayer K, Holmes K, Villareal M: Minimally invasive direct coronary bypass surgery. AORN J 66(6):1012–1037, 1997

21. Oetker-Black S, Teeters D, Cukr P, Rininger S: Self-efficacy enhanced preoperative instruction. AORN J 66(5):854–864, 1997

22. Cupples S: Effects of timing and reinforcement of preoperative education on knowledge of patients having coronary artery bypass surgery. Heart Lung 20:654–660, 1991

23. Czar ML: Perceived learning needs of patients with coronary artery disease using a questionnaire assessment tool. Heart Lung 26:109–117, 1997

24. Hankela S, Kiikkala I: Intraoperative nursing care as experienced by surgical patients. AORN J 63(2):435–442, 1997

25. Carr JA, Powers MJ: Stressors associated with coronary artery bypass surgery. Nurs Res Nurs Health 14:173–178, 1991

26. Lynn-McHale DJ: Preoperative ICU tours: Are they helpful? Am J Crit Care 6(2):106–115, 1997

27. Vaca K: Nursing care of patients undergoing thoracoscopic minimally invasive bypass grafting. Am J Crit Care 6(2):281–286, 1997

28. Moore SM: Development of discharge information for recovery after coronary artery bypass surgery. Appl Nurs Res 7(4):170–177, 1994

29. Scott-Conner C, Dawson DL: Operative Anatomy. Philadelphia, JB Lippincott Co, 1993, pp 633–635

30. Conant P, Miller SK: Techniques in coronary artery bypass. Point of View 35(3):17–21, 1997

31. Wollan DL: Removal of epicardial pacing wires: an expanded role for nurses. Prog Cardiovasc Nurs 10(4):21–26, 1995

32. Thomson SC: Chest tube removal after cardiac surgery. Crit Care Nurse 17(1):34–38, 1997

33. Davis CJ, Filipi CJ: A history of endoscopic surgery. In Arrugui ME, Fitzgibboms RJ Jr, Katkhouda J, McKernan JB, Reich H, eds: Principles of Laparoscopic Surgery: Basic and Advanced Techniques. New York, Springer-Verlag, 1995, pp 3–20

34. Langer BL, Taylor BR: Biliary tract procedures. In: American College of Surgeons: Care of the Surgical Patient, Chap 11, Surgical Techniques. New York, Scientific American Medicine, 1997, pp 1–17

35. Smith DA: Hernia repair. In Meeker MM, Rothrock JC, eds: Alexander's Care of the Patient in Surgery, 11th ed. St Louis, CV Mosby, in press

36. Rusch V: Thoracoscopy. In: American College of Surgeons: Care of the Surgical Patient. Surgical Technique Supplement no.2. New York, Scientific American Medicine, 1993

37. Salvino C, Pulawski G, Geis P: The use of laparoscopy in trauma. In Arregui ME, et al, eds: Principles of Laparoscopic Surgery: Basic and Advanced Techniques. New York, Springer-Verlag, 1995, pp 379–395

38. Kessler R: Modern diagnostic and therapeutic thoracoscopy. In Hunter JG, Sackier JM eds: Minimally Invasive Surgery. New York, McGraw-Hill, 1993, pp 329–337

39. Abboud PA, Malet PF, Berlin JA: Predictors of common bile duct stones prior to cholecystectomy: A meta-analysis. AHCPR Res Highlights 204:8, 1997

40. Fried G: Laparoscopic cholecystectomy. In: American College of Surgeons: Care of the Surgical Patient. Surgical Technique Supplement no.4. New York, Scientific American Medicine, 1994

41. Leahy PF: Low anterior resection. In Ballantyne GH, Leahy PF, Modlin IM, eds: Laparoscopic Surgery. Philadelphia, WB Saunders Co, 1994, pp 575–582

42. Flowers JL, Zucker KA, Bailey RW: Complications. In Ballantyne GH, Leahy PF, Modlin IM, eds. Laparoscopic Surgery. Philadelphia, WB Saunders Co, 1994, pp 77–91

43. Wehlage MB: Anesthetic implications of laparoscopy, thoracoscopy, and hysteroscopy. In Arregui ME, et al, eds: Principles of Laparoscopic Surgery: Basic and Advanced Techniques. New York, Springer-Verlag, 1995, pp 79–85

44. Milsom PJ: Closed and open techniques of trocar insertion. In Ballantyne GH, Leahy PF, Modlin IM, eds: Laparoscopic Surgery. Philadelphia, WB Saunders Co, 1994, pp 97–106

45. Svenberg J: Pathophysiology of pneumoperitoneum. In Ballantyne GH, Leahy PF, Modlin IM, eds: Laparoscopic Surgery. Philadelphia, WB Saunders Co, 1994, pp 61–68

46. Odell RC: Laparoscopic electrosurgery. In Hunter JG, Sackiler JM, eds: Minimally Invasive Surgery. New York, McGraw-Hill, 1993, pp 33–41

47. Kirshenbaum G, Temple DR: Active electrode monitoring in laparoscopy: A surgeon's perspective. Surg Serv Management 2(2):46–49, 1996

48. Tucker RD, Voyles R: Laparoscopic electrosurgical complications and their prevention. AORN J 62(1):51–71, 1995

49. Szabo Z: Laparoscopic suturing and tissue approximation. In Hunter JG, Sackier JM, eds: Minimally Invasive Surgery. New York, McGraw-Hill, 1993, pp 141–154

50. Cooperman AM: Complications of laparoscopic surgery. In Arregui ME, et al, eds: Principles of Laparoscopic Surgery: Basic and Advanced Techniques. New York, Springer-Verlag, 1995, pp 71–76

51. Bolufer JM, Delgado F, Blanes F, Martinez-Abad M, Canos JI, Martin J, Oliver MJ: Injury in laparoscopic surgery. Surg Laparosc Endosc 5(4):318–323, 1996

52. Conlon KC, Curtin J: A simple technique for the closure of laparoscopic trocar wounds. J Am Coll Surg 181:565–566, 1995

53. Haimovici H: Vascular Surgery: Principles and Techniques. Connecticut, Appleton & Lange, 1989, pp 100–120

54. Laurendeau F: French contribution to vascular surgery. Can J Surg 31:221–223, 1988

55. Hlozek CC, Zacharias WM: The RN first assistant's role during inferior epigastric artery harvesting. AORN J 65:26–29, 1997

56. Groetzsch GA: RN first assisting—1997 Canadian update. Can OR Nurs J 15:13–17, 1997

57. Owings JT, Kennedy JP, Blaisdell FW: Injuries to the extremities. In: American College of Surgeons: Care of the Surgical Patient, section IX, chap 4. New York, Scientific American Medicine, 1997, pp 11-1–11-16

58. Quinn J, Wells G, Sutcliffe T, Jarmuske M, Maw J, Stiell I, Johns P: A randomized trial comparing octylcyanoacrylate tissue adhesive and sutures in the management of lacerations. JAMA 277:1527–1530, 1997

59. Larsen LL, Thurston NE: Research utilization: Development of a central venous catheter procedure. Appl Nurs Res 10(1):44–51, 1997

60. Liston SM: Stent-graft placement procedures for descending thoracic aortic aneurysms. AORN J 66:433–444, 1997

61. Clinical pathways: CareMaps used in perioperative patient care. OR Manager 13:18–20, 1997

62. Colburn MD, Moore WS: Cerebrovascular disease. In Ritchie WP, Steele G, Dean RH, eds: General Surgery. Philadelphia, JB Lippincott, 1995, p 598

63. Code of ethics for nursing. Washington, DC, American Nurses Association, 1998

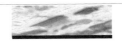

I

AORN Official Statement on RN First Assistants

Preamble

Perioperative nursing practice has historically included the role of the RN as assistant at surgery. As early as 1980, documents issued by the American College of Surgeons supported the appropriateness for qualified RNs to first assist.

AORN officially recognized this role as a component of perioperative nursing in 1983 and adopted the first Official Statement on RN First Assistants (RNFA) in 1984. All state boards of nursing recognize the RNFA role as being within the scope of nursing practice.

AORN's official statement delineates the definition, scope of practice, qualifications, educational requirements, and clinical privileges that must be met by the perioperative nurse who practices as an RNFA. AORN further recognizes the need for appropriate compensation/reimbursement to RNs who fulfill this role in providing perioperative patient care.

Definition of RN First Assistant

The RN first assistant at surgery collaborates with the surgeon and the health care team in performing a safe operation with optimal outcomes for the patient. The RN first assistant practices perioperative nursing and must have acquired the necessary knowledge, skills, and judgment specific to clinical practice. The RN first assistant practices in collaboration with and at the direction of the surgeon during the intraoperative phase of the perioperative experience. The RN first assistant does not concurrently function as the scrub nurse.

Scope of Practice

The scope of practice of the nurse performing as first assistant is a part of perioperative nursing practice. Perioperative nursing is a specialized area of practice. The activities included in first assisting are further refinements of perioperative nursing practice which are executed within the context of the nursing process. The observable nursing behaviors are based on an extensive body of scientific knowledge. These intraoperative nursing behaviors may include:

- handling tissue,
- providing exposure,
- using instruments,
- suturing, and
- providing hemostasis.

These behaviors may vary depending on patient populations, practice environments, services provided, accessibility of human and fiscal resources, institutional policy, and state nurse practice acts.

The decision by an RN to practice as a first assistant must be made voluntarily and deliberately, with an understanding of the professional accountability that the role entails.

QUALIFICATIONS OF THE RN FIRST ASSISTANT

Qualifications for RN first assistants should include, but not be limited to:

- certification in perioperative nursing (CNOR);
- documentation of proficiency in perioperative nursing practice as both a scrub and circulating nurse;
- ability to apply principles of asepsis and infection control;
- knowledge of surgical anatomy, physiology, pathophysiology, and operative technique related to the operative procedures in which the RN assists;
- ability to perform cardiopulmonary resuscitation;
- ability to perform effectively in stressful and emergency situations;
- ability to recognize safety hazards and initiate appropriate preventive and corrective action;
- ability to perform effectively and harmoniously as a member of the operative team;
- ability to demonstrate skill in behaviors unique to the RN first assistant (as defined);
- meets requirements of statutes, regulations, and institutional policies relevant to RN first assistants; and
- successful completion of the RNFA program that meets the AORN Recommended Education Standards for RN First Assistant Programs.

PREPARATION FOR THE RN FIRST ASSISTANT

The complexity of knowledge and skill required to effectively care for recipients of operating room nursing services compels nurses to be well educated and to continue their education beyond generic nursing programs.[1]

Perioperative nurses who wish to practice as RN first assistants must develop a set of cognitive, psychomotor, and affective behaviors that demonstrate accountability and responsibility for identifying and meeting the needs of the recipients of their nursing services.

Development of this set of behaviors begins with and builds upon the education program leading to licensure as an RN, which provides basic knowledge, skills, and attitudes essential to the practice of perioperative nursing. Further preparation for the RN first assistant includes perioperative nursing practice with diversified experience in scrubbing and circulating. This should culminate in the nurse achieving certification as a CNOR. Additional preparation is then acquired through completion of an RNFA program which meets the AORN Recommended Education Standards for RN First Assistant Programs.

These programs should consist of curricula that address all of the content areas of the modules in the Core Curriculum for the RN First Assistant, take place in, or in collaboration with, institutions approved by the appropriate regional accrediting body for higher education,[2] and award college/university credits and a certificate upon satisfactory completion of all requirements.

ESTABLISHMENT OF CLINICAL PRIVILEGES FOR THE RN FIRST ASSISTANT

To determine if an RN qualifies for clinical privileges as a first assistant, an approval process must be established by the institution in which the individual will practice.

The process for granting clinical privileges should include mechanisms for:

- assessing individual qualifications for practice,
- assessing continuing proficiency,
- evaluating annual performance,
- assessing compliance with relevant institutional and departmental policies,
- defining lines of accountability,
- retrieving documentation of participation as first assistant, and
- establishing systems for peer review.

Each RN first assistant demonstrates behaviors that progress on a continuum from basic competency to excellence. Once having met the educational and experiential requirements, the RNFA is encouraged to achieve and maintain certification (CRNFA) for this specific role.

Submitted: 3/84
Adopted: 3/5/84
House of Delegates, Atlanta
Proposed Revision to Board: 9/92
Adopted: 3/4/93
House of Delegates, Anaheim, California
Proposed Revision to Board: 11/97
Adopted: 4/2/98
House of Delegates, Orlando, Florida

Notes

1. "A model for perioperative nursing practice," in *AORN Standards, Recommended Practices, and Guidelines* (Denver: Association of Operating Room Nurses, Inc, 1997) 77.
2. Academic accreditation is awarded by the six regional Associations of Colleges and Schools: Middle States, New England, North Central, Northwest, Southern, and Western.

Suggested Reading

American College of Surgeons. "Statements on principles." *Socioeconomic Factbook for Surgery 1996-1997*. Chicago: American College of Surgeons, 1996.

Association of Operating Room Nurses, Inc. *Core Curriculum for the RN First Assistant*. Denver: Association of Operating Room Nurses, Inc, 1994.

Association of Operating Room Nurses, Inc. "Perioperative patient care quality." *1997-1998 Chapter Resource Manual*. Denver: Association of Operating Room Nurses, Inc, 1997.

"Competency statements in perioperative nursing." In *AORN Standards, Recommended Practices, and Guidelines*. Denver: Association of Operating Room Nurses, Inc, 1997, 81.

Joint Commission on Accreditation of Healthcare Organizations. *Comprehensive Accreditation Manual for Hospitals*. Oakbrook Terrace, Ill: Joint Commission on Accreditation of Healthcare Organizations, 1996.

"Medicare and Medicaid programs: Revisions to conditions of participation for hospitals-HCFA; Final rule," *Federal Register* 59 (Dec 13, 1994) 64141-64153.

"Standards of perioperative nursing." In *AORN Standards, Recommended Practices, and Guidelines* (Denver: Association of Operating Room Nurses, Inc, 1997) 105.

II

AORN RECOMMENDED EDUCATION STANDARDS FOR RN FIRST ASSISTANT PROGRAMS

Please note: *When choosing an RNFA program, prospective students are advised to use these recommended education standards to evaluate each program under consideration. Although programs meeting these standards are considered to be of high quality, there is no formal approval or accreditation process in place. Therefore, any claim that a program is "approved" or "accredited" by AORN or the RNFA Specialty Assembly is inaccurate.*

I. PROGRAM OVERVIEW

The RN first assistant (RNFA) program is designed to provide the experienced perioperative nurse with the advanced preparation necessary to assume the role of the first assistant. These programs are equivalent to one year of formal, academic post-basic nursing study and should consist of curricula that address all of the content areas of the modules in the *Core Curriculum for the RN First Assistant*,[1] take place in colleges and universities approved by appropriate regional accrediting bodies for higher education, and award college credits and degrees or certificates of RNFA status upon satisfactory completion of all requirements.

Using a multidisciplinary faculty and a variety of instructional methodologies, these programs focus on expanded perioperative nursing concepts and nursing behaviors using the nursing process as the basis for providing nursing care to patients experiencing surgical intervention. Based on the *Core Curriculum for the RN First Assistant*, the structured didactic and supervised clinical learning activities prepare the perioperative nurse with the cognitive, psychomotor, and affective behaviors necessary to assume the role of the first assistant.

AORN's official statement on the role of the RN first assistant should be recognized by all schools offering RN first assistant programs.

II. Target Audience

Registered nurses who practice perioperative nursing.

III. Preadmission Requirements

A. General

General preadmission requirements are facility-determined and may include:

1. Complete physical exam or current health record.
2. Complete dental exam or current dental record.
3. Current tetanus immunization (within a 10-year period).
4. Mantoux test (PPD). If Mantoux test is positive, a chest x-ray is required.
5. Hepatavax form—either copy of Hepatavax record or signed statement refusing Hepatavax.
6. Completed application and tuition fee.
7. Curriculum vitae or resume.
8. Photograph.

B. Specific, Didactic

Specific didactic requirements may include the following.

1. Must be a registered nurse, graduated from an accredited school of nursing.
2. Must be licensed to practice as a registered nurse in the state in which the clinical internship will be accomplished.
3. Must provide proof of RN licensure.
4. Experience: The RNFA candidate must have a minimum of two years of recent perioperative nursing experience. This experience must include demonstrated competency in the scrubbing, circulating, or first assisting roles of the intraoperative nursing dimension.
5. CNOR: Must be CNOR, or CNOR eligible with CNOR status obtained before a certificate of program completion awarded. All students must submit verification of CNOR status.
6. CPR: Cardiopulmonary resuscitation (CPR) or basic cardiac life support certification (BCLS) required, advanced cardiac life support (ACLS) preferred.
7. Recommendations: Must submit two letters of recommendation that validate:
   a. One's proficiency in the roles of scrubbing, circulating, or first assisting.
   b. One's ability to perform effectively in stressful and emergency situations.
   c. One's ability to perform effectively and harmoniously as a team member.
   d. One's ability to perform effectively as a leader.

C. Specific, Clinical

Specific clinical requirements may include the following.

1. Must successfully complete all requirements of didactic component of course before beginning the supervised clinical internship.
2. Must provide proof of current personal professional liability insurance specific for RN first assistants.
3. Must provide proof of current CPR, BCLS, or ACLS certification.

IV. Structured Didactic Component

A. Content Overview

The didactic component is designed to provide the RNFA candidate with the intellectual concepts and the manual techniques necessary to assume the role of first assisting. Emphasis is placed upon the RNFA's independent nursing behaviors, which encompass preoperative assessment, postoperative evaluation, and patient education. Nursing diagnosis is stressed as the basis for planning, implementing, and evaluating outcomes of patient care.

The expanded functions unique to the RN first assistant during surgical intervention are emphasized as the RNFA candidate is prepared to assume responsibility in advanced surgical assisting skills such as providing exposure, tissue handling, suturing, providing hemostasis, and using surgical instruments. The collaborative and interdependent relationships of the surgeon-physician, nurse, and patient are stressed. The combination of this intellectual knowledge and manual dexterity prepares the qualified perioperative nurse with the essential skills necessary to function in this expanded professional role. Objectives are based on the *Core Curriculum for the RN First Assistant.*

B. Faculty

Minimum faculty requirements should include:

1. Master's-prepared or ARNP perioperative nurse.
2. Registered nurse who is both a CNOR and RNFA/CRNFA.
3. Board-certified surgeon.

C. Length of Program

The structured, didactic component should be a minimum of one academic semester of study, including student assignments, classroom instruction, and laboratory practicum.

D. Teaching Methodologies

Teaching methodologies should include, but not be limited to, lecture, discussion, independent study requirements, audiovisual aids, demonstrating/return demonstration, and laboratory practicums on suturing and knot-tying.

E. Evaluation Methodologies

Evaluation methodologies should include, but not be limited to, written examinations, laboratory practicums, nursing care plans, and required independent learning assignments.

F. TEXTBOOKS

1. *Required texts* should be
   Core Curriculum for the RN First Assistant
   The current edition of *AORN Standards, Recommended Practices, and Guidelines*[2]
   A clinical surgery text of choice
   A physical assessment text of choice
   An anatomy and physiology text of choice
2. *Recommended textbooks* should include
   The RN First Assistant: An Expanded Perioperative Nursing Role[3]
   A perioperative nursing text of choice
   A nursing process/nursing diagnosis text of choice
   A diagnostic test information text of choice.

V. SUPERVISED CLINICAL INTERNSHIP

A. CONTENT OVERVIEW

The RNFA clinical internship exists for the purpose of offering the necessary clinical preparation for perioperative nurses in assuming the expanded role of first assisting. This is a supervised clinical learning experience and is mutually planned by both the student and his or her primary mentor to cover a wide variety of surgical interventions dependent upon individual learning needs. Each student should have an active part in determining objectives, identifying learning resources, and evaluating attainment of goals for his or her individual learning needs.

The primary mentor for this internship should be a surgeon who has agreed to fulfill the mentoring role and who will assist the student in acquiring the knowledge and developing the skills necessary to adequately assist the surgeon and patient during surgical intervention. When feasible, an RNFA/CRNFA also should be appointed as a mentor for the clinical internship.

B. FACULTY

Minimum faculty requirements should include:

1. A surgeon in the student's primary area of practice.
2. RNFA program faculty.

C. LENGTH OF PROGRAM

The supervised clinical internship should be a minimum of one academic semester of study, with an institution-determined number of clinical hours specific to the role of the RN first assistant.

D. TEACHING METHODOLOGIES

Teaching methodologies should include, but not be limited to, physician-supervised clinical activities, assigned independent learning activities, self-evaluative learning diary, clinical case study project, and surgical intervention participation log.

E. Evaluation Methodologies

Evaluation methodologies should include, but not be limited to, completion of assigned independent learning activities, self-evaluative learning diary, clinical case study project, surgical intervention participation log, and mentor evaluations.

Students must satisfactorily complete all requirements. The RNFA program faculty reviews all documentation and the surgeon/RNFA preceptor provides a summative evaluation and recommendation based on all required learning activities.

> These recommended education standards were developed by the RN First Assistant Specialty Assembly in July 1994 and were approved by the AORN Board of Directors in November 1994.
>
> Originally published March 1995, AORN Journal. Revised November 1995.
>
> Revised October 1996; approved by the AORN Board of Directors in November 1996.

Notes

1. R E Vaiden, V J Fox, J C Rothrock, eds, *Core Curriculum for the RN First Assistant* (Denver: Association of Operating Room Nurses, Inc, 1994).
2. Association of Operating Room Nurses, *AORN Standards, Recommended Practices, and Guidelines* (Denver: Association of Operating Room Nurses, Inc, 1997).
3. J C Rothrock, *The RN First Assistant: An Expanded Perioperative Role*, second ed (Philadelphia: J B Lippincott Co, 1993).

III

DIAGNOSTIC STUDIES
AND THEIR MEANING

ABBREVIATIONS

CONVENTIONAL UNITS

kg	= kilogram	mM	= millimole
gm	= gram	nM	= nanomole
mg	= milligram	mOsm	= milliosmole
μg	= microgram	mm	= millimeter
μμg	= micromicrogram	μ	= micron or micrometer
ng	= nanogram	mm Hg	= millimeters of mercury
pg	= picogram	U	= unit
dL	= 100 milliliters	mU	= milliunit
mL	= milliliter	μU	= microunit
cu mm	= cubic millimeter	mEq	= milliequivalent
fL	= femtoliter	IU	= International Unit
		mIU	= milliInternational Unit

SI UNITS

g	= gram
L	= liter
d	= day
h	= hour
mol	= mole
mmol	= millimole
μmol	= micromole
nmol	= nanomole
pmol	= picomole

REFERENCE RANGES—HEMATOLOGY*

Determination	REFERENCE RANGE		Clinical Significance
	Conventional Units	*SI Units*	
A$_2$ hemoglobin	1.5%–3.5% of total hemoglobin	Mass fraction: 0.015–0.035 of total hemoglobin	Increased in certain types of thalassemia
Bleeding time	1–9 min	2–8 min	Prolonged in thrombocytopenia, defective platelet function, and aspirin therapy

(continued)

REFERENCE RANGES—HEMATOLOGY* (*continued*)

Determination	REFERENCE RANGE		Clinical Significance
	Conventional Units	*SI Units*	
Factor V assay (pro-accelerin factor)	60%–140%		
Favor VIII assay (anti-hemophiliac factor)	50%–200%		Deficient in classical hemophilia
Factor IX assay (plasma thromboplastin component)	75%–125%		Deficient in Christmas disease (pseudohemophilia)
Factor X (Stuart factor)	60%–140%		Deficient in Stuart clotting defect
Fibrinogen	200–400 mg/dL	2–4 g/dL	Increased in pregnancy, infections accompanied by leukocytosis, nephrosis
			Decreased in severe liver disease, abruptio placentae
Fibrin split products	Less than 10 mg/L	Less than 10 mg/L	Increased in disseminated intravascular coagulation
Fibrinolysins (whole blood clot lysis time)	No lysis in 24 h		Increased activity associated with massive hemorrhage, extensive surgery, transfusion reactions
Partial thromboplastin time (activated)	20–45 sec		Prolonged in deficiency of fibrinogen, factors II, V, VIII, IX, X, XI, and XII, and in heparin therapy
Prothrombin consumption	Over 20 sec		Impaired in deficiency of factors VIII, IX, and X
Prothrombin time INR	9.5–12 sec 1.0		Prolonged by deficiency of factors I, II, V, VIII, and X, fat malabsorption, severe liver disease, coumarin-anticoagulant therapy. INR used to standardize the prothombin time and anticoagulation therapy
Erythrocyte count	Males: 4,600,000–6,200,000/cu mm	$4.6–6.2 \times 10^{12}$/L	Increased in severe diarrhea and dehydration, polycythemia, acute poisoning, pulmonary fibrosis
	Females: 4,200,000–5,400,000/cu mm	$4.2–5.4 \times 10^{12}$/L	Decreased in all anemias, in leukemia, and after hemorrhage, when blood volume has been restored
Erythrocyte indices			
Mean corpuscular volume (MCV)	80–94 (cu µ)	80–90 fL	Increased in macrocytic anemias; decreased in microcytic anemia
Mean corpuscular hemoglobin (MCH)	27–32 µµg/cell	27–32 pg	Increased in macrocytic anemias; decreased in microcytic anemia
Mean corpuscular hemoglobin concentration (MCHC)	33%–38%	Concentration fraction: 0.33–0.38	Decreased in severe hypochromic anemia

(continued)

REFERENCE RANGES—HEMATOLOGY* (*continued*)

| Determination | REFERENCE RANGE | | Clinical Significance |
	Conventional Units	*SI Units*	
Reticulocytes	0.5%–1.5% of red cells	Number fraction: 0.005–0.015	Increased with any condition stimulating increase in bone marrow activity (ie, infection, blood loss [acute and chronic]); following iron therapy in iron deficiency anemia, polycythemia rubra vera Decreased with any condition depressing bone marrow activity, acute leukemia, late stage of severe anemias
Erythrocyte sedimentation rate (ESR)—Westergren method	Males under 50 yr: <15mm/h	<15mm/h	Increased in tissue destruction, whether inflammatory or degenerative; during menstruation and pregnancy; and in acute febrile diseases
	Males over 50 yr: <20 mm/h	<20 mm/h	
	Females under 50 yr: <20 mm/h	<20 mm/h	
	Females over 50 yr: <30 mm/h	<30 mm/h	
Erythrocyte sedimentation ratio—Zeta centrifuge	41%–50% in both sexes	Fraction: 0.41–0.54	Significance similar to ESR
Hematocrit	Males:42%–50%	Volume fraction: 0.42–0.5	Decreased in severe anemias, anemia of pregnancy, acute massive blood loss
	Females: 40%–48%	Volume fraction: 0.4–0.48	Increased in erythrocytosis of any cause, and in dehydration or hemoconcentration associated with shock
Hemoglobin	Males: 13–18 g/dL	2.02–2.79 mmol/L	Decreased in various anemias, pregnancy, severe or prolonged hemorrhage, and with excessive fluid intake
	Females: 12–16 gm/dL	1.86–2.48 mmol/L	
			Increased in polycythemia, chronic obstructive pulmonary disease, failure of oxygenation because of congestive heart failure, and normally in people living at high altitudes
Hemoglobin F	Less than 2% of total hemoglobin	Mass fraction: <0.02	Increased in infants and children, and in thalassemia and many anemias
Leukocyte alkaline phosphatase	Score of 40–100		Increased in polycythemia vera, myelofibrosis, and infections Decreased in chronic granulocytic leukemia, paroxysmal nocturnal hemoglobinuria, hypoplastic marrow, and viral infections, particularly infectious mononucleosis

(*continued*)

REFERENCE RANGES—HEMATOLOGY* (*continued*)

Determination	REFERENCE RANGE		Clinical Significance
	Conventional Units	*SI Units*	
Leukocyte count	Total: 5,000–10,000/cu mm	5–10×10^9/L	Elevated in acute infectious diseases, predominantly in the neutrophilic fraction with bacterial diseases, and in the lymphocytic and monocytic fractions in viral diseases
Neutrophils	60%–70%	Number fraction: 0.6–0.7	
Eosinophils	1%–4%	Number fraction: 0.01–0.04	
Basophils	0%–0.5%	Number fraction: 0.00–0.05	Elevated in acute leukemia, following menstruation, and following surgery or trauma
Lymphocytes	20%–30%	Number fraction: 0.2–0.3	Depressed in aplastic anemia, agranulocytosis, and by toxic agents such as chemotherapeutic agents used in treating malignancy
Monocytes	2%–6%	Number fraction: 0.02–0.06	
			Eosinophils elevated in collagen disease, allergy, intestinal parasitosis
Osmotic fragility of red cells	Increased if hemolysis occurs in over 0.5% NaCl Decreased if hemolysis is incomplete in 0.3% NaCl		Increased in congenital spherocytosis, idiopathic acquired hemolytic anemia, isoimmune hemolytic disease, ABO hemolytic disease of newborn Decreased in sickle cell anemia, thalassemia
Platelet count	100,000–400,000/cu mm	0.1–0.4×10^{12}/L	Increased in malignancy, myeloproliferative disease, rheumatoid arthritis, and postoperatively; about 50% of patients with unexpected increase of platelet count will be found to have a malignancy Decreased in thrombocytopenic purpura, acute leukemia, aplastic anemia, and during cancer chemotherapy, infections, and drug reactions

*Laboratory values vary according to the techniques used in different laboratories.

REFERENCE RANGES—SERUM, PLASMA, AND WHOLE BLOOD CHEMISTRIES

Determination	NORMAL ADULT REFERENCE RANGE		CLINICAL SIGNIFICANCE	
	Conventional Units	*SI Units*	*Increased*	*Decreased*
Acetoacetate	0.2–1.0 mg/dL	19.6–98 μmol/L	Diabetic acidosis Fasting	
Acetone	0.3–2.0 mg/dL	51.6–344.0 μmol/L	Toxemia of pregnancy Carbohydrate-free diet High-fat diet	
Acid, total phosphatase	0–11 UL	0–11 UL	Carcinoma of prostate Advanced Paget's disease Hyperparathyroidism Gaucher's disease	
Acid, phosphatase, prostatic—RIA	0–10 ng/mL Borderline: 2.5–3.3 IU/L	0–10 μg/L	Carcinoma of prostate	
Alkaline phosphatase	Adults: 30–115 mU/mL	30–115 μ/L	Conditions reflecting increased osteoblastic activity of bone Rickets Hyperparathyroidism Liver disease	
Alkaline phosphatase, thermostable fraction	Thermostable fraction >35%: hepatic disease and combined disease with predominant hepatic component Thermostable fraction between 25% and 35%: combined hepatic and skeletal disease Thermostable fraction <25%: skeletal disease with increased osteoblastic activity		Hepatic disease	

(continued)

REFERENCE RANGES—SERUM, PLASMA, AND WHOLE BLOOD CHEMISTRIES (*continued*)

| Determination | NORMAL ADULT REFERENCE RANGE | | CLINICAL SIGNIFICANCE | |
	Conventional Units	*SI Units*	*Increased*	*Decreased*
Adrenocorticotropic hormone (ACTH) (plasma)—RIA	Less than 50 pg/mL	Less than 50 mg/L	Pituitary-dependent Cushing's syndrome Ectopic ACTH syndrome Primary adrenal atrophy	Adrenocortical tumor Adrenal insufficiency secondary to hypopituitarism
Aldolase	3–8 Sibley-Lehninger U/dL at 37°C	22–59 mU/L at 37°C	Hepatic necrosis Granulocytic leukemia Myocardial infarction Skeletal muscle disease	
Aldosterone (plasma)—RIA	Supine: 3–10 ng/dL Upright: 5–30 ng/dL Adrenal vein: 200–800 ng/dL	0.08–0.30 nmol/L 0.14–0.90 nmol/L 5.54–22.16 nmol/L	Primary aldosteronism (Conn's syndrome) Secondary aldosteronism	Addison's disease
Alpha-1-antitrypsin	200–400 mg/dL	2–4 g/L		Certain forms of chronic lung and liver disease in young adults
Alpha-1-fetoprotein	None detected		Hepatocarcinoma Metastatic carcinoma of liver Germinal cell carcinoma of the testicle or ovary Fetal neural tube defects—elevation in maternal serum	
Alpha-hydroxybutyric dehydrogenase	Up to 140 U/mL	Up to 140 U/L	Myocardial infarction Granulocytic leukemia Hemolytic anemias Muscular dystrophy	
Ammonia (plasma)	40–80 μg/dL (enzymatic method); varies considerably with method	22.2–44.3 μmol/L	Severe liver disease Hepatic decompensation	

(*continued*)

REFERENCE RANGES—SERUM, PLASMA, AND WHOLE BLOOD CHEMISTRIES (*continued*)

Determination	NORMAL ADULT REFERENCE RANGE		CLINICAL SIGNIFICANCE	
	Conventional Units	*SI Units*	*Increased*	*Decreased*
Amylase	60–160 Somogyi U/dL	111–296 U/L	Acute pacreatitis Mumps Duodenal ulcer Carcinoma of head of pancreas Prolonged elevation with pseudocyst of pancreas Increased by drugs that constrict pancreatic duct sphincters: morphine, codeine, cholinergics	Chronic pancreatitis Pancreatic fibrosis and atrophy Cirrhosis of liver Pregnancy (2nd and 3rd trimesters)
Arsenic	6–20 µg/dL; if 50 µg/dL, suspect toxicity	0.78–2.6 µmol/L	Accidental or intentional poisoning Excessive occupational exposure	
Ascorbic acid (vitamin C)	0.4–1.5 mg/dL	23–85 µmol/L	Large doses of ascorbic acid as a prophylactic against the common cold	
Bilirubin	Total: 0.1–1.2mg/dL	1.7–20.5 µmol/L	Hemolytic anemia (indirect)	
	Direct: 0.1–0.2 mg/dL	1.7–3.4 µmol/L	Biliary obstruction and disease	
	Indirect: 0.1–1 mg/dL	1.7–17.1 µmol/L	Hepatocellular damage (hepatitis) Pernicious anemia Hemolytic disease of newborn	
Blood gases Oxygen, arterial (whole blood):				
Partial pressure (PaO$_2$)	95–100 mm Hg	12.64–13.30 kPa	Polycythemia	Anemia
Saturation (SaO$_2$)	94%–100%	Volume fraction: 0.94–1	Anhydremia	Cardiac decompensation Chronic obstructive pulmonary disease

(continued)

REFERENCE RANGES—SERUM, PLASMA, AND WHOLE BLOOD CHEMISTRIES (*continued*)

Determination	NORMAL ADULT REFERENCE RANGE		CLINICAL SIGNIFICANCE	
	Conventional Units	*SI Units*	*Increased*	*Decreased*
Carbon dioxide, arterial (whole blood): partial pressure ($PaCO_2$)	35–45 mm Hg	4.66–5.9 kPa	Respiratory acidosis Metabolic alkalosis	Respiratory alkalosis Metabolic acidosis
pH (whole blood arterial)	7.35–7.45	7.35–7.45	Vomiting Hyperpnea Fever Intestinal obstruction	Uremia Diabetic acidosis Hemorrhage Nephritis
Calcitonin	Basal: nondetectable 400 pg/mL	400 ng/L	Medullary carcinoma of the thyroid Some nonthyroid tumors Zollinger-Ellison syndrome	
Calcium	8.5–10.5 mg/dL	2.123–2.625 mmol/L	Tumor or hyperplasia of parathyroid Hypervitaminosis D Multiple myeloma Nephritis with uremia Malignant tumors Sarcoidosis Hyperthyroidism Skeletal immobilization Excess calcium intake: milk-alkali syndrome	Hypoparathyroidism Diarrhea Celiac disease Vitamin D deficiency Acute pancreatitis Nephrosis After parathyroidectomy
CO_2, venous	Adults 24–32 mEq/L Infants: 18–24 mEq/L	24–32 mmol/L 18–24 mmol/L	Tetany Respiratory disease Intestinal obstruction Vomiting	Acidosis Nephritis Eclampsia Diarrhea Anesthesia
Carcinoembryonic antigen (CEA)—RIA	0–2.5 ng/mL (nonsmoker) 0–5 mg/mL (smoker)	0–2.5 µg/L (nonsmoker) 0–5 µg/L (smoker)	The repeatedly high incidence of this antigen in cancers of the colon, rectum, pancreas, and stomach suggests that CEA levels may be useful in the therapeutic monitoring of these conditions	

(continued)

REFERENCE RANGES—SERUM, PLASMA, AND WHOLE BLOOD CHEMISTRIES (*continued*)

| Determination | NORMAL ADULT REFERENCE RANGE | | CLINICAL SIGNIFICANCE | |
	Conventional Units	*SI Units*	*Increased*	*Decreased*
Catecholamines (plasma)—RIA	Epinephrine, random: up to 90 pg/mL	Up to 490 pmol/L	Pheochromocytoma	
	Norepinephrine, random 100–550 pg/mL	590–3240 pmol/L		
	Dopamine, random up to 130 pg/mL	Up to 850 pmol/L		
Ceruloplasmin	30–80 mg/dL	300–800 mg/L		Wilson's disease (hepatolenticular degeneration)
Chloride	95–105 mEq/L	95–105 mmol/L	Nephrosis Nephritis Urinary obstruction Cardiac decompensation Anemia	Diabetes Diarrhea Vomiting Pneumonia Heavy metal poisoning Cushing's syndrome Burns Intestinal obstruction Febrile conditions
Cholesterol	150–200 mg/dL	3.9–5.2 mmol/L	Lipemia Obstructive jaundice Diabetes Hypothyroidism	Pernicious anemia Hemolytic anemia Hyperthyroidism Severe infection Terminal states of debilitating disease
Cholesterol esters	60%–70% of total	Fraction of total cholesterol 0.6–0.7		The esterified fraction decreases in liver diseases
Cholinesterase	Serum: 0.6–1.6 delta pH	0.6–1.6 U	Nephrosis Exercise	Nerve gas intoxication (greater effect on red cell activity)
	Red cells: 0.6–1 delta pH	0.6–1 U		Insecticides, organic phosphates (greater effect on plasma activity)
Chorionic gonadotropin, beta subunit—RIA	0–5 IU/L	0–5 IU/L	Pregnancy Hydatidiform mole Choriocarcinoma	
Complement, human C_3	70–150 mg/dL	880–2520 mg/L	Some inflammatory diseases, acute myocardial infarction, cancer	Acute glomerulonephritis Disseminated lupus erythematosus with renal involvement

(*continued*)

REFERENCE RANGES—SERUM, PLASMA, AND WHOLE BLOOD CHEMISTRIES (*continued*)

	NORMAL ADULT REFERENCE RANGE		CLINICAL SIGNIFICANCE	
Determination	*Conventional Units*	*SI Units*	*Increased*	*Decreased*
Complement C_4	16–45 mg/dL	140–510 mg/L	Some inflammatory diseases, acute myocardial infarction, cancer	Often decreased in immunologic disease, especially with active systemic lupus erythematosus Hereditary angioneuritic edema
Complement, total (hemolytic)	90%–94% complement	25–70 U/mL	Some inflammatory diseases	Acute glomerulonephritis Epidemic meningitis Subacute bacterial endocarditis
Copper	70–165 µg/dL	11–25.9 µmol/L	Cirrhosis of liver Pregnancy	Wilson's disease
Cortisol—RIA	8 AM: 7–25 µg/dL 4 PM: 2–9 µg/dL	193–690 nmol/L 55–248 nmol/L	Stress: infectious disease, surgery, burns, etc. Pregnancy Cushing's syndrome Pancreatitis Eclampsia	Addison's disease Anterior pituitary hypofunction
C-peptide reactivity	1.5–10 ng/mL	1.5–10 µg/L	Insulinoma	Diabetes
Creatine	0.2–0.8 mg/mL	15.3–61 µmol/L	Pregnancy Skeletal muscle necrosis or atrophy Starvation Hyperthyroidism	
Creatine phosphokinase (CPK)	Males 50–325 mU/mL Females: 50–250 mU/mL	50–325 U/L 50–250 U/L	Myocardial infarction Skeletal muscle diseases Intramuscular injections Crush syndrome Hypothyroidism Alcohol withdrawal delirium Alcoholic myopathy Cerebrovascular disease	
Creatine phosphokinase isoenzymes	MM band present (skeletal muscle); MB band absent (heart muscle)		MB band increased in myocardial infarction, ischemia	

(continued)

REFERENCE RANGES—SERUM, PLASMA, AND WHOLE BLOOD CHEMISTRIES (*continued*)

	NORMAL ADULT REFERENCE RANGE		CLINICAL SIGNIFICANCE	
Determination	*Conventional Units*	*SI Units*	*Increased*	*Decreased*
Creatinine	0.7–1.4 mg/dL	62–124 μmol/L	Nephritis Chronic renal disease	Kidney diseases
Creatinine clearance	100–150 mL of blood cleared of creatinine per min	1.67–2.5 mL/s		
Cryoglobulins, qualitative	Negative		Multiple myeloma Chronic lymphocytic leukemia Lymphosarcoma Systemic lupus erythematosus Rheumatoid arthritis Infective subacute endocarditis Some malignancies Scleroderma	
11-Deoxycortisol	1 μg/dL	<0.029 μmol/L	Hypertensive form of virilizing adrenal hyperplasia due to an 11-β-hydroxylase defect	
Dibucaine number	Normal: 70%–85% inhibition Heterozygote: 50%–65% inhibition Homozygote: 16%–25% inhibition			Important in detecting carriers of abnormal cholinesterase activity who are susceptible to succinylcholine anesthetic shock
Dihydrotestosterone	Males: 50–210 ng/dL Females: none detectable	1.72–7.22 nmol/L		Testicular feminization syndrome
Estradiol—RIA	Females: Follicular: 10–90 pg/mL Midcycle: 100–500 pg/mL Luteal: 50–240 pg/mL Follicular phase: 2–20 ng/dL Midcycle: 12–40 ng/dL Luteal phase: 10–30 ng/dL Postmenopausal: 1–5 ng/dL Males: 0.5–5 ng/dL	37–370 pmol/L 367–1835 pmol/L 184–881 pmol/L	Pregnancy	Depressed or failure to peak—ovarian failure

(continued)

REFERENCE RANGES—SERUM, PLASMA, AND WHOLE BLOOD CHEMISTRIES (*continued*)

Determination	NORMAL ADULT REFERENCE RANGE		CLINICAL SIGNIFICANCE	
	Conventional Units	*SI Units*	*Increased*	*Decreased*
Estriol—RIA	Nonpregnant females: <0.5 ng/mL	<1.75 nmol/L	Pregnancy	Depressed or failure to peak—ovarian failure
	Pregnant females:			
	1st trimester: up to 1 ng/mL	Up to 3.5 nmol/L		
	2nd trimester: 0.8–7 ng/mL	2.8–24.3 nmol/L		
	3rd trimester: 5–25 ng/mL	17.4–86.8 nmol/L		
Estrogens, total—RIA	Females: cycle days:		Pregnancy	Fetal distress
	Day 1–10: 61–394 pg/mL	61–394 ng/L	Measured on a daily basis, can be used to evaluate response of hypogonadotrophic, hypoestrogenic women to human menopausal or pituitary gonadotropin	Ovarian failure
	Day 11–20: 122–437 pg/mL	122–437 ng/L		
	Day 21–30: 156–350 pg/mL	156–350 ng/L		
	Males: 40–115 pg/mL	40–115 ng/L		
Estrone—RIA	Females:			Depressed or failure to peak—ovarian failure
	Day 1–10: 4.3–18 ng/dL	15.9–66.6 pmol/L		
	Day 11–20: 7.5–19.6 ng/dL	27.8–72.5 pmol/L		
	Day 21–30: 13–20 ng/dL	48.1–74 pmol/L		
	Males: 2.5–7.5 ng/dL	9.3–27.8 pmol/L		
Ferritin—RIA	Males: 29–438 ng/mL	29–438 µg/L	Nephritis	Iron deficiency
	Females: 9–219 ng/mL	9–219 µg/L	Hemochromatosis	
			Certain neoplastic diseases	
			Acute myelogenous leukemia	
			Multiple myeloma	
Folic acid—RIA	2.5–20 ng/mL	6–46 nmol/L		Megaloblastic anemias of infancy and pregnancy
				Inadequate diet
				Liver disease
				Malabsorption syndrome
				Severe hemolytic anemia

(*continued*)

REFERENCE RANGES—SERUM, PLASMA, AND WHOLE BLOOD CHEMISTRIES (*continued*)

| Determination | NORMAL ADULT REFERENCE RANGE | | CLINICAL SIGNIFICANCE | |
	Conventional Units	*SI Units*	*Increased*	*Decreased*
Follicle stimulating hormone (FSH)— RIA	Males: 2–10 mIU/mL Females:		Menopause and primary ovarian failure	Pituitary failure
	Follicular phase: 5–20 mIU/mL	5–20 IU/L		
	Peak of middle cycle: 12–30 mIU/mL	12–30 IU/L		
	Luteinic phase: 5–15 mIU/mL	5–15 IU/L		
	Menopausal females: 40–200 mIU/mL	40–200 IU/L		
Galactose	<5 mg/dL	<0.28 mmol/L		Galactosemia
Gamma glutamyl transpeptidase	Males: <45 IU/L Females: <30 IU/L	45 U/L 30 U/L	Hepatobiliary disease Anicteric alcoholics Drug therapy damage Myocardial infarction Renal infarction	
Gastrin—RIA	Fasting: 50–155 pg/mL	50–155 ng/L	Zollinger-Ellison syndrome Peptic ulceration of the duodenum	
	Postprandial: 80–170 pg/mL	80–107 ng/L		
	Zollinger-Ellison syndrome: 200– over 2000 pg/mL	200-over 2000 ng/L	Pernicious anemia	
	Pernicious anemia: 130–2260 pg/mL (mean 912)	130–2260 ng/L (mean 912)		
Glucose	Fasting: 60–110 mg/dL Postprandial (2 h): 65–140 mg/dL	3.3–6.05 mmol/L 3.58–7.7 mmol/L	Diabetes Nephritis Hyperthyroidism Early hyperpituitarism Cerebral lesions Infections Pregnancy Uremia	Hyperinsulinism Hypothyroidism Late hyperpituitarism Pernicious vomiting Addison's disease Extensive hepatic damage
Glucose tolerance (oral)	Features of a normal response:		(Flat or inverted curve)	(High or prolonged curve)

(continued)

REFERENCE RANGES—SERUM, PLASMA, AND WHOLE BLOOD CHEMISTRIES (*continued*)

| Determination | NORMAL ADULT REFERENCE RANGE | | CLINICAL SIGNIFICANCE | |
	Conventional Units	*SI Units*	*Increased*	*Decreased*
	1. Normal fasting between 60–110 mg/dL 2. No sugar in urine 3. Upper limits of normal: Fasting = 125 1 hour = 190 2 hours = 140 3 hours = 125	3.3–6.05 mmol/L 6.88 mmol/L 10.45 mmol/L 7.70 mmol/L 6.88 mmol/L	Hyperinsulinism Adrenal cortical insufficiency (Addison's disease) Anterior pituitary hypofunction Hypothyroidism Sprue and celiac diseases	Diabetes Hyperthyroidism Primary adrenal cortical tumor or hyperplasia Severe anemia Certain central nervous system disorders
Glucose-6-phosphate dehydrogenase (red cells)	Screeing: Decolorization in 20–100 min Quantitative: 1.86–2.5 IU/mL RBC	 1860–2500 U/L		Drug-induced hemolytic anemia Hemolytic disease of newborn
Glycoprotein (alpha-1-acid)	40–110 mg/dL	400–1100 mg/L	Neoplasm Tuberculosis Diabetes complicated by degenerative vascular disease Pregnancy Rheumatoid arthritis Rheumatic fever Infectious liver disease Lupus erythematosus	
Growth hormone—RIA	<10 ng/mL	<10 mg/L	Acromegaly	Failure to stimulate with arginine or insulin—hypopituitarism
Haptoglobin	50–250 mg/dL	0.5–2.5 g/L	Pregnancy Estrogen therapy Chronic infections Various inflammatory conditions	Hemolytic anemia Hemolytic blood transfusion reaction
Hemoglobin (plasma)	0.5–5 mg/dL	5–50 mg/L	Transfusion reactions Paroxysmal nocturnal hemoglobinuria Intravascular hemolysis	

(continued)

REFERENCE RANGES—SERUM, PLASMA, AND WHOLE BLOOD CHEMISTRIES (*continued*)

| Determination | NORMAL ADULT REFERENCE RANGE | | CLINICAL SIGNIFICANCE | |
	Conventional Units	*SI Units*	*Increased*	*Decreased*
Hemoglobin A1 (Glycohemoglobin)	Nondiabetics & diabetics whose control of glucose is: Good: 4.4%–8.2% Fair: 8.3%–9.2% Poor: >9.2%			
Hexosaminidase, total	Controls: 333–375 nM/mL/h	333–375 μmol/L/h	Sandhoff's disease	
Hexosaminidase A	Controls: 49%–68% of total Heterozygotes: 26%–45% of total Tay–Sachs disease: 0%–4% of total Diabetics: 39%–59% of total	Fraction of total: 0.49–0.68 0.26–0.45 0–0.04 0.39–0.59		Tay-Sachs disease and heterozygotes
High-density lipoprotein cholesterol (HDL cholesterol)	Males: 35–70 mg/dL Females: 35–85 mg/dL	0.91–1.81 mmol/L 0.91–220 mmol/L		HDL cholesterol is lower in patients with increased risk for coronary heart disease

Age (yr)	Males (mg/dL)	Females (mg/dL)	Males (mmol/L)	Females (mmol/L)
0–19	30–65	30–70	0.78–1.68	0.78–1.81
20–29	35–70	35–75	0.91–1.81	0.91–1.94
30–39	30–65	35–80	0.78–1.68	0.91–2.07
40–49	30–65	40–85	0.78–1.68	1.04–2.2
50–59	30–65	35–85	0.78–1.68	0.91–2.2
60–69	30–65	35–85	0.78–1.68	0.91–2.2

Determination	*Conventional Units*	*SI Units*	*Increased*	*Decreased*
17-Hydroxy-progesterone—RIA	Males: 0.4–4 ng/mL Females: 0.1–3.3 ng/mL Children: 0.1–0.5 ng/mL	1.2–12 nmol/L 0.3–10 nmol/L 0.3–1.5 nmol/L	Congenital adrenal hyperplasia Pregnancy Some cases of adrenal or ovarian adenomas	
Immunoglobulin A	Adults: 50–300 mg/dL (in children the normals are lower and vary with age)	0.5–3 g/L	Gamma A myeloma Wiskott-Aldrich syndrome Autoimmune disease Hepatic cirrhosis	Ataxia telangiectasis Agammaglobulinemia Hypogammaglobulinemia, transient Dysgammaglobulinemia Protein-losing enteropathies

(continued)

REFERENCE RANGES—SERUM, PLASMA, AND WHOLE BLOOD CHEMISTRIES (*continued*)

Determination	NORMAL ADULT REFERENCE RANGE		CLINICAL SIGNIFICANCE	
	Conventional Units	*SI Units*	*Increased*	*Decreased*
Immunoglobulin D	0–30 mg/dL	0–300 mg/L	IgD multiple myeloma Some patients with chronic infectious diseases	
Immunoglobulin E	20–740 ng/mL	20–740 µg/L	Allergic patients and those with parasitic infections	
Immunoglobulin G	Adults: 565–1765 mg/dL	6.35–14 g/L	IgG myeloma Following hyper-immunization Autoimmune disease states Chronic infections	Congenital and ac-quired hypogam-maglobulinemia IgA myelomas, Waldenström's (IgM) macroglob-ulinemia Some malabsorp-tion syndromes Extensive protein loss
Immunoglobulin M	Adults: 55–375 mg/dL	0.4–2.8 g/L	Waldenström's macroglobu-linemia Parasitic infections Hepatitis	Agammaglobuline-mias Some IgG and IgA myelomas Chronic lymphatic leukemia
Insulin—RIA	5–25 µU/mL	0.2–1 µg/L	Insulinoma Acromegaly	Diabetes mellitus
Iron	50–160 µg/dL	9–29 µmol/L	Pernicious anemia Aplastic anemia Hemolytic anemia Hepatitis Hemochromatosis	Iron-deficiency ane-mia
Iron-binding capacity	IBC: 150–235 µg/dL TIBC: 230–410 µg/dL % Saturation: 20–50	26.9–42.1 µmol/L 41–73 µmol/L Fraction of total iron-binding ca-pacity: 0.2–0.5	Iron deficiency anemia Acute and chronic blood loss Hepatitis	Chronic infectious diseases Cirrhosis
Isocitric dehydro-genase	50–180 U	0.83–3 U/L	Hepatitis: cirrhosis Obstructive jaundice Metastatic carcin-oma of the liver Megaloblastic anemia	

(continued)

REFERENCE RANGES—SERUM, PLASMA, AND WHOLE BLOOD CHEMISTRIES (*continued*)

Determination	NORMAL ADULT REFERENCE RANGE		CLINICAL SIGNIFICANCE	
	Conventional Units	*SI Units*	*Increased*	*Decreased*
Lactic acid (whole blood)	Venous: 5–20 mg/dL Arterial: 3–7 mg/dL	0.6–2.2 mmol/L 0.3–0.8 mmol/L	Increased muscular activity Congestive heart failure Hemorrhage Shock Some varieties of metabolic acidosis Some febrile infections May be increased in severe liver disease	
Lactic dehydrogenase (LDH)	100–225 mU/mL	100–225 U/L	Untreated pernicious anemia Myocardial infarction Pulmonary infarction Liver disease	
Lactic dehydrogenase isoenzymes				
Total lactic dehydrogenase	100–225 mU/mL	100–225 U/L Fraction of total LDH:	LDH-1 and LDH-2 are increased in myocardial infarction, megaloblastic anemia, and hemolytic anemia	
LDH-1	20%–35%	0.2–0.35		
LDH-2	25%–40%	0.25–0.4		
LDH-3	20%–30%	0.2–0.3		
LDH-4	0–20%	0–0.2		
LDH-5	0–25%	0–0.25	LDH-4 and LDH-5 are increased in pulmonary infarction, congestive heart failure, and liver disease	
Lead (whole blood)	Up to 40 μg/dL	Up to 2 μmol/L	Lead poisoning	
Leucine aminopeptidase	80–200 U/mL	19.2–48 U/L	Liver or biliary tract diseases Pancreatic disease Metastatic carcinoma of liver and pancreas Biliary obstruction	
Lipase	0.2–1.5 U/mL	55–417 U/L	Acute and chronic pancreatitis Biliary obstruction Cirrhosis Hepatitis Peptic ulcer	

(*continued*)

REFERENCE RANGES—SERUM, PLASMA, AND WHOLE BLOOD CHEMISTRIES (*continued*)

Determination	NORMAL ADULT REFERENCE RANGE		CLINICAL SIGNIFICANCE	
	Conventional Units	*SI Units*	*Increased*	*Decreased*
Lipids, total	400–1,000 mg/dL	4–10 g/L	Hypothyroidism Diabetes Nephrosis Glomerulonephritis Hyperlipoproteinemias	Hyperthyroidism

Lipoprotein Phenotype: Summary of Findings in the Primary Hyperlipoproteinemias

Type	Frequency	Appearance	Triglyceride	Cholesterol	LIPOPROTEIN STAINING				Secondary Causes
					Beta	*Pre-Beta*	*Alpha*	*Chylomicrons*	
Normal		Clear	Normal	Normal	Moderate	Zero to moderate	Moderate	Weak	
I	Very rare	Creamy	Markedly increased	Normal to moderately increased	Weak	Weak	Weak	Markedly increased	Dysglobu-linemia
II	Common	Clear	Normal to slightly increased	Slightly to markedly increased	Strong	Zero to strong	Moderate	Weak	Hypothyroid-ism, myeloma, hepatic syndrome, macroglob-ulinemia, and high dietary cholesterol
III	Uncommon	Clear, cloudy or milky	Increased	Increased	Broad intense band	Extends into beta	Moderate	Weak	
IV	Very common	Clear, cloudy, or milky	Slightly to markedly increased	Normal to slightly increased	Weak to moderate	Moderate to strong	Weak to moderate	Weak	Hypothyroidism, diabetes mellitus, pancreatitis, glycogen storage diseases, nephrotic syndrome, myeloma, pregnancy, and oral contraceptives
V	Rare	Cloudy to creamy	Markedly increased	Increased	Weak	Moderate	Weak	Strong	Diabetes mellitus, pancreatitis, and alcoholism

Types I and II are fat induced; types III and IV are carbohydrate induced; type V is fat and carbohydrate induced.

Determination	NORMAL ADULT REFERENCE RANGE		CLINICAL SIGNIFICANCE	
	Conventional Units	*SI Units*	*Increased*	*Decreased*
Lithium	Usual maintenance level: 0.5–1 mEq/L	0.5–1 mmol/L		

(continued)

REFERENCE RANGES—SERUM, PLASMA, AND WHOLE BLOOD CHEMISTRIES (*continued*)

Determination	NORMAL ADULT REFERENCE RANGE		CLINICAL SIGNIFICANCE	
	Conventional Units	*SI Units*	*Increased*	*Decreased*
Low-density lipopro-tein cholesterol (LDL cholesterol)	mg/dL <130 (desirable) 130–159 (borderline) >160 (high risk)		LDL cholesterol is higher in pa-tients with in-creased risk for coronary heart disease	
Luteinizing hor-mone—RIA	Males 4.9–15 mIU/mL Females: Follicular phase: 2–3 mIU/mL Ovulatory peak: 40–200 mIU/mL Luteal phase: 0–20 mIU/mL Postmenopausal: 35–120 mIU/mL	4.9–15 mg/L 0.5–6.9 mg/L 9.2–46 mg/L 0–5 mg/L 8–27.5 mg/L	Pituitary tumor Ovarian failure	Depressed or fail-ure to peak—pi-tuitary failure
Lysozyme (muramidase)	2.8–8 µg/mL	2.8–8 mg	Certain types of leukemia (acute monocytic leukemia) Inflammatory states and infections	Acute lymphocytic leukemia
Magnesium	1.3–2.4 mEq/L	0.7–1.2 mmol/L	Excess ingestion of magnesium-containing ant-acids	Chronic alcoholism Severe renal dis-ease Diarrhea Defective growth
Manganese	0.04–1.4 µg/dL	72.9–255 nmol/L		
Mercury	Up to 10 µg/dL	Up to 0.5 µmol/L	Mercury poisoning	
Myoglobin—RIA	Up to 85 ng/mL	Up to 85 µg/mL	Myocardial infarction Muscle necrosis	
5′ Nucleotidase	3.2–11.6 IU/L	3.2–11.6 U/L	Hepatobiliary disease	
Osmolality	280–300 mOsm/kg	280–300 mmol/L	Useful in the study of elec-trolyte and water balance	Inappropriate se-cretion of antidi-uretic hormone
Parathyroid hormone	160–350 pg/mL	160–350 ng/L	Hyperparathyroid-ism	
Phenylalanine	1.2–3.5 mg/dL 1st week 0.7–3.5 mg/dL thereafter	0.07–0.21 mmol/L 0.04–0.21 mmol/L	Phenylketonuria	

(*continued*)

REFERENCE RANGES—SERUM, PLASMA, AND WHOLE BLOOD CHEMISTRIES (*continued*)

Determination	NORMAL ADULT REFERENCE RANGE		CLINICAL SIGNIFICANCE	
	Conventional Units	*SI Units*	*Increased*	*Decreased*
Phosphohexose isomerase	20–90 IU/L	20–90 U/L	Malignancy Disease of heart, liver, and skeletal muscles	
Phospholipids	125–300 mg/dL	1.25–3 g/L	Diabetes Nephritis	
Phosphorus, inorganic	2.5–4.5 mg/dL	0.8–1.45 mmol/L	Chronic nephritis Hypoparathyroidism	Hyperparathyroidism Vitamin D deficiency
Potassium	3.8–5 mEq/L	3.8–5 mmol/L	Addison's disease Oliguria Anuria Tissue breakdown or hemolysis	Diabetic acidosis Diarrhea Vomiting
Progesterone—RIA	Follicular phase: up to 0.8 ng/mL Luteal phase: 10–20 ng/mL End of cycle: <1 ng/mL Pregnant: up to 50 ng/mL in 20th week	2.5 nmol/L 31.8–63.6 nmol/L <3 nmol/L Up to 160 nmol/L	Useful in evaluation of menstrual disorders and infertility and in the evaluation of placental function during pregnancies complicated by toxemia, diabetes mellitus, or threatened miscarriage	
Prolactin—RIA	6–24 ng/mL	6–24 µg/L	Pregnancy Functional or structural disorders of the hypothalamus Pituitary stalk section Pituitary tumors	
Prostate-specific antigen	<4 ng/mL		Prostatic cancer, benign prostatic hyperplasia, prostatitis	
Protein, total Albumin Globulin	6–8 gm/dL 3.5–5 gm/dL 1.5–3 gm/dL	60–80 g/L 35–50 g/L 15–30 g/L	Hemoconcentration Shock Multiple myeloma (globulin fraction) Chronic infections (globulin fraction) Liver disease (globulin)	Malnutrition Hemorrhage Loss of plasma from burns Proteinuria

(continued)

REFERENCE RANGES—SERUM, PLASMA, AND WHOLE BLOOD CHEMISTRIES (*continued*)

Determination	NORMAL ADULT REFERENCE RANGE		CLINICAL SIGNIFICANCE	
	Conventional Units	*SI Units*	*Increased*	*Decreased*
Protein				
Electrophoresis (cellulose acetate)		35–50 g/L 2–4 g/L		
Albumin	3.5–5 gm/dL	6–10 g/L		
Alpha-1 globulin	0.2–0.4 gm/dL	6–12 g/L		
Alpha-2 globulin	0.6–1 gm/dL	7–15 g/L		
Beta globulin	0.6–1.2 gm/dL			
Gamma globulin	0.7–1.5 gm/dL			
Protoporphyrin erythrocyte (whole blood)	15–100 µg/dL	0.27–1.80 µmol/L	Lead toxicity Erythropoietic porphyria	
Pyridoxine	3.6–18 ng/mL			A wide spectrum of clinical conditions, such as mental depression, peripheral neuropathy, anemia, neonatal seizures, and reactions to certain drug therapies
Pyruvic acid (whole blood)	0.3–0.7 mg/dL	34–80 µmol/L	Diabetes Severe thiamine deficiency Acute phase of some infections, possibly secondary to increased glycogenolysis and glycolysis	
Renin (plasma)—RIA	Normal diet: Supine: 0.3–1.9 ng/mL/h Upright: 0.6–3.6 ng/mL/h Low salt diet: Supine: 0.9–4.5 ng/mL/h Upright: 4.1–9.1 ng/mL/h	0.08–0.52 ng/L/S 0.16–1.00 µg/L/S 0.25–1.25 µg/L/S 1.13–2.53 µg/L/S	Renovascular hypertension Malignant hypertension Untreated Addison's disease Primary salt-losing nephropathy Low-salt diet Diuretic therapy Hemorrhage	Frank primary aldosteronism Increased salt intake Salt-retaining steroid therapy Antidiuretic hormone therapy Blood transfusion
Sodium	135–145 mEq/L	135–145 mmol/L	Hemoconcentration Nephritis Pyloric obstruction	Alkali deficit Addison's disease Myxedema
Sulfate (inorganic)	0.5–1.5 mg/dL	0.05–0.15 mmol/L	Nephritis Nitrogen retention	

(continued)

REFERENCE RANGES—SERUM, PLASMA, AND WHOLE BLOOD CHEMISTRIES (*continued*)

| Determination | NORMAL ADULT REFERENCE RANGE | | CLINICAL SIGNIFICANCE | |
	Conventional Units	*SI Units*	*Increased*	*Decreased*
Testosterone—RIA	Females: 25–100 ng/dL Males: 300–800 ng/dL	0.9–3.5 nmol/L 10.5–28 nmol/L	Females: Polycystic ovary Virilizing tumors	Males: Orchidectomy for neoplastic disease of the prostate or breast Estrogen therapy Klinefelter's syndrome Hypopituitarism Hypogonadism Hepatic cirrhosis
T_3 (triiodothyronine) uptake	25%–35%	Relative uptake fraction: 0.25–0.35	Hyperthyroidism Thyroxine-binding globulin (TBG) deficiency Androgens and anabolic steroids	Hypothyroidism Pregnancy TBG excess Estrogens and antiovulatory drugs
T_3, total circulating—RIA	75–200 ng/dL	1.15–3.1 nmol/L	Pregnancy Hyperthyroidism	Hypothyroidism
T_4 (thyroxine)—RIA	4.5–11.5 µg/dL	58.5–150 nmol/L	Hyperthyroidism Thyroiditis Elevated thyroxine-binding proteins caused by oral contraceptives Pregnancy	Primary and pituitary hypothyroidism Idiopathic involvement Cases of diminished thyroxine-binding proteins caused by androgenic and anabolic steroids Hypoproteinemia Nephrotic syndrome
T_4, free	1–2.2 ng/dL	13–30 pmol/L	Euthyroid patients with normal free thyroxine levels may have abnormal T_3 and T_4 levels caused by drug preparations	
Thyroid-stimulating hormone (TSH)—RIA		0.3–5 m/IU/L	Hypothyroidism	Hyperthyroidism
Thyroid-binding globulin	10–26 µg/dL	100–260 µg/L	Hypothyroidism Pregnancy Estrogen therapy Oral contraceptives Genetic and idiopathic	Androgens and anabolic steroids Nephrotic syndrome Marked hypoproteinemia Hepatic disease

(continued)

REFERENCE RANGES—SERUM, PLASMA, AND WHOLE BLOOD CHEMISTRIES (*continued*)

Determination	NORMAL ADULT REFERENCE RANGE		CLINICAL SIGNIFICANCE	
	Conventional Units	*SI Units*	*Increased*	*Decreased*
Transaminase, serum glutamic-oxaloacetate (SGOT, aspartate aminotransferase)	7–40 U/mL	4–20U/L	Myocardial infarction Skeletal muscle disease Liver disease	
Transaminase, serum glutamic-oxaloacetate (SGPT, alanine aminotransferase)	10–40 U/mL	5–20 U/L	Same conditions as SGOT, but increase is more marked in liver disease than SGOT	
Transferrin	230–320 mg/dL	2.3–3.2 g/L	Pregnancy Iron-deficiency anemia due to hemorrhaging Acute hepatitis Polycythemia Oral contraceptives	Pernicious anemia in relapse Thalassemic and sickle cell anemia Chromatosis Neoplastic and hepatic diseases
Triglycerides	10–150 mg/dL	0.10–1.65 mmol/L	See *Lipoprotein Phenotype*	
Tryptophan	1.4–3 mg/dL	68.6–147 nmol/L		Tryptophan-specific malabsorption syndrome
Tyrosine	0.5–4 mg/dL	27.6–220.8 mmol/L	Tyrosinosis	
Urea nitrogen (BUN)	10–20 mg/dL	3.6–7.2 mmol/L	Acute glomerulonephritis Obstructive uropathy Mercury poisoning Nephrotic syndrome	Severe hepatic failure Pregnancy
Uric acid	2.5–8 mg/dL	0.15–0.5 mmol/L	Gouty arthritis Acute leukemia Lymphomas treated by chemotherapy Toxemia of pregnancy	Xanthinuria Defective tubular reabsorption
Viscosity	1.4–1.8 relative to water at 37°C (98.6°F)		Patients with marked increases of the gamma globulins	
Vitamin A	50–220 μg/dL	1.75–7.7 μmol/L	Hypervitaminosis A	Vitamin A deficiency Celiac disease Sprue Obstructive jaundice Giardiasis Parenchymal hepatic disease

(continued)

REFERENCE RANGES—SERUM, PLASMA, AND WHOLE BLOOD CHEMISTRIES (*continued*)

Determination	NORMAL ADULT REFERENCE RANGE		CLINICAL SIGNIFICANCE	
	Conventional Units	*SI Units*	*Increased*	*Decreased*
Vitamin B₁ (thiamine)	1.6–4 µg/dL	47.4–135.7 nmol/L		Anorexia Beriberi Polyneuropathy Cardiomyopathies
Vitamin B₆ (pyridoxal phosphate)	3.6–18 ng/mL	14.6–72.8 nmol/L		Chronic alcoholism Malnutrition Uremia Neonatal seizures Malabsorption, such as celiac syndrome
Vitamin B₁₂—RIA	130–785 pg/mL	100–580 pmol/L	Hepatic cell damage and in association with the myeloproliferative disorders (the highest levels are encountered in myeloid leukemia)	Strict vegetariansim Alcoholism Pernicious anemia Total or partial gastrectomy Ileal resection Sprue and celiac disease Fish tapeworm infestation
Vitamin E	0.5–2 mg/dL	11.6–46.4 µmol/L		Vitamin E deficiency
Xylose absorption test	2 hr, 30–50 mg/dL	2–3.35 mmol/L		Malabsorption syndrome
Zinc	55–150 µg/dL	7.65–22.95 µmol/L	Zinc is essential for the growth and propagation of cell cultures and the functioning of several enzymes	

RIA = by radioimmunoassay.

REFERENCE RANGES—IMMUNODIAGNOSTIC TESTS

Determination	Normal Value	Clinical Significance
Acetylcholine receptor binding antibody	Negative or <0.03 nmol/L	Considered to be diagnostic for myasthenia gravis in patients with symptoms.
Anti-ds-DNA antibody	<70 U by enzyme-linked immunosorbent assay (ELISA) <1:20 by indirect fluorescence	Valuable in supporting diagnosis or monitoring disease activity and prognosis of systemic lupus erythematosus (SLE).
Antiglomerular basement membrane antibody	Negative or less than 10 U	Primarily used in the differential diagnosis of glomerular nephritis induced by antiglomerular basement membrane antibodies from other types of glomerular nephritis.
Anti-insulin antibody	<3% binding of labeled beef and pork insulin by patient's serum; or <9 mIU/L	Helpful in determining the best therapeutic agent in diabetics and the cause of allergic manifestations. Also used to identify insulin resistance.
Antimitochondrial antibody and anti–smooth muscle antibody	<1:5 and <1:20, respectively	Increased in cirrhosis, autoimmune disease, thyroiditis, pernicious anemia.
Antinuclear antibody	Negative, <1:20	Increased in SLE, chronic hepatitis, scleroderma, leukemia, and mononucleosis.
Anti–parietal cell antibody	Negative, <1:20	Helpful in diagnosing chronic gastric disease and differentiating autoimmune pernicious anemia from other megloblastic anemias.
Antiribonucleoprotein antibody	Negative	Helpful in differential diagnosis of systemic rheumatic disease.
Antiscleroderma antibody	Negative	Highly diagnostic for scleroderma.
Anti-Smith antibody	Negative	Highly diagnostic of SLE.
Anti-SS-A anti-SS-B antibody	Negative	SS-A antibodies are found in Sjögren's syndrome alone or associated with lupus. SS-B antibodies are associated with primary Sjögren's syndrome.
Antithyroglobulin and antimicrosomal antibodies	<1:100 titer by gelatin or hemagglutination	Presence and concentration is important in evaluation and treatment of various thyroid disorders, such as Hashimoto's thyroiditis and Graves' disease. May indicate previous autoimmune disorders.
CA 15-3 tumor marker	<22 IU/mL	Increased in metastatic breast cancer.
CA 19-9 tumor marker	<37 IU/mL	Increased in pancreatic, hepatobiliary, gastric, and colorectal cancer; gallstones.
CA 125	0–35 IU/mL	Increased in colon, upper gastrointestinal (GI), ovarian, and other gynecologic cancers; pregnancy, peritonitis.
Cold agglutinins	<1:16	Increased in mycoplasma pneumonia, viral illness, mononucleosis, multiple myeloma, scleroderma.
C-reactive protein	<0.8 mg/dL	Increase indicates active inflammation.
Hepatitis A virus antibodies, IgM (HAV-Ab/IgM)	Negative	Positive in acute-stage hepatitis A; develops early in disease.

(continued)

REFERENCE RANGES—IMMUNODIAGNOSTIC TESTS (*continued*)

Determination	Normal Value	Clinical Significance
Hepatitis A virus antibodies, IgG (HAV-Ab/IgG)	Negative	Positive if previous exposure and immunity to hepatitis A.
Hepatitis B surface antigen (HBsAg)	Negative	Positive in acute-stage hepatitis B.
Hepatitis B surface antibody (HBsAb)	Negative	Positive if previous exposure and immunity to hepatitis B.
Infectious mononucleosis tests (monospot, mono-test, heterophile antigen test, Epstein–Barr virus (EBV), antiviral capsid antigen IgM and IgG)	Negative, <1:80	Positive monospot and monotest are presumptive; positive EBV IgM and IgG indicate acute and recent or past infection, respectively.
Lyme disease titer	Negative, <1:256 by indirect fluorescent antibody method <0.8 by ELISA	Positive results help diagnose Lyme disease. False positive may occur with high rheumatoid factor titers or syphilis. Positive ELISA confirmed by Western blot test.
Pyroglobulin test	Negative	These abnormal proteins may be associated with myeloma, lymphoma, polycythemia vera, and SLE.
Rheumatoid factor	Negative or less than 60 IU/mL	Elevated in rheumatoid arthritis, lupus, endocarditis, tuberculosis, syphilis, sarcoidosis, cancer.
T and B cell lymphocyte surface markers T-helper/T-suppressor ratio	T and B surface markers: Percent T cells (CD2) 60%–88% Percent helper cells (CD4) 34%–67% Percent suppressor cells (CD8) 10%–42% Percent B cells (CD19) 3%–21% Absolute counts: Lymphocytes 0.66–4.60 thou/mL T cells 644–2201 cells/mL Helper cells 493–1191 cells/mL Suppressor T cells 182–785 cells/mL B cells 92–392 cells/mL Lymphocyte ratio: T_H/T_S ratio > 1	Done to evaluate immune system by identifying the specific cells involved in the immune response. Valuable in diagnosis of lymphocytic leukemia, lymphoma, and immunodeficiency diseases including acquired immunodeficiency syndrome, and in the assessment of patient response to chemotherapy and radiation.

REFERENCE RANGES—URINE CHEMISTRY

| Determination | NORMAL ADULT REFERENCE RANGE | | CLINICAL SIGNIFICANCE | |
	Conventional Units	SI Units	Increased	Decreased
Acetone and acetoacetate	Zero		Uncontrolled diabetes Starvation	
Acid muco-polysaccharides	Negative		Hurler syndrome Marfan syndrome Morquio-Ullrich disease	

Aldosterone	Normal salt:
	  Normal: 4–20 µg/24 h
	  Renovascular: 10–40 µg/24 h
	  Tumor: 20–100 µg/24 h
		11.1–55.5 nmol/24 h
		27.7–111 nmol/24 h
		55.4–277 nmol/24 h
			Primary aldoster-onism (adren-ocortical tumor)
			Secondary aldo-steronism
			Salt depletion
			Postassium loading
			ACTH in large doses
			Cardiac failure
			Cirrhosis with ascites formation
			Nephrosis
			Pregnancy	

Alpha amino nitrogen	50–200 mg/24 h	3.6–14.3 mmol/24 h	Leukemia Diabetes Phenylketonuria Other metabolic diseases	
Amylase	35–260 units excreted per h	6.5–48.1 U/h	Acute pancreatitis	
Arylsulfatase A	>2.4 U/mL			Metachromatic leukodystrophy
Bence-Jones protein	None detected		Myeloma	
Calcium	<150 mg/24 h	<3.75 mmol/24 h	Hyperparathy-roidism Vitamin D intoxication Fanconi's syndrome	Hypoparathyroidism Vitamin D deficiency
Catecholamines	Total: 0–275 µg/24 h Epinephrine: 10%–40% Norepinephrine: 60%–90%	0–275 µg/24 h Fraction total: 0.10–8.4 Fraction total: 0.60–0.90	Pheochromocy-toma Neuroblastoma	
Chorionic gona-dotrophin, qualitative (pregnancy test)	Negative		Pregnancy Chorionepithe-lioma Hydatidiform mole	

(continued)

REFERENCE RANGES—URINE CHEMISTRY (*continued*)

Determination	NORMAL ADULT REFERENCE RANGE		CLINICAL SIGNIFICANCE	
	Conventional Units	*SI Units*	*Increased*	*Decreased*
Copper	20–70 μg/24 h	0.32–1.12 μmol/24 h	Wilson's disease Cirrhosis Nephrosis	
Coproporphyrin	50–300 μg/24 h	0.075–0.45 μmol/24 h	Poliomyelitis Lead poisoning Porphyria hepatica Porphyria erythropoietica Porphyria cutanea tarda	
Cortisol, free	20–90 μg/24 h	55.2–248.4 nmol/d	Cushing's syndrome	
Creatine	0–200 mg/24 h	0–1.52 mmol/24 h	Muscular dystrophy Fever Carcinoma of liver Pregnancy Hyperthryoidism Myositis	
Creatinine	0.8–2 gm/24 h	7–17.6 mmol/24 h	Typhoid fever Salmonella infections Tetanus	Muscular atrophy Anemia Advanced degeneration of kidneys Leukemia
Creatinine clearance	100–150 mL of blood cleared of creatinine per min	1.67–2.5 mL/s		Measures glomerular filtration rate Renal diseases
Cystine and cysteine	10–100 mg/24 h	0.08–0.83 mmol/24 h	Cystinuria	
Delta aminolevulinic acid	0–0.54 mg/dL	0–40 μmol/L	Lead poisoning Porphyria hepatica Hepatitis Hepatic carcinoma	
11-Desoxycortisol	20–100 μg/24 h	0.6–2.9 μmol/d	Hypertensive form of virilizing adrenal hyperplasia due to an 11-beta hydroxylase defect	

Estriol (placental)	**Weeks of pregnancy**	**μm/24 h**	**nmol/24 h**	Decreased values occur with fetal distress of many conditions, including preeclampsia, placental insufficiency, and poorly controlled diabetes mellitus
	12	<1	<3.5	
	16	2–7	7–24.5	
	20	4–9	14–32	
	24	6–13	21–45.5	
	28	8–22	28–77	
	32	12–43	42–150	
	36	14–45	49–158	
	40	19–46	66.5–160	

(continued)

REFERENCE RANGES—URINE CHEMISTRY (*continued*)

Determination	NORMAL ADULT REFERENCE RANGE		CLINICAL SIGNIFICANCE	
	Conventional Units	*SI Units*	*Increased*	*Decreased*

Estrogens, total (fluormetric)	Females:
	  Onset of menstruation: 4–25 µg/24 h
	  Ovulation peak: 28 µg/24 h
	  Luteal peak: 22–105 µg/24 h
	  Menopausal: 1.4–19.6 µg/24 h
	Males: 5–18 µg/24 h
		4–25 µg/24 h
		
		28 µg/24 h
		
		22–105 µg/24 h
		
		1.4–19.6 µg/24 h
		
		5–18 µg/24 h
			Hyperestrogenism due to gonadal or adrenal neoplasm	Primary or secondary amenorrhea

Etiocholanolone	Males: 1.9–6 mg/24 h Females: 0.5–4 mg/24 h	6.5–20.6 µmol/24 h 1.7–13.8 µmol/24 h	Adrenogenital syndrome Idiopathic hirsutism	

Follicle-stimulating hormone—RIA	Females:
	  Follicular: 5–20 IU/24 h
	  Luteal: 5–15 IU/24 h
	  Midcycle: 15–60 IU/24 h
	  Menopausal: 50–100 IU/24 h
	Males: 5–25 IU/24 h
		5–20 IU/d
		
		5–15 IU/d
		
		15–60 IU/d
		
		50–100 IU/d
		
		5–25 IU/d
			Menopause and primary ovarian failure	Pituitary failure

Glucose	Negative		Diabetes mellitus Pituitary disorders Intracranial pressure Lesion in floor of 4th ventricle	
Hemoglobin and myoglobin	Negative		Extensive burns Transfusion of incompatible blood Myoglobin increased in severe crushing injuries to muscles	
Homogentisic acid, qualitative	Negative		Alkaptonuria Ochronosis	
Homovanillic acid	Up to 15 mg/24 h	Up to 82 µmol/d	Neuroblastoma	
17-hydroxycortico-steroids	2–10 mg/24 h	5.5-27.5 µmol/d	Cushing's disease	Addison's disease Anterior pituitary hypofunction
5-Hydroxyindole-acetic acid, qualitative	Negative		Malignant carcinoid tumors	

(*continued*)

REFERENCE RANGES—URINE CHEMISTRY (*continued*)

Determination	NORMAL ADULT REFERENCE RANGE		CLINICAL SIGNIFICANCE	
	Conventional Units	*SI Units*	*Increased*	*Decreased*
Hydroxyproline	15–43 mg/24 h	0.11–0.33 μmol/d	Paget's disease Fibrous dysplasia Osteomalacia Neoplastic bone disease Hyperparathyroidism	
17-ketosteroids, total	Males: 10–22 mg/24 h Females: 6–16 mg/24 h	35–76 μmol/d 21–55 μmol/d	Interstitial cell tumor of testes Simple hirsutism, occasionally Adrenal hyperplasia Cushing's syndrome Adrenal cancer, virilism Adrenoblastoma	Thyrotoxicosis Female hypogonadism Diabetes mellitus Hypertension Debilitating disease of mild to moderate severity Eunuchoidism Addison's disease Panhypopituitarism Myxedema Nephrosis
Lead	Up to 150 μg/24 h	Up to 60 μmol/24 h	Lead poisoning	
Luteinizing hormone	Males: 5–18 IU/24 h Females: 　Follicular phase: 2–25 IU/24 h 　Ovulatory peak: 30–95 IU/24 h 　Luteal phase: 2–20 IU/24 h 　Postmenopausal: 40–110 IU/24 h	 2–25 IU/d 30–95 IU/d 2–20 IU/d 40–110 IU/d	Pituitary tumor Ovarian failure	Depressed or failure to peak—pituitary failure
Metanephrines, total	Less than 1.3 mg/24 h	Less than 6.5 μmol/d	Pheochromocytoma; a few patients with pheochromocytoma may have elevated urinary metanephrines but normal catecholamines and vanillylmandelic acid (VMA)	
Osmolality	Males: 390–1090 mM/kg Females: 300–1090 mM/kg	390–1090 mmol/kg 300–1090 mmol/kg	Useful in the study of electrolyte and water balance	

(continued)

REFERENCE RANGES—URINE CHEMISTRY (*continued*)

Determination	NORMAL ADULT REFERENCE RANGE		CLINICAL SIGNIFICANCE	
	Conventional Units	*SI Units*	*Increased*	*Decreased*
Oxalate	Up to 40 mg/24 h	Up to 456 μmol/d	Primary hyper-oxaluria	
Phenylpyruvic acid qualitative	Negative		Phenylketonuria	
Phosphorous, inorganic	0.8–1.3 gm/24 h	26–42 mmol/24 h	Hyperparathy-roidism Vitamin D intoxication Paget's disease Metastatic neo-plasm to bone	Hypoparathyroidism Vitamin D deficiency
Porphobilinogen, qualitative	Negative		Chronic lead poisoning Acute porphyria Liver disease	
Porphobilinogen, quantitative	0–1 mg/24 h	0–4.4 μmol/24 h	Acute porphyria Liver disease	
Porphyrins, qualitative	Negative		See porphyrins, quantitative	
Porphyrins, quanti-tative (copro-porphyrin and uroporphyrin)	Coproporphyrin: 50–160 μg/24 h Uroporphyrin: up to 50 μg/24 h	0.075–0.24 μmol/24 h Up to 0.06 μmol/24 h	Porphyria hepatica Porphyria eryth-ropoietica Porphyria cutanea tarda Lead poisoning (only copro-porphyrin increased)	
Potassium	40–65 mEq/24 h	40–65 mmol/24 h	Hemolysis	
Pregnanediol	Females: Proliferative phase: 0.5–1.5 mg/24 h Luteal phase: 2–7 mg/24 h Menopause: 0.2–1 mg/24 h Pregnancy:	1.6–4.8 μmol/24 h 6–22 μmol/24 h 0.6–3.1 μmol/24 h	Corpus luteum cysts When placental tissue remains in the uterus following par-turition Some cases of adrenocortical tumors	Placental dysfunction Threatened abortion Intrauterine death

Weeks of gestation	mg/24 h	μmol/24 h
10–12	5–15	15.6–47
12–18	5–25	15.6–78.0
18–24	15–33	47.0–103.0
24–28	20–42	62.4–131.0
28–32	27–47	84.2–146.6
Males: 0.1–2 mg/24 h		0.3–6.2 μmol/24 h

(continued)

REFERENCE RANGES—URINE CHEMISTRY (*continued*)

Determination	NORMAL ADULT REFERENCE RANGE		CLINICAL SIGNIFICANCE	
	Conventional Units	*SI Units*	*Increased*	*Decreased*
Pregnanetriol	0.4–2.4 mg/24 h	1.2–7.1 μmol/24 h	Congenital adrenal androgenic hyperplasia	
Protein	Up to 100 mg/24 h	Up to 100 mg/24 h	Nephritis Cardiac failure Mercury poisoning Bence-Jones protein in multiple myeloma Febrile states Hematuria	
Sodium	130–200 mEq/24 h	130–200 mmol/ 24 h	Useful in detecting gross changes in water and salt balance	
Titratable acidity	20–40 mEq/24 h	20–40 mmol/24 h	Metabolic acidosis	Metabolic alkalosis
Urea nitrogen	9–16 gm/24 h	0.32–0.57 mol/L	Excessive protein catabolism	Impaired kidney function
Uric acid	250–750 mg/24 h	1.48–4.43 mmol/24 h	Gout	Nephritis
Urobilinogen	Random urine: <0.25 mg/dL 24-hour urine: up to 4 mg/24 h	<0.42 mol/24 h Up to 6.76 μmol/24 h	Liver and biliary tract disease Hemolytic anemias	Complete or nearly complete biliary obstruction Diarrhea Renal insufficiency
Uroporphyrins	Up to 50 μg/24 h	Up to 0.06 μmol/24 h	Porphyria	
Vanillylmandelic acid (VMA)	0.7–6.8 mg/24 h	3.5–34.3 μmol/ 24 h	Pheochromocytoma Neuroblastoma Coffee, tea, aspirin, bananas, and several different drugs	
Xylose absorption test (5-hour)	16%–33% of ingested xylose	Fraction absorbed: 0.16–0.33		Malabsorption syndromes
Zinc	0.15–1.2 mg/24 h	2.3–18.4 μmol/ 24 h	Zinc is an essential nutritional element	

REFERENCE RANGES—CEREBROSPINAL FLUID (CSF)

| Determination | NORMAL ADULT REFERENCE RANGE | | CLINICAL SIGNIFICANCE | |
	Conventional Units	SI Units	Increased	Decreased
Albumin	15–30 mg/dL	150–300 mg/L	Certain neurological disorders Lesion in the choroid plexus or blockage of the flow of CSF Damage to the blood–central nervous system (CNS) barrier	
Cell count	0–5 mononuclear cells per cu mm	$0-5 \times 10^6$/L	Bacterial meningitis Neurosyphilis Anterior poliomyelitis Encephalitis lethargica	
Chloride	100–130 mEq/L	100–300 mmol/L	Uremia	Acute generalized meningitis Tuberculous meningitis
Glucose	50–75 mg/dL	2.75–4.13 mmol/L	Diabetes mellitus Diabetic coma Epidemic encephalitis Uremia	Acute meningitis Tuberculous meningitis Insulin shock
Glutamine	6–15mg/dL	0.41–1 mmol/L	Hepatic encephalopathies, including Reye's syndrome Hepatic coma Cirrhosis	
IgG	0–6.6 mg/dL	0–66 mg/L	Damage to the blood–CNS barrier Multiple sclerosis Neurosyphilis Subacute sclerosing panencephalitis Chronic phases of CNS infections	
Lactic acid	<24 mg/dL	<2.7 mmol/L	Bacterial meningitis Hypocapnia Hydrocephalus Brain abscesses Cerebral ischemia	
Lactic dehydrogenase	$\frac{1}{10}$ that of serum	Activity fraction: 0.1 of serum	CNS disease	

REFERENCE RANGES—CEREBROSPINAL FLUID (CSF) (*continued*)

Determination	NORMAL ADULT REFERENCE RANGE		CLINICAL SIGNIFICANCE	
	Conventional Units	*SI Units*	*Increased*	*Decreased*
Protein:			Acute meningitides	
Lumbar	15–45 mg/dL	150–450 mg/L	Tubercular meningitis	
Cisternal	15–25 mg/dL	150–250 mg/L	Neurosyphilis	
Ventricular	5–15 mg/dL	50–150 mg/L	Poliomyelitis	
			Guillain-Barré syndrome	
Protein electrophoresis (cellulose acetate)	% of total:	Fraction:	An increase in the level of albumin alone can be the result of a lesion in the choroid plexus or a blockage of the flow of CSF. An elevated gamma globulin value with a normal albumin level has been reported in multiple sclerosis, neurosyphilis, subacute sclerosing panencephalitis, and the chronic phase of CNS infections. If the blood–CNS barrier has been damaged severely during the course of these diseases, the CSF albumin level may also be elevated.	
Prealbumin	3–7	0.03–0.07		
Albumin	56–74	0.56–0.74		
Alpha$_1$ globulin	2–6.5	0.02–0.065		
Alpha$_2$ globulin	3–12	0.03–0.12		
Beta globulin	8–18.5	0.08–0.185		
Gamma globulin	4–14	0.04–0.14		

MISCELLANEOUS VALUES

Determination	Normal Value	CLINICAL SIGNIFICANCE	
		Conventional Units	SI Units
Acetaminophen	Zero	Therapeutic level = 10–20 µg/mL	10–20 mg/L
Aminophylline (theophylline)	Zero	Therapeutic level = 10–20 µg/mL	10–20 mg/L
Bromide	Zero	Therapeutic level = 5–50 mg/dL	50–500 mg/L
Carbamazepine	Zero	Therapeutic level = 8–12 µg/mL	34–51 µmol/L
Carbon monoxide	0%–2%	Symptoms with >20% saturation	
Chlordiazepoxide	Zero	Therapeutic level = 1–3 µg/mL	1–3 mg/L
Diazepam	Zero	Therapeutic level = 0.5–2.5 µg/dL	5–25 µg/L
Digitoxin	Zero	Therapeutic level = 5–30 ng/mL	5–30 µg/L
Digoxin	Zero	Therapeutic level = 0.5–2 ng/mL	0.5–2 µg/L

Ethanol	0%–0.01%	Legal intoxication level = 0.10% or above
		  0.3%–0.4% = marked intoxication
		  0.4%-0.5% = alcoholic stupor	

Gentamicin	Zero	Therapeutic level = 4–10 µg/mL	4–10 mg/L
Lithium	Zero	Therapeutic level = 0.6–1.2 mEq/L	0.6–1.2 mmol/L
Methanol	Zero	May be fatal in concentration as low as 10 mg/dL	100 mg/L
Phenobarbital	Zero	Therapeutic level = 15–40 µg/mL	10–20 mg/L
Phenytoin	Zero	Therapeutic level = 10–20 µg/mL	10–20 mg/L
Primidone	Zero	Therapeutic level = 5–12 µg/mL	5–12 mg/L
Quinidine	Zero	Therapeutic level = 0.2–0.5 mg/dL	2–5 mg/L
Salicylate	Zero	Therapeutic level = 2–25 mg/dL Toxic level = >30 mg/dL	20–250 mg/L 300 mg/L

(Source: Nettina S. Appendix I: Diagnostic studies and their meaning. In The Lippincott Manual of Nursing Practice, 6th ed. Philadelphia, Lippincott–Raven, 1996.)

Index